Infections in Children

Editors

JENNIFER E. SCHUSTER
JASON G. NEWLAND

INFECTIOUS DISEASE CLINICS OF NORTH AMERICA

www.id.theclinics.com

Consulting Editor
HELEN W. BOUCHER

March 2018 • Volume 32 • Number 1

ELSEVIER

1600 John F. Kennedy Boulevard • Suite 1800 • Philadelphia, Pennsylvania, 19103-2899.

http://www.theclinics.com

INFECTIOUS DISEASE CLINICS OF NORTH AMERICA Volume 32, Number 1
March 2018 ISSN 0891–5520, ISBN-13: 978-0-323-58156-1

Editor: Kerry Holland
Developmental Editor: Donald Mumford

Infectious Disease Clinics of North America (ISSN 0891–5520) is published in March, June, September, and December by Elsevier Inc., 360 Park Avenue South, New York, NY 10010-1710. Periodicals postage paid at New York, NY and additional mailing offices. Subscription prices are $319.00 per year for US individuals, $629.00 per year for US institutions, $100.00 per year for US students, $379.00 per year for Canadian individuals, $785.00 per year for Canadian institutions, $428.00 per year for international individuals, $785.00 per year for international institutions, and $200.00 per year for Canadian and international students. To receive student rate, orders must be accompanied by name of affiliated institution, date of term, and the *signature* of program/residency coordinator on institution letterhead. Orders will be billed at individual rate until proof of status is received. Foreign air speed delivery is included in all *Clinics* subscription prices. All prices are subject to change without notice. **POSTMASTER**: Send address changes to *Infectious Disease Clinics of North America,* Elsevier Health Sciences Division, Subcription Customer Service, 3251 Riverport Lane, Maryland Heights, MO 63043. **Customer Service: 1-800-654-2452 (US). From outside of the US and Canada, call 1-314-447-8871. Fax: 1-314-447-8029. E-mail: JournalsCustomerService-usa@elsevier.com (print support) or JournalsOnlineSupport-usa@elsevier.com (online support).**

Infectious Disease Clinics of North America is also published in Spanish by Editorial Inter-Médica, Junin 917, 1er A 1113, Buenos Aires, Argentina.

Reprints. For copies of 100 or more, of articles in this publication, please contact the Commercial Reprints Department, Elsevier Inc., 360 Park Avenue South, New York, New York 10010-1710. Tel. 212-633-3874, Fax: 212-633-3820, E-mail: reprints@elsevier.com.

Infectious Disease Clinics of North America is covered in *MEDLINE/PubMed (Index Medicus), Current Contents/Clinical Medicine, Science Citation Alert, SCISEARCH,* and *Research Alert.*

Contributors

CONSULTING EDITOR

HELEN W. BOUCHER, MD, FIDSA, FACP
Director, Infectious Diseases Fellowship Program, Division of Geographic Medicine and Infectious Diseases, Tufts Medical Center, Associate Professor of Medicine, Tufts University School of Medicine, Boston, Massachusetts, USA

EDITORS

JENNIFER E. SCHUSTER, MD, MSCI
Assistant Professor of Pediatrics, Division of Pediatric Infectious Diseases, Children's Mercy Kansas City, Kansas City, Missouri, USA

JASON G. NEWLAND, MD, MEd
Associate Professor, Department of Pediatrics, Division of Infectious Diseases, Washington University School of Medicine in St. Louis, St. Louis Children's Hospital, St Louis, Missouri, USA

AUTHORS

MARK J. ABZUG, MD
Professor, Department of Pediatrics, University of Colorado, Children's Hospital Colorado, Aurora, Colorado, USA

MONICA I. ARDURA, DO, MSCS
Associate Professor, Department of Pediatrics, Pediatric Infectious Diseases, The Ohio State University, Medical Director, Host Defense Program, Nationwide Children's Hospital, Columbus, Ohio, USA

SANDRA ARNOLD, MD, MSc
Professor, Department of Pediatrics, The University of Tennessee Health Science Center, Le Bonheur Children's Hospital, Memphis, Tennessee, USA

DAVID F. BUTLER, MD
Fellow, Department of Pediatrics, Division of Pediatric Critical Care Medicine, Seattle Children's Hospital, University of Washington School of Medicine, Seattle, Washington, USA

ANGELA J.P. CAMPBELL, MD, MPH
Influenza Division, National Center for Immunization and Respiratory Diseases, Centers for Disease Control and Prevention, Atlanta, Georgia, USA

ELLEN G. CHADWICK, MD
Professor of Pediatrics, Northwestern University Feinberg School of Medicine, Ann & Robert H. Lurie Children's Hospital of Chicago, Chicago, Illinois, USA

LARA DANZIGER-ISAKOV, MD, MPH
Professor of Pediatrics, Division of Infectious Diseases, Cincinnati Children's Hospital
Medical Center, Cincinnati, Ohio, USA

STEPHANIE C. DE SILVA, MD
Chief Resident, Department of Pediatrics, Washington University in St. Louis, St Louis,
Missouri, USA

SAMUEL R. DOMINGUEZ, MD, PhD
Associate Professor, Department of Pediatrics, University of Colorado, Children's
Hospital Colorado, Aurora, Colorado, USA

MARC FISCHER, MD, MPH
Chief, Surveillance and Epidemiology Activity, Arboviral Diseases Branch, Centers for
Disease Control and Prevention, Fort Collins, Colorado, USA

MARK D. GONZALEZ, PhD, D(ABMM)
Associate Director of Clinical Microbiology, Department of Pathology, Children's
Healthcare of Atlanta, Atlanta, Georgia, USA

LISA A. GROHSKOPF, MD, MPH
Influenza Division, National Center for Immunization and Respiratory Diseases, Centers
for Disease Control and Prevention, Atlanta, Georgia, USA

ARON J. HALL, DVM, MSPH
Division of Viral Diseases, Centers for Disease Control and Prevention, Atlanta, Georgia,
USA

DAVID TAYLOR HENDRIXSON, MD
Department of Pediatrics, Division of Infectious Diseases, Washington University in
St. Louis, St. Louis Children's Hospital, St Louis, Missouri, USA

SARAH HESTON, MD
Department of Pediatrics, The University of Tennessee Health Science Center,
Le Bonheur Children's Hospital, Memphis, Tennessee, USA

NATASHA M. KAFAI, BS
Medical Scientist Training Program, Washington University School of Medicine in
St. Louis, St Louis, Missouri, USA

SOPHIE E. KATZ, MD
Division of Infectious Diseases, Monroe Carell Jr. Children's Hospital at Vanderbilt,
Department of Pediatrics, Vanderbilt University School of Medicine, Nashville,
Tennessee, USA

KATHRYN E. KYLER, MD
Fellow, Pediatric Hospital Medicine, Department of Pediatrics, Children's Mercy Kansas
City, University of Missouri-Kansas City, Kansas City, Missouri, USA

LATANIA K. LOGAN, MD, MS
Associate Professor, Department of Pediatrics, Rush Medical College, Rush University
Medical Center, Chicago, Illinois, USA

RUSSELL J. McCULLOH, MD
Director of Research, Pediatric Hospital Medicine, Associate Professor, Department of
Pediatrics, Children's Mercy Kansas City, Associate Professor, Department of Internal
Medicine, University of Missouri-Kansas City, Kansas City, Missouri, USA

ERIN McELVANIA, PhD, D(ABMM)
Director of Clinical Microbiology, Department of Pathology, NorthShore University Health System, Evanston, Illinois, USA

RACHEL L. MEDERNACH, MD
Internal Medicine-Pediatric Resident Physician, Department of Pediatrics, Rush Medical College, Rush University Medical Center, Chicago, Illinois, USA

KEVIN MESSACAR, MD
Assistant Professor, Department of Pediatrics, University of Colorado, Children's Hospital Colorado, Aurora, Colorado, USA

WILLIAM J. MULLER, MD, PhD
Associate Professor of Pediatrics, Northwestern University Feinberg School of Medicine, Ann & Robert H. Lurie Children's Hospital of Chicago, Chicago, Illinois, USA

ANGELA L. MYERS, MD, MPH
Associate Professor of Pediatrics, Director, Travel Medicine, Director, Pediatric Infectious Diseases Fellowship Training Program, Division of Pediatric Infectious Diseases, Children's Mercy Kansas City, University of Missouri-Kansas City School of Medicine, Kansas City, Missouri, USA

JASON G. NEWLAND, MD, MEd
Associate Professor, Department of Pediatrics, Division of Infectious Diseases, Washington University School of Medicine in St. Louis, St. Louis Children's Hospital, St Louis, Missouri, USA

AUDREY R. ODOM JOHN, MD, PhD
Associate Professor, Department of Pediatrics and Molecular Microbiology, Washington University School of Medicine in St. Louis, St Louis, Missouri, USA

FELICIA A. SCAGGS HUANG, MD
Clinical Fellow, Division of Infectious Diseases, Cincinnati Children's Hospital Medical Center, Cincinnati, Ohio, USA

ELIZABETH SCHLAUDECKER, MD, MPH
Assistant Professor, Division of Infectious Diseases, Cincinnati Children's Hospital Medical Center, Cincinnati, Ohio, USA

JENNIFER E. SCHUSTER, MD, MSCI
Assistant Professor of Pediatrics, Division of Pediatric Infectious Diseases, Children's Mercy Kansas City, Kansas City, Missouri, USA

MINESH P. SHAH, MD, MPH
Division of Viral Diseases, Centers for Disease Control and Prevention, Atlanta, Georgia, USA

INDI TREHAN, MD, MPH, DTM&H
Medical Director, Lao Friends Hospital for Children, Luang Prabang, Lao PDR; Associate Professor, Department of Pediatrics, Washington University in St. Louis, St Louis, Missouri, USA; Former Clinical Lead, Maforki Ebola Holding and Treatment Centre, Port Loko, Sierra Leone

KENNETH L. TYLER, MD
Louise Baum Endowed Chair of Neurology and Chairman, Department of Neurology, Professor of Medicine and Immunology-Microbiology, University of Colorado, Aurora, Colorado, USA

DEREK J. WILLIAMS, MD, MPH
Division of Hospital Medicine, Monroe Carell Jr. Children's Hospital at Vanderbilt, Department of Pediatrics, Vanderbilt University School of Medicine, Nashville, Tennessee, USA

JOHN V. WILLIAMS, MD
Professor of Pediatrics, Children's Hospital of Pittsburgh of UPMC, University of Pittsburgh School of Medicine, Pittsburgh, Pennsylvania, USA

Contents

Preface: Old and New Infections of Childhood   xiii

Jennifer E. Schuster and Jason G. Newland

The Growing Threat of Antibiotic Resistance in Children   1

Rachel L. Medernach and Latania K. Logan

> Antimicrobial resistance is a global public health threat and a danger that continues to escalate. These menacing bacteria are having an impact on all populations; however, until recently, the increasing trend in drug-resistant infections in infants and children has gone relatively unrecognized. This article highlights the current clinical and molecular data regarding infection with antibiotic-resistant bacteria in children, with an emphasis on transmissible resistance and spread via horizontal gene transfer.

New Developments in Rapid Diagnostic Testing for Children   19

Mark D. Gonzalez and Erin McElvania

> The advent of new diagnostics assays for Group A Streptococcus, influenza, and respiratory syncytial virus now provide rapid results with increased sensitivity and specificity. Molecular testing is no longer confined to the walls of the laboratory but moving to the patient in the form of point-of-care tests. In addition, multiplex syndromic panels are allowing broad testing of pathogens associated with a single clinical presentation. This article focuses specifically on rapid diagnostic tests for pathogens most affecting children. Rapid and accurate pathogen detection in children may result in decreased time to optimal antimicrobial treatment and improved patient outcomes.

Current Concepts in the Evaluation and Management of Bronchiolitis   35

Kathryn E. Kyler and Russell J. McCulloh

> Bronchiolitis is a lower respiratory tract illness caused by viral infection in children 2 years and younger, frequently associated with wheezing on physical examination. It is a common cause of hospitalization, particularly in patients with risk factors for more serious disease. The diagnosis can be made based on clinical signs and symptoms alone, and care is generally supportive with a focus on safely doing less for symptomatic children. Bronchodilators, systemic steroids, and other therapies have been shown to have no significant effect on hospitalization rates, length of stay, or symptom duration.

Pediatric Community-Acquired Pneumonia in the United States: Changing Epidemiology, Diagnostic and Therapeutic Challenges, and Areas for Future Research   47

Sophie E. Katz and Derek J. Williams

> Community-acquired pneumonia (CAP) is one of the most common serious infections in childhood. This article focuses on pediatric CAP in

the United States and other industrialized nations, specifically highlighting the changing epidemiology of CAP, diagnostic and therapeutic challenges, and areas for further research.

Emerging Respiratory Viruses in Children   65

Jennifer E. Schuster and John V. Williams

Respiratory viral infections are a leading cause of pediatric disease. Emerging respiratory viruses can cause outbreaks with significant morbidity and mortality or circulate routinely. The rapid identification of pathogens, epidemiologic tracing, description of symptoms, and development of preventative and therapeutic measures are crucial to limiting the spread of these viruses. Some emerging viruses, such as rhinovirus C and influenza C, circulate yearly but were previously undetected owing to limited diagnostic methods. Although some pathogens have a geographic focus, globalization dictates that providers be aware of all emerging diseases to recognize outbreaks and diagnose and treat patients.

Updates on Influenza Vaccination in Children   75

Angela J.P. Campbell and Lisa A. Grohskopf

Influenza vaccination is recommended for all children 6 months and older who do not have contraindications. This article provides an overview of information concerning burden of influenza among children in the United States; US-licensed influenza vaccines; vaccine immunogenicity, effectiveness, and safety; and recent updates relevant to the use of these vaccines in pediatric populations. Influenza antiviral medications are discussed. Details concerning vaccine-related topics may be found in the current US Centers for Disease Control and Prevention/Advisory Committee on Immunization Practices recommendations for use of influenza vaccines (https://www.cdc.gov/vaccines/hcp/acip-recs/vacc-specific/flu.html). Additional information on influenza antivirals is located at https://www.cdc.gov/flu/professionals/antivirals/index.htm.

Pediatric Considerations for Postexposure Human Immunodeficiency Virus Prophylaxis   91

William J. Muller and Ellen G. Chadwick

Exposures that carry the risk of transmission of blood-borne disease are rare in pediatrics but cause great anxiety in patients and families. Specialists in pediatric infectious diseases are often asked about initial antimicrobial prophylaxis in these cases. Guidelines for nonoccupational postexposure prophylaxis for human immunodeficiency virus have evolved as new formulations and medications become available and greater experience is obtained in assessing relative risks of different exposures and relative costs and benefits for different interventions. This article discusses the evidence behind recent updates to Centers for Disease Control and Prevention guidelines for nonoccupational postexposure prophylaxis for human immunodeficiency virus, focusing on application in the pediatric population.

Norovirus Illnesses in Children and Adolescents   103

Minesh P. Shah and Aron J. Hall

Norovirus is a leading cause of childhood vomiting and diarrhea in the United States and globally. Although most illnesses caused by norovirus are self-resolving, severe outcomes may occur from dehydration, including hospitalization and death. A vast majority of deaths from norovirus occur in developing countries. Immunocompromised children are at risk for more severe outcomes. Treatment of norovirus illness is focused on early correction of dehydration and maintenance of fluid status and nutrition. Hand hygiene, exclusion of ill individuals, and environmental cleaning are important for norovirus outbreak prevention and control, and vaccines to prevent norovirus illness are currently under development.

Changing Epidemiology of *Haemophilus influenzae* in Children   119

David F. Butler and Angela L. Myers

Haemophilus influenzae remains a common cause of illness in children throughout the world. Before the introduction of vaccination, *H influenzae* type b (Hib) disease was the leading cause of bacterial meningitis in young children and a frequent cause of pneumonia, epiglottitis, and septic arthritis. Clinicians should remain diligent in counseling parents on the dangers of Hib and provide vaccination starting at 2 months of age. The epidemiology of invasive *H influenzae* disease is shifting. It is imperative that clinicians recognize the changing epidemiology and antibiotic resistance patterns for *H influenzae* to optimize care in hospital and ambulatory settings.

Syphilis in Children   129

Sarah Heston and Sandra Arnold

Syphilis, caused by *Treponema pallidum*, is transmitted both sexually and transplacentally. Untreated syphilis is a progressive disease that may result in death or disability in children and adults. Syphilis diagnosis requires 2-stage serologic testing for nontreponemal and treponemal antibodies. Congenital syphilis diagnosis requires careful review of maternal testing and treatment, comparison of maternal and neonatal nontreponemal antibody titers, and clinical evaluation of the neonate. In this article, the authors present the current epidemiology of syphilis and the clinical manifestations, diagnosis, and management of syphilis as they relate to pediatric practice, specifically, congenital syphilis and acquired syphilis in adolescents and pregnant women.

Encephalitis in US Children   145

Kevin Messacar, Marc Fischer, Samuel R. Dominguez, Kenneth L. Tyler, and Mark J. Abzug

Encephalitis is an uncommon but severe disease characterized by neurologic dysfunction with central nervous system inflammation. Children with encephalitis should receive supportive care and empiric therapies for common and treatable causes while prioritizing diagnostic evaluation for common, treatable, and high-risk conditions. Even with an extensive diagnostic workup, an infectious cause is identified in less than half of cases, suggesting a role for postinfectious or noninfectious processes.

Fever in the Returning Traveler   163

Felicia A. Scaggs Huang and Elizabeth Schlaudecker

Millions of children travel annually, whether they are refugees, international adoptees, visitors, or vacationers. Although most young travelers do well, many develop a febrile illness during or shortly after their trips. Approaching a fever in the returning traveler requires an appropriate index of suspicion to diagnose and treat in a timely manner. As many as 34% of patients with recent travel history are diagnosed with routine infections, but serious infections such as malaria, enteric fever, and dengue fever should be on the differential diagnosis because of the high morbidity and mortality in children.

Malaria in Children   189

Natasha M. Kafai and Audrey R. Odom John

Malaria remains widespread throughout the planet, and increasing global travel continues to lead to imported cases of malaria in travelers, including children. This article provides an overview of pediatric malaria, including its epidemiology, clinical features, diagnosis, treatment, and prevention in travelers.

Management of Ebola Virus Disease in Children   201

Indi Trehan and Stephanie C. De Silva

The West African outbreak of 2013 to 2016 was the largest Ebola epidemic in history. With tens of thousands of patients treated during this outbreak, much was learned about how to optimize clinical care for children with Ebola. In anticipation of inevitable future outbreaks, a firsthand summary of the major aspects of pediatric Ebola case management in austere settings is presented. Emphasis is on early and aggressive critical care, including fluid resuscitation, electrolyte repletion, antimicrobial therapy, and nutritional supplementation.

Zika Virus Infection in Children   215

David Taylor Hendrixson and Jason G. Newland

Zika virus is a mosquito-borne *Flavivirus* responsible for symptomatic and asymptomatic infections in humans. Zika was first identified in Africa as a cause of sporadic febrile illness. Beginning in 2015, Zika virus infection was identified in Brazil and linked with several symptomatic infections. Notably, congenital infections were observed with marked neurologic abnormalities. Diagnosis relies on the detection of Zika virus by real-time polymerase chain reaction or by the presence of anti-Zika antibodies. Treatment of this viral illness remains supportive; however, proactive screening and interventions are indicated in the treatment of infants with symptomatic congenital infection.

Infections in Children on Biologics   225

Lara Danziger-Isakov

Biologics target various pathways to modify immunologic activity. Biologic use to treat pediatric patients continues to expand, but limited data exist regarding infectious complications of these agents, especially for newer agents. Infectious events reported in the literature for pediatric patients indicate that a variety of bacterial, mycobacterial, viral, and fungal infections can occur. Further pediatric-specific reports are needed to fill knowledge gaps in the complications related to these agents.

Overview of Infections Complicating Pediatric Hematopoietic Cell Transplantation   237

Monica I. Ardura

Hematopoietic cell transplants (HCTs) are increasingly being performed in children for the treatment of malignant and nonmalignant diseases. Infections remain an important cause of morbidity and mortality after HCT, where the type and timing of infection is influenced by host, transplant, and pathogen-related factors. Herein, an overview of the epidemiology of infections is presented and organized by timing before and after HCT, understanding that infection may occur at any time point until there is successful immune reconstitution.

INFECTIOUS DISEASE CLINICS OF NORTH AMERICA

FORTHCOMING ISSUES

June 2018
Overcoming Barriers to Eliminate Hepatitis C
Camilla S. Graham and Stacey B. Trooskin, *Editors*

September 2018
Management of Infections in Solid Organ Transplant Recipients
Sherif Beniameen Mossad, *Editor*

December 2018
Device-Associated Infections
Vivian H. Chu, *Editor*

RECENT ISSUES

December 2017
Infections in Older Adults
Robin L.P. Jump and David H. Canaday, *Editors*

September 2017
Complex Infectious Disease Issues in the Intensive Care Unit
Naomi P. O'Grady and Sameer S. Kadri, *Editors*

March 2017
Legionnaire's Disease
Cheston B. Cunha and Burke A. Cunha, *Editors*

Preface

Old and New Infections of Childhood

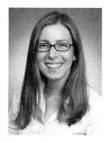 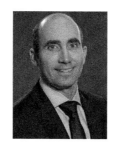

Jennifer E. Schuster, MD, MSCI   Jason G. Newland, MD, MEd
Editors

Childhood infections range from mild, common diseases to severe, unusual pathogens, and they are a leading cause of morbidity and mortality worldwide. Although mortality from infectious diseases is rare in North America, the field of infectious diseases continues to evolve. In the first year of life, a child could suffer as many as one infection per month, and the care of children with infectious diseases is a common part of a clinician's job. The plethora of pathogens that can impact children is ever changing and expanding as old pathogens evolve over time and emerging pathogens develop.

In this issue of *Infectious Disease Clinics of North America*, a wide range of pediatric infectious diseases topics that will be helpful to primary care physicians and subspecialists are presented by leading experts in the field. Older pathogens and diseases, such as *Haemophilus influenzae*, syphilis, norovirus, and encephalitis, are reviewed, including changing epidemiology and improved testing strategies. Globalization dictates that pediatric providers know how to evaluate fever in the returning traveler and recognize newly emerging pathogens, such as Zika virus, Ebola, and emerging respiratory viruses, as well as older pathogens, such as malaria, that cause disease outside of their local region. Antimicrobial resistance and hosts with altered immune systems, such as those undergoing hematopoietic stem cell transplant and those on biologic medications, present new challenges for seasoned physicians. New guidelines for the management of common pediatric infectious diseases, such as community-acquired pneumonia and bronchiolitis, are based on new evidence, including rapid diagnostics and cost-effectiveness. Prevention of infectious diseases in pediatrics is still tantamount, and we review updates to influenza vaccine recommendations as well as human immunodeficiency virus postexposure prophylaxis, two areas with increasing pediatric data. Last, we highlight new rapid diagnostics to aid in the care of the pediatric patient with an infectious disease.

Infect Dis Clin N Am 32 (2018) xiii–xiv
https://doi.org/10.1016/j.idc.2017.12.001
id.theclinics.com

We are honored for the opportunity to assemble such an outstanding group of experts in the field of pediatric infectious diseases. We want to thank Donald Mumford for guiding us through this process. We are grateful to all the authors of this issue for the significant time and effort that they have spent in providing such outstanding, educational contributions.

Jennifer E. Schuster, MD, MSCI
Division of Pediatric Infectious Diseases
Children's Mercy Kansas City
2401 Gillham Road
Kansas City, MO 64108, USA

Jason G. Newland, MD, MEd
Division of Pediatric Infectious Diseases
Washington University in St. Louis School of Medicine
Campus Box 8116
660 South Euclid Avenue
St Louis, MO 63110, USA

E-mail addresses:
jeschuster@cmh.edu (J.E. Schuster)
jgnewland@wustl.edu (J.G. Newland)

The Growing Threat of Antibiotic Resistance in Children

Rachel L. Medernach, MD, Latania K. Logan, MD, MS*

KEYWORDS

- Drug resistance • Child • Epidemiology • Infection • Bacteria • Public health
- Genetic structures • β-Lactamases

KEY POINTS

- Antimicrobial resistance is a significant public health threat and a global crisis. Infections with antibiotic-resistant organisms are associated with significant morbidity and mortality.
- Antibiotic-resistant infections are increasing in children nationally and globally. This is primarily due to the selective pressure created by the broad use of antibiotics.
- Understanding the mechanisms that lead to antimicrobial resistance is critical in the development of strategies for infection prevention and control of spread.

INTRODUCTION TO ANTIBIOTIC RESISTANCE

Antibiotic resistance is one of the most significant public health threats of our time. Although antibiotic-resistant bacteria have existed for millions of years, these organisms were most often confined to the environment. What has led to resistance in bacteria being at the forefront of medicine over the past 70 years is the selective pressure created by the broad use of antibiotics in agriculture, livestock, veterinary and human medical practices.[1] The result has been an expansion of multidrug-resistant organisms (MDROs) on a global level in all people, including children, and these MDROs (predominantly gram-negative bacilli [GNB], *Staphylococcus aureus*, and *Enterococcus* sp) are associated with significant morbidity and mortality in affected individuals.[2]

Disclosure Statement: The authors have no disclosures relevant to this article.
Financial Disclosure: The authors have no financial disclosures relevant to this article.
Funding Source: This work was directly supported by the National Institute of Allergy and Infectious Diseases at the National Institutes of Health (grant K08AI112506 to L.K. Logan).
Conflicts of Interest: The authors have no conflicts of interest relevant to this article.
Department of Pediatrics, Rush Medical College, Rush University Medical Center, 1710 W. Harrison Street, Suite 710 POB, Chicago, IL 60612, USA
* Corresponding author. Department of Pediatrics, Section of Pediatric Infectious Diseases, Rush Medical College, Rush University Medical Center, 1620 West Harrison Street, Suite 951 Jelke, Chicago, IL 60612.
E-mail address: Latania_Logan@rush.edu

Infect Dis Clin N Am 32 (2018) 1–17
https://doi.org/10.1016/j.idc.2017.11.001
0891-5520/18/© 2017 Elsevier Inc. All rights reserved.
id.theclinics.com

This article provides a brief overview of select antibiotic-resistant bacteria, with a focus on the US epidemic, and the current clinical and molecular data regarding infection with organisms known to have significant clinical impact on children.

THE GENETICS OF ANTIBIOTIC RESISTANCE

Antibiotic resistance emerged as protective survival mechanisms in environmental (soil) bacteria millions of years ago, principally as de novo nucleic acid mutations in the bacterial chromosome. Mutations can alter resistance phenotypes and remain an important mechanism of resistance in several bacterial species.[3] The current pandemic of antibiotic-resistant organisms, however, stems from an evolution of spread occurring through horizontal gene transfer, and the acquisition of exogenous DNA encoding antibiotic resistance determinants, which possess the ability to mobilize (**Fig. 1**).[3] Horizontal gene transfer occurs via 3 main mechanisms: transduction (via vectors such as bacteriophages), transformation (mainly by homologous recombination), and conjugation; the latter involves transfer of DNA via physical cell-to-cell contact (mating) and is the most significant contributor to the dissemination of antibiotic resistance among bacteria.[4,5]

Plasmids are transmitted between organisms vertically, during bacterial division, and horizontally and serve as the scaffold for a complex set of genetic elements important in transmissible resistance (**Table 1**). The classification of these extrachromosomal genetic elements containing antibiotic resistance genes has become more

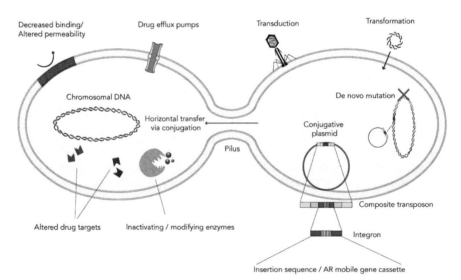

Fig. 1. Mechanisms of antibiotic resistance and horizontal gene transfer. The four main systems of antibiotic resistance are highlighted: encoding enzymes that modify or degrade antibiotics; genes that modify the molecular targets for antibiotics; genes that decrease permeability through cell wall or outer membrane changes; and alterations that increase active drug efflux. The 3 main mechanisms of horizontal gene transfer are transduction (via vectors such as bacteriophages), transformation (mainly by homologous recombination), and conjugation; the latter involves transfer of DNA via physical cell-to-cell contact (mating) and is the most significant contributor to the dissemination of antibiotic resistance. The conjugative plasmid is enlarged to show the complex set of genetic elements important in transmissible resistance. AR, antibiotic resistance.

Table 1
Mobile genetic elements and the transmission of antibiotic resistance

Element	Description
Plasmid	Extrachromosomal genetic element. Able to replicate independently of organism's chromosome
Transposon	Mobile segment of nucleic acid requiring integration into the organism's chromosome or into a plasmid to propagate
Composite transposon	Transposon including 2 insertion sequences that contain information necessary for movement, and flank a segment of DNA (such as antibiotic resistance and conjugative genes); move as a unit
Insertion sequence	Simple element containing terminal inverted repeats and an integrase, allowing insertion into a chromosome or plasmid; reorganizes target site
Integron	Segment of DNA containing an integrase for incorporation of antibiotic resistance genes and a promoter for expression of resistance determinants; insert into plasmids or transposons

Data from Cherry J, Demmler-Harrison GJ, Kaplan SL, et al. Feigin and Cherry's Textbook of Pediatric Infectious Diseases. 8th edition. Philadelphia: Elsevier, in press; and Ambler RP. The structure of beta-lactamases. Philos Trans R Soc Lond B Biol Sci 1980;289:321–31.

challenging in the wake of whole-genome sequencing, which types according to phylogenetic relatedness and is able to define relatedness in the presence of multiple plasmids in organisms. Traditional classification schemes, however, exploit backbone loci associated with replication (replicon typing including incompatibility [*Inc*] grouping) or plasmid mobility (MOB typing).[6]

Although plasmids have the ability to replicate independently from an organism's chromosome, other mobile segments of nucleic acid, such as transposons (also known as jumping genes) must be integrated into an organism's chromosome or a plasmid to propagate. Composite transposons (Tn), have 2 insertion sequences (containing the information necessary for movement), which flank a segment of DNA (such as antibiotic resistance genes as well as conjugative genes also known as integrative and conjugative elements) and can move as a unit.[7] Insertion sequences are simple elements composed of terminal inverted repeats on each end and an integrase that allows the ability to insert themselves into chromosomes or plasmids and reorganize the target site. Other mobile genetic elements (MGEs) important in the transfer of antibiotic resistance include integrons, which are segments of DNA inserted in plasmids or transposons and contain an integrase important in the incorporation of antibiotic resistance gene cassettes as well as a promoter required for expression of resistance determinants.[8] Integrons are organized into classes and most integrons harboring antibiotic resistance genes belong to class 1.[9]

Specific mechanisms of antibiotic resistance may be intrinsic or acquired and are facilitated through 4 main systems: encoding enzymes that modify or degrade antibiotics; genes that modify the molecular targets for antibiotics; genes that decrease permeability through cell wall or outer membrane changes; or alterations, which increase active drug efflux (see **Fig. 1**). The interplay between bacterial chromosomal mutations and gene rearrangements, promiscuous plasmids moving freely between genera, and the clonal expansion of pathogenic strains has resulted in efficient transmission of antibiotic resistance genes and has led to the rapid and sustained dissemination of multidrug-resistant (MDR) bacteria in the community and in health care settings (**Fig. 2**).

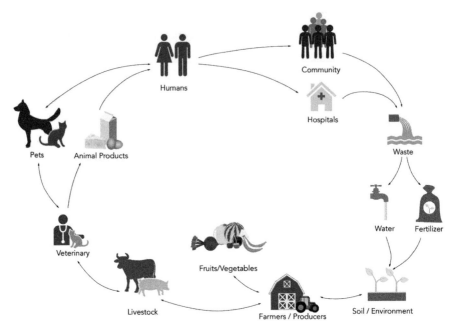

Fig. 2. The chain of transmission of antibiotic resistance. Antibiotic resistance at the human–animal–environment interface is exceptionally complex. The driver of antibiotic resistance in bacteria is mainly due to the selective pressure created by the broad use of antibiotics in agriculture, livestock, veterinary, and human medical practices. With a continuum of transmission routes and vehicles of resistance, each reservoir of resistance serves a perpetual source for antibiotic-resistant bacteria into the other reservoirs within the chain of transmission.

OVERVIEW ON THE EPIDEMIOLOGY OF ANTIBIOTIC RESISTANCE IN GRAM-POSITIVE BACTERIA
Staphylococcus aureus

Strains of *Staphylococcus aureus* resistant to methicillin (MRSA) were first recognized as a clinical threat in adult patient populations in the 1960s. MRSA infections were uncommon in the pediatric population until the 1990s, when infections (primarily skin and soft tissue) were noted in adults and children without prior health care contact,[10] and strains were subsequently named community-associated MRSA (CA-MRSA). As CA-MRSA infections increased, healthcare-associated (HA-MRSA) infections continued to burden hospitalized patients, resulting in divergent epidemiology of MRSA infections in health care settings. During the early period of the community epidemic, HA-MRSA and CA-MRSA strains were separate entities; however, recent molecular analyses of patients with MRSA infections have shown that CA-MRSA strains are now a common cause of MRSA infections acquired in health care settings, blurring the distinction.[11]

With both CA-MRSA and HA-MRSA, the main alteration conferring resistance is a single penicillin-binding protein (PBP), labeled PBP2a, encoded by the *mec* gene.[12] PBPs are located on bacterial cell surface and catalyze transglycosylation and transpeptidation, thereby providing protection.[12] The *mec* gene is located on an MGEs referred to as the *staphylococcal cassette chromosome mec (SCCmec)* genetic element, and to date at least 11 *SCCmec* types have been reported. HA-MRSA strains often have gene cassettes conferring resistance to multiple classes of antibiotics, thereby limiting therapy to more expensive antibiotics and/or those with more concerning safety profiles. In North America, HA-MRSA strains classically feature *SCCmec* types I to III, whereas CA-MRSA commonly feature *SCCmec* type IV.

To further differentiate the epidemiology of circulating MRSA strains, bacterial nomenclature organizes MRSA into clonal complexes based on DNA fingerprint patterns by pulsed-field gel electrophoresis. CA-MRSA strains in North America commonly belong to the USA300 group, and HA-MRSA more commonly belong to the USA100 and USA800 groups.[13] USA300 strains often have a smaller amount of genetic material in their *SCCmec* sequences, which allow for low-cost replication and ease of dissemination of genetic material to susceptible isolates. As a result, USA300 strains have great potential to cause significant resistant and invasive infections.[14]

Studies regarding CA-MRSA in US children generally highlight the rapid increase in infections from the mid-1990s until 2005 to 2006, with a subsequent decrease in infection rates thereafter.[15] There is significant geographic variation, however, and although both pediatric HA-MRSA and CA-MRSA rates have mostly stabilized, some regions have noted continued increases in CA-MRSA infection.[16–18]

Trimethoprim-sulfamethoxazole (TMP/SMX) and clindamycin are often used in the treatment of CA-MRSA; and although resistance to TMP/SMX has remained relatively uncommon, clindamycin resistance in both CA-MRSA and methicillin-sensitive *S aureus* (MSSA) has increased over the past decade. A recent study from the US Military Health System found CA-MRSA clindamycin resistance increased from 9.3% in 2005 to 16.7% in 2014.[15] Similar increases in MSSA clindamycin resistance have been reported.[19]

To help eradicate MRSA carriage and control spread, infection prevention measures involve the application of mupirocin ointment into the anterior nares, often in conjunction with chlorhexidine baths to further reduce colonization burden. Although decolonization campaigns have successfully reduced MRSA infection rates, resistance to mupirocin and chlorhexidine have begun to emerge. The increase in mupirocin resistance is primarily facilitated by the plasmid-based *mupA* gene, which confers resistance by encoding a novel RNA synthetase. Chlorhexidine resistance genes, known as *qacA*/B, are also plasmid-mediated and encode efflux pumps. Studies of pediatric mupirocin resistance rates range from 2% in isolates in St. Louis and the northwestern US to 19% of MRSA isolates in the southern US.[20,21] MRSA resistance to chlorhexidine remains uncommon. Resistance to chlorhexidine was approximately 1% in an outpatient pediatric study in St. Louis.[20]

Streptococcus pyogenes

Streptococcus pyogenes clinical isolates are universally susceptible to penicillin; however, macrolides are occasionally used to treat infections, particularly in patients with severe penicillin allergy. Macrolide-resistant strains of *Streptococcus pyogenes* emerged in the clinical setting in the 1980s, as a result of selective pressure after a dramatic increase in the prescription of macrolides for upper respiratory infections.[22,23] Two main mechanisms of macrolide resistance are employed by *Streptococcus pyogenes*. The first mechanism involves methylation of the 23S ribosomal RNA by *erm* genes, which causes coresistance to macrolide, lincosamide, and streptogramin (MLS) antibiotics (MLS phenotype). MLS resistance may be constitutive or inducible. The second, and more common mechanism, is an active efflux pump related to enzymes encoded for by *mef* genes (M phenotype). M and MLS phenotypes are often distinguished by using double-disk diffusion testing evaluating clindamycin (lincosamide) susceptibility in the presence of erythromycin resistance.[22,23]

In the US, current resistance to macrolides has been estimated at approximately 5%, which is a 2-fold increase compared with 1990s. The clinical significance of this resistance has become apparent, because there have been cases of children treated with macrolides for *Streptococcus pyogenes* pharyngitis who went on to develop acute rheumatic fever.[22,23] Overall, macrolide resistance in pediatric *Streptococcus pyogenes* isolates differs drastically geographically, from reported rates of 2.6% in Germany to as high as 95% in studies of Chinese children.[23] Correspondingly, the prevalence of macrolide resistance seems to correlate with regional utilization rates of macrolides.

Streptococcus pneumoniae

Similar to *Staphylococcus aureus, Streptococcus pneumoniae* confers resistance to penicillins through PBPs. Unlike MRSA, however, where resistance is primarily due to dissemination of clonal strains, circulating penicillin-resistant *Streptococcus pneumoniae* are much more heterogeneous.[24] Like *Streptococcus pyogenes, Streptococcus pneumoniae* is able to express the M and MLS phenotypes conferring resistance to macrolides and clindamycin.[25]

Internationally, penicillin and macrolide resistance were increasing at the turn of the twenty-first century. Infection rates overall, including with penicillin-resistant serotypes, significantly decreased after the introduction of pneumococcal vaccines. Early US studies noted an initial decrease in pneumococcal activity after the introduction of 7-valent vaccine (PCV7),[26] with residual high resistance by serotypes not covered by PCV7. The 13-valent vaccine (PCV13) coverage of serotype 19A led to a decrease in one of the most pathogenic (and resistant) circulating serotypes, and since 2010, there has been an overall downward trend in nonsusceptible invasive pneumococcal infections. Regional differences in circulating antibiotic-resistant *Streptococcus pneumoniae* remain; however, this resistance does not seem related to a dominant nonvaccine serotype.[27]

Enterococcus Species

Antibiotic resistance in *Enterococcus* species (*E faecalis and E faecium*) became a significant problem in health care settings during the 1980s, when the organisms began displaying high level resistance to vancomycin. Genes responsible for vancomycin resistance (known as *van* genes) are located on plasmids and/or transposons and alter the peptidoglycan synthesis pathway. *Enterococcus* isolates are notoriously hardy organisms, withstanding conventional cleaning methods, and are able to survive on surfaces for several days. This has led to the spread of vancomycin-resistant *Enterococcus* (VRE) in health care settings.[28]

While VRE remain stable residents of adult ICUs, these resistant organisms have increased in pediatric inpatient settings. A study of VRE in US children described VRE rates of 53 cases per million in 1997, which increased to 120 cases per million by 2012. A majority of affected children had a history of prolonged health care and antibiotic exposures.[28]

NOTABLE ANTIBIOTIC RESISTANCE IN ATYPICAL ORGANISMS
Mycoplasma pneumoniae

Since the turn of the century, there has been an increase in reports of macrolide-resistant *Mycoplasma pneumoniae* infections. Resistance to macrolides is due to a point mutation in the 23S ribosome, which leads to poor antibiotic binding.

Resistance trends in *M pneumoniae* isolates differ globally. In Asian countries where macrolides are commonly prescribed, *Mycoplasma* resistance to macrolides may be as high as 90%.[29] Macrolide resistance in *M pneumoniae* has remained relatively low in the US, although resistance may be on the rise. A recent study examining *M pneumoniae* isolates from 6 US centers caring for children found macrolide resistance rates to be approximately 13%.[30] The treatment of macrolide-resistant *Mycoplasma* infections often involves tetracyclines or quinolones, which have limited indications in children due to side-effect profiles. Therefore, surveillance of macrolide-resistant *M pneumoniae* may become increasingly important.

OVERVIEW OF THE EPIDEMIOLOGY OF ANTIBIOTIC RESISTANCE IN GRAM-NEGATIVE BACTERIA

Fluoroquinolone Resistance

Resistance to fluoroquinolone antibiotics (FQR) is commonly mediated by mutations in the genes encoding gyrase or topoisomerase enzymes (gyrA/parC), alteration in porins, and efflux pumps. This is mainly chromosomally based resistance in the non–lactose-fermenting GNB, such as *Pseudomonas* and *Acinetobacter* species. FQR genes can be carried on plasmids (PMFQR) and is common to Enterobacteriaceae. PMFQR is associated with agricultural and veterinary use of antibiotics, and mechanisms include acetyltransferases, efflux pumps, and pentapeptide proteins. FQR may be high level in isolates where PMFQR and chromosomal mechanisms are both present.[31]

There is a paucity of data regarding FQR GNB infections in the pediatric population, and although quinolones are not commonly used in younger children, FQR is still a problem because they are prescribed in adolescents, for MDR GNB infections, and for the treatment of select conditions. Available data suggest that FQR in GNB ranges between 5% and 14% at major US medical centers.[32] Moreover, this uptrend may be reflective of increasing PMFQR in MDR Enterobacteriaceae recovered from children nationally and globally.[33,34] Studies from Asia have noted significant PMFQR in Enterobacteriaceae infections in children, ranging from 10% in Korea to 23% in China with an increase in prevalence over time.[35,36]

β-Lactam Resistance

Among the first noteworthy pediatric clinical impacts of β-lactam resistance due to β-lactamases (enzymes that breakdown β-lactams) in GNB was the recognition of ampicillin-resistant *Haemophilus influenzae* meningitis in 1974.[37]

Since that time, the increase in β-lactam usage and introduction of broad-spectrum β-lactams has been met with continued adaptations in GNB, where the number of β-lactamase genes (encoding β-lactamases) in GNB has now surpassed 2100.[9,38,39] Originally these β-lactamase genes were narrow spectrum and chromosomally based; however, the current pandemic of β-lactamase-producing Enterobacteriaceae (Ent) is due to the rapid increase in transmissible extended-spectrum β-lactamase (ESBL) and carbapenemase genes.

β-Lactamase genes are organized into 2 classification systems based on their amino acid motifs (structure) in the Ambler classification and by their substrate and inhibitor functions in the Bush-Jacoby-Medeiros classification system (**Table 2**). Organisms carrying ESBL genes were first recognized in 1983 in Germany, when a single nucleotide polymorphism resulted in a transferable SHV gene.[42] SHV-type and TEM-type ESBLs harboring GNB were the main source of transmissible β-lactam resistance until the emergence of CTX-M–type ESBLs in the mid-1990s. These CTX-M–carrying bacteria were found in health care settings and in persons without significant health care exposure, which led to the label of CTX-M as community-acquired

Table 2 Classification schema of β-lactamase genes			
Ambler Class	**A**	**B**	**C**	**D**
Bush-Jacoby classification	2a, 2b, 2be, 2br, 2ber, 2c, 2ce, 2e, 2f	3a, 3b	1, 1e	2d, 2de, 2df
Notable enzyme types	ESBLs—TEM, SHV, CTX-M, PER, VEB	—	—	ESBLs—OXA
	Carbapenemases —KPC	Carbapenemases —IMP, VIM, NDM	AmpC cephalosporinases —CMY, DHA, FOX, ACT, MIR	Carbapenemases —OXA

Data from Refs.[39–41]

ESBL. The CTX-M pandemic is mainly associated with a clonal lineage of *Escherichia coli* (known as ST131). These clonal strains, in particular the clade C, ST131-H30 *E coli* strains, are MDR and harbor additional plasmids yielding resistance to aminoglycosides, TMP/SMX, and fluoroquinolones. Transmissible AmpC resistance remains much less common than ESBLs in clinical GNB isolates and is most commonly CMY-2.[43] Other plasmid-based AmpCs, however, have been found in Enterobacteriaceae recovered from children.[44]

Carbapenemases are categorized by their molecular structures and belong to Ambler class A, B, or D.[39,45] Classes A and D carbapenemases require serine at their active site whereas class B, the metallo-β-lactamases (MBLs), require zinc for β-lactam hydrolysis. MBLs is inhibited by metal-chelating agents such as ethylenediaminetetraacetic acid.[39,46]

Most notable of the class A carbapenemases are the *Klebsiella pneumoniae* carbapenemases (KPCs), and strains harboring KPC genes commonly have acquired resistance to multiple (≥3) antibiotic classes, making them MDROs.[47] The global spread of KPC-Ent is primarily due to clonal expansion of strains of *K pneumoniae* belonging to clonal complex 258 and, more specifically, ST258 strains harboring a KPC-2 or KPC-3 gene found on a Tn3-based transposon, Tn4401.[44,48] The propagation of KPC genes, however, is much more complex, and the major circulating ST258 *K pneumoniae* strains comprise 2 distinct genetic clades (I and II). Additionally, strains of multiple sequence types have been associated with KPC carriage and are linked to a diverse group of plasmids.[44,47,48]

The class D oxacillin-hydrolyzing (OXA) β-lactamases are a heterogeneous group of enzymes found in *Acinetobacter* spp and, increasingly, in Enterobacteriaceae.[40] The spread of OXA-48–producing Enterobacteriaceae is most commonly associated with an IncL/M-type plasmid with integration of the OXA-48 gene through the acquisition of a Tn1999 composite transposon.[40,41]

The class B MBLs are a complex group, and notable transmissible MBL genes include active on imipenem (IMP), New-Delhi MBL (NDM), and Verona integron-encoded MBL (VIM).[47,48] VIM-type and IMP-type MBLs are often embedded in class 1 integrons and are associated with plasmids or transposons, which enable spread.[49] The NDM-type MBL are of major global concern because they have widely disseminated in Enterobacteriaceae in less than a decade. It has been theorized that the most common circulating NDM-type MBL gene (NDM-1) evolved from *Acinetobacter baumannii*.[50] NDM-type MBL genes have been found in multiple epidemic clones, and it is thought that the rapid and dramatic dissemination of NDM MBLs is facilitated by the genetic elements' bacterial promiscuity.[48]

THE CLINICAL IMPACT OF ANTIBIOTIC RESISTANCE IN GRAM-NEGATIVE BACILLI, BY ORGANISM
Acinetobacter Species

Acinetobacter are a complex genus of very resilient organisms that are resistant to desiccation and thereby survive on dry surfaces for several months.[51] The major driver of poor outcomes in *Acinetobacter* infections is antibiotic resistance, and *A baumannii* harbor a major resistance genomic island comprising 45 resistance genes, facilitating resistance to multiple antibiotic classes.[52] β-Lactam resistance is due to multiple mechanisms, including chromosomal, plasmid-encoded, or transposon-encoded β-lactamases. This, in combination with active efflux systems, reduced outer membrane proteins, the absence of PBP2, and transposon-mediated aminoglycoside, sulfonamide, tetracycline resistance mechanisms have resulted in a perfect storm of highly resistant bacterial populations reported globally.[52]

In the pediatric population, most of the published literature on *A baumannii* infections is single-centered, cohort studies and report that risk factors include solid malignancy, renal disease, and male gender.[53] Although patients with *A baumannii* infections are commonly hospitalized, infections may develop in the outpatient setting in children with central lines or receiving at home ventilator care.[53]

In adults, carbapenem-resistant (CR) *A baumannii* (CRAB) is increasing and has been linked to OXA genes. There are few data on pediatric CRAB; however, in children, this CR phenotype may be most often due to a combination of intrinsic resistance mechanisms and selection pressure. This is based on unpublished data on trends of *A baumannii* infections in US children between 1999 and 2012, which found that most CRAB isolates from children were typically not MDR, which is often the case for OXA-harboring CRAB (L. Logan, personal communication, 2017). An alternate possibility is that *A baumannii* recovered from children represent another species of less virulent *Acinetobacter*, because until recently it was difficult for microbiology laboratories to differentiate *A baumannii* from *Acinetobacter calcoaceticus*.[52]

Pseudomonas aeruginosa

Similar to *Acinetobacter* species, *P aeruginosa* often feature multiple resistance mechanisms and are able to survive in harsh environments. *P aeruginosa* have resistance mechanisms that include intrinsic, chromosomally encoded β-lactamase enzymes, quorum-sensing proteins, efflux pumps, structural topoisomerase mutations, porin alterations, and reduced outer membrane permeability.[52,54] The acquisition of MGE that harbor genes encoding for carbapenemases, aminoglycoside-modifying enzymes, and FQR determinants additionally contribute to the expression of MDR phenotypes among isolates.[52]

A recent analysis of more than 87,000 non-cystic fibrosis *P aeruginosa* isolates recovered from US children ages 1 year to 17 years was notable for an increase in MDR *P aeruginosa* from 15.4% to 26% between 1999 and 2012. Additionally, carbapenem resistance increased from 9.4% to 20%. The study noted that both MDR and CR infections were more common in the ICU setting, among children aged 13 years to 17 years, in respiratory specimens, and in the West North Central region. Of added concern, resistance to other antibiotic classes (aminoglycosides, fluoroquinolones, cephalosporins, and piperacillin-tazobactam) also increased during the study period.[54] As with *Acinetobacter* infections, these data emphasize the importance of aggressive infection prevention strategies and antimicrobial stewardship programs (ASPs) to help combat antimicrobial resistance.

ENTEROBACTERIACEAE

This section focuses on the etiology of increasing β-lactam resistance in Enterobacteriaceae and the challenges clinicians face relating to these emerging threats.

Extended-Spectrum β-Lactamase–Producing Enterobacteriaceae

In the US, the prevalence of ESBL-producing Enterobacteriaceae (ESBL-Ent) infections in the pediatric population has dramatically increased in the past decade and is related to the current pandemic of ESBL-Ent infections due to the dissemination of MDR ST131 CTX-M-producing E coli strains.[44,50]

The acquisition of ESBL-Ent significantly varies by region, age, health care exposure, organism, and ESBL genotype. In health care settings, international studies describe an increase in ESBL-Ent colonization and infection in the neonatal population, and younger gestational age, prolonged mechanical ventilation, low birth weight, and antibiotic use are risk factors for infection in this population.[55] US data suggest, however, that the highest pediatric age risk group is 1 year to 5 years.[56] Outside the neonatal period, risk factors for ESBL-Ent infections are more similar to the adult population and include antibiotic exposure, chronic medical conditions, health care exposure, and recurrent infections.[57,58] Neurologic conditions may be a risk factor unique to children.[9] A majority of published data, however, have not differentiated risk factors for ESBL-Ent infection by genotype.[34,59]

AmpC Cephalosporinase-Producing Enterobacteriaceae

In a study of 4 pediatric medical centers in 3 US regions, AmpC genes were present in 29% of extended-spectrum cephalosporin-resistant (ESC-R) E coli and Klebsiella sp isolates, and 87% of the AmpC phenotype was due to presence of a CMY-2 gene. Most CMY-2–producing isolates were recovered from the West region.[60] This contrasted to findings in a 6-center Chicago area study, where the prevalence of AmpC genes in ESC-R isolates from children was 14.2%, and the ACT/MIR-type AmpC genes predominated (78%).[44]

Carbapenem Resistance in Enterobacteriaceae

GNB that feature resistance to carbapenems typically accomplish resistance in 1 of 2 ways: structural mutations (alteration of porins) along with the production of other β-lactamases (such as ESBL or AmpC) or by producing carbapenemases.[48]

Risk factors for carbapenem resistance in Enterobacteriaceae (CRE) infection in children include medical comorbidities, prolonged hospitalizations, immunosuppression, and prior antibiotic use.[61] These data are mainly from small studies of critically ill and immunosuppressed patients in the pediatric ICU or transplant units.[58,62] Moreover, most pediatric studies of CRE have used phenotypic data to assess risk factors, and mechanistic data are scant. A recent multicentered case-case-control study of KPC-Ent in Chicago children found specific factors associated with KPC-Ent infection included pulmonary and neurologic comorbidities, gastrointestinal and pulmonary devices, and exposure to carbapenems and aminoglycosides. A majority of strains available for genotyping were non-ST258 KPC-Ent strains, which differ from adults.[63]

At the turn of the twenty-first century, CRE infections in the US were rare in the pediatric population. An analysis examining more than 300,000 Enterobacteriaceae isolates from children ages 0 to 18 years, however, noted an increase in CRE over time. In 1999 to 2000, there were zero pediatric CRE infections, which rose to 0.47% by the end of the study period in 2011 to 2012.[64] The largest increase occurred in Enterobacter species, which increased from 0% being CRE in 1999 to

5.2% in 2012, followed by *Klebsiella* sp and *E coli*, which increased from 0% to 1.7% and 0.14% CRE, respectively. The prevalence of MBL-Ent considerably varies by region, and countries such as India have a high prevalence of NDM-producing Enterobacteriaceae infections in neonates and children. Recently, MBL-producing Enterobacteriaceae have emerged in US children. These data are alarming because several children, especially infants, were found to be silently colonized with these organisms, and studies have shown that children may remain colonized with MDR Enterobacteriaceae for months to years.[65,66]

Controlling the Spread of Carbapenem Resistance in Enterobacteriaceae in Pediatric Healthcare Settings

The importance of understanding the genetic background in CRE isolates cannot be underscored; yet, most clinical laboratories do not have the capability of genotyping isolates in real time to affect clinical practice. Because of this, there is a need for CRE prevention guidance using phenotypic data. We herein propose a conceptual algorithm to aid in the decision process for managing CRE in the US pediatric health care setting (**Fig. 3**). It is important to note that in the discussion of transmissible resistance, the reference is person-to-person rather than organism-to-organism transmission. Also, bacteria do not follow algorithms and may have both transmissible and nontransmissible elements contributing to their resistance phenotype.

Using pediatric data, a potential way to distinguish transmissible versus nontransmissible CR is by organism. For nontransmissible CRE, the most common organism is *Enterobacter*, and the CR phenotype is due to expression of a chromosomal AmpC cephalosporinase in combination with a porin channel alteration.[61] *Enterobacter* may

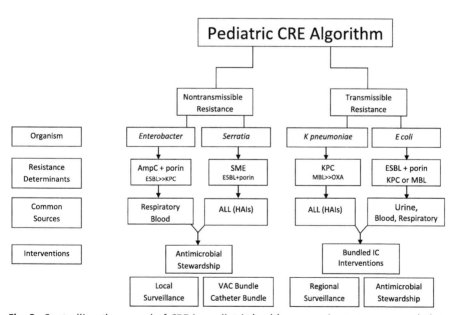

Fig. 3. Controlling the spread of CRE in pediatric health care settings—a conceptual algorithm. Size of text in each box represents the relative amount or frequency of the element. ALL, all sources; AmpC, AmpC cephalosporinases; Catheter Bundle, aimed at reducing device-related infections; HAIs, healthcare–associated infections; IC, infection control; Porin, outer membrane porin channel alteration; SME, *Serratia marcescens* enzyme; VAC, ventilator-associated complication.

harbor transmissible ESBL and/or carbapenemase genes, however, although this is less common. Common sources for CR *Enterobacter* are the respiratory tract and secondarily from blood, typically in children located in an ICU.[64] CR *Serratia marcescens* most often are expressing a chromosomally based carbapenemase known as *S marcescens* enzyme and cause health care–associated infections in critically ill patients.[67] CRE infections due to nontransmissible resistance mechanisms are frequently related to antibiotic usage and resultant selection pressure, and risk factors include mechanical ventilation and devices. Therefore, interventions should focus on Antimicrobial Stewardship Programs (ASPs) and targeted bundle interventions, such as a ventilator-associated complication bundle and reducing device-related infections.[68,69] Molecular characterization and surveillance are critical at the local level, because increases in CRE, particularly if focused in certain units or patient populations, may be due to transmissible resistance mechanisms.

With transmissible resistance and carbapenemase-producing Enterobacteriaceae (CPE), the most common organism is *K pneumoniae*. The most common carbapenemase gene in the US is KPC, and infection most often occurs in a child who is critically ill and/or has chronic comorbidities.[61] MBL-Ent and OXA-Ent have been recovered from US children and may be associated with outbreaks or travel to endemic regions.[48,65] *E coli* is the second most common organism to harbor carbapenemases; however, the CR phenotype in *E coli* may also be due to a transmissible ESBL or AmpC gene in combination with a porin mutation. Carbapenemase-producing and ESBL *E coli* are most often from urinary sources. For CPE, the focus is on halting spread. Therefore, bundled infection control interventions are critical. Additionally, studies have shown that ASPs in combination with bundled infection control interventions can further reduce CPE colonization and infection.[70] Antibiotics, especially those that disturb the anaerobic microflora and/or lacking significant activity against CPE, are thought to promote intestinal CPE colonization and prolong carriage.[71] Lastly, in hospitals with significant rates of CPE, local and regional surveillance, along with interfacility communication, is of great importance in controlling spread.[72]

EMERGING THREATS
Colistin Resistance

In children, reports of side effects of polymyxins (polymyxin B and colistin) are high, with 22% of children experiencing nephrotoxicity and 4% experienced neurotoxicity in a multicentered, pediatric case series.[73] Because of this, polymyxins are reserved for use in MDR GNB infections and after less toxic options have been exhausted.

Resistance to polymyxins is mainly chromosomal based, and is associated with mutations in the PmrAB or PhoPQ 2-component systems or with alterations of the *mgrB* gene.[74] In 2016, however, the first reports of plasmid-mediated colistin resistance in Enterobacteriaceae (known as mcr-1) were published, and the mcr-1 gene was associated with multiple plasmid backbones.[75] Colistin therapy has been used for agricultural and veterinary purposes for many years, and resistance has been linked to animal sources. To date, 3 mobile colistin resistance genes have been detected (mcr-1 to mcr-3), mainly in *E coli*.[76] Plasmid-mediated colistin resistance in the pediatric population is thought to be rare, with only single reports of children colonized with plasmid-mediated colistin-resistant *E coli* recovered from stool samples in China.[77]

SUMMARY

Antibiotic resistance in bacteria continues to evolve and represent an ever-increasing danger in all populations, including children. Recognition of this global public health threat through molecular and clinical epidemiologic studies, along with dedicated surveillance, may allow for timely strategies in prevention and treatment. Opportunities to mitigate spread of these dangerous organisms are numerous, and multifaceted approaches should focus on education and training, bundled infection prevention measures, antibiotic stewardship programs, and addressing modifiable risk factors for infection. A heightened awareness and targeted resources by national and international programs, especially those dedicated to the health of children, are essential to halt the spread of these menacing pathogens in our most vulnerable population.

ACKNOWLEDGMENTS

We thank Mr Sworup Ranjit for creation of the illustrations. We would like to thank Dr Robert A. Weinstein for thoughtful comments. This content is solely the responsibility of the authors and does not necessarily represent the official views of the National Institutes of Health.

REFERENCES

1. White DG, Zhao S, Sudler R, et al. The isolation of antibiotic-resistant salmonella from retail ground meats. N Engl J Med 2001;345:1147–54.
2. Toleman MA, Walsh TR. Combinatorial events of insertion sequences and ICE in Gram-negative bacteria. FEMS Microbiol Rev 2011;35:912–35.
3. Woodford N, Ellington MJ. The emergence of antibiotic resistance by mutation. Clin Microbiol Infect 2007;13:5–18.
4. Balcazar JL. Bacteriophages as vehicles for antibiotic resistance genes in the environment. PLoS Pathog 2014;10:e1004219.
5. Domingues S, Nielsen KM, da Silva GJ. Various pathways leading to the acquisition of antibiotic resistance by natural transformation. Mob Genet Elem 2012;2:257–60.
6. Orlek A, Stoesser N, Anjum MF, et al. Plasmid classification in an era of whole-genome sequencing: application in studies of antibiotic resistance epidemiology. Front Microbiol 2017;8:182.
7. Partridge SR. Analysis of antibiotic resistance regions in Gram-negative bacteria. FEMS Microbiol Rev 2011;35:820–55.
8. Mahillon J, Chandler M. Insertion sequences. Microbiol Mol Biol Rev 1998;62:725–74.
9. Cherry J, Demmler-Harrison GJ, Kaplan SL, et al. Feigin and Cherry's textbook of pediatric infectious diseases. 8th edition. Philadelphia: Elsevier, in press.
10. Herold BC, Immergluck LC, Maranan MC, et al. Community-acquired methicillin-resistant Staphylococcus aureus in children with no identified predisposing risk. JAMA 1998;279:593–8.
11. Popovich KJ, Weinstein RA, Hota B. Are community-associated methicillin-resistant Staphylococcus aureus (MRSA) strains replacing traditional nosocomial MRSA strains? Clin Infect Dis 2008;46:787–94.
12. Sauvage E, Kerff F, Terrak M, et al. The penicillin-binding proteins: structure and role in peptidoglycan biosynthesis. FEMS Microbiol Rev 2008;32:234–58.
13. Tong SY, Davis JS, Eichenberger E, et al. Staphylococcus aureus infections: epidemiology, pathophysiology, clinical manifestations, and management. Clin Microbiol Rev 2015;28:603–61.
14. Thurlow LR, Joshi GS, Richardson AR. Virulence strategies of the dominant USA300 lineage of community-associated methicillin-resistant Staphylococcus aureus (CA-MRSA). FEMS Immunol Med Microbiol 2012;65:5–22.

15. Sutter DE, Milburn E, Chukwuma U, et al. Changing susceptibility of *Staphylococcus aureus* in a US pediatric population. Pediatrics 2016;137:e20153099.

16. David MZ, Daum RS, Bayer AS, et al. *Staphylococcus aureus* bacteremia at 5 US academic medical centers, 2008-2011: significant geographic variation in community-onset infections. Clin Infect Dis 2014;59:798–807.

17. Iwamoto M, Mu Y, Lynfield R, et al. Trends in invasive methicillin-resistant *Staphylococcus aureus* infections. Pediatrics 2013;132:e817–24.

18. Logan LK, Healy SA, Kabat WJ, et al. A prospective cohort pilot study of the clinical and molecular epidemiology of Staphylococcus aureus in pregnant women at the time of group B streptococcal screening in a large urban medical center in Chicago, IL. Virulence 2013;4:654–8.

19. Gandra S, Braykov N, Laxminarayan R. Is methicillin-susceptible Staphylococcus aureus (MSSA) sequence type 398 confined to Northern Manhattan? Rising prevalence of erythromycin- and clindamycin-resistant MSSA clinical isolates in the United States. Clin Infect Dis 2014;58:306–7.

20. Fritz SA, Hogan PG, Camins BC, et al. Mupirocin and chlorhexidine resistance in Staphylococcus aureus in patients with community-onset skin and soft tissues infections. Antimicrob Agents Chemother 2013;57:559–68.

21. McNeil JC, Hulten KG, Kaplan SL, et al. Mupirocin resistance in Staphylococcus aureus causing recurrent skin and soft tissue infections in children. Antimicrob Agents Chemother 2011;55:2431–3.

22. Green MD, Deall B, Marcon MJ, et al. Multicentre surveillance of the prevalence and molecular epidemiology of macrolide resistance among pharyngeal isolates of group A Streptococci in the USA. J Antimicrob Chemother 2006;57:1240–3.

23. Logan L, McAuley J, Shulman S. Macrolide treatment failure in Streptococcal pharyngitis resulting in acute rheumatic fever. Pediatrics 2012;129:e798–802.

24. Hakenbeck R, Briese T, Chalkley L, et al. Antigenic variation of penicillin-binding proteins from penicillin-resistant clinical strains of Streptococcus pneumoniae. J Infect Dis 1991;164:313–9.

25. Stephens DS, Zughaier SM, Whitney CG, et al. Incidence of macrolide resistance in Streptococcus pneumoniae after introduction of the pneumococcal conjugate vaccine: population-based assessment. Lancet 2005;365:855–63.

26. Tanz RR, Shulman ST, Shortridge VD. Community-based surveillance in the United States of macrolide-resistant pediatric pharyngeal group A Streptococci during 3 respiratory disease seasons. Clin Infect Dis 2004;39(12):1794–801.

27. Tomczyk S, Lynfield R, Schaffner W, et al. Prevention of antibiotic-nonsusceptible invasive pneumococcal disease with the 13-valent pneumococcal conjugate vaccine. Clin Infect Dis 2016;62:1119–25.

28. Adams DJ, Eberly MD, Goudie A, et al. Rising vancomycin-resistant Enterococcus infections in hospitalized children in the United States. Hosp Pediatr 2016;6:404–11.

29. Meyer Sauteur PM, van Rossum AM, Vink C. Mycoplasma pneumoniae in children: carriage, pathogenesis, and antibiotic resistance. Curr Opin Infect Dis 2014;27:220–7.

30. Zheng X, Lee S, Selvarangan R, et al. Macrolide-resistant Mycoplasma pneumoniae, United States. Emerg Infect Dis 2015;21:1470–2.

31. Hawkey PM. Mechanisms of quinolone action and microbial response. J Antimicrob Chemother 2003;51(Suppl 1):29–35.

32. Jackson MA, Schutze GE, Committee on infectious diseases. The use of systemic and topical fluoroquinolones. Pediatrics 2016;138:e20162706.

33. Logan LK, Hujer AM, Marshall SM, et al. Fluoroquinolone Resistance (FQR) Mechanisms in Extended-Spectrum Beta-Lactamase producing Enterobacteriaceae (Ent) Isolates from Children. ASM Microbe 2016, Boston, MA, June 16–20, 2016.

34. Medernach RL, Rispens JR, Marshall SH, et al. Resistance mechanisms and factors associated with plasmid-mediated fluoroquinolone resistant (PMFQR) Enterobacteriaceae (Ent) infections in children. ASM Microbe 2017, New Orleans, LA, June 1–5, 2017.

35. Xue G, Li J, Feng Y, et al. High prevalence of plasmid-mediated quinolone resistance determinants in Escherichia coli and Klebsiella pneumoniae isolates from pediatric patients in China. Microb Drug Resist 2017;23:107–14.

36. Kim NH, Choi EH, Sung JY, et al. Prevalence of plasmid-mediated quinolone resistance genes and ciprofloxacin resistance in pediatric bloodstream isolates of Enterobacteriaceae over a 9-year period. Jpn J Infect Dis 2013;66:151–4.

37. Tomeh MO, Starr SE, McGowan JE Jr, et al. Ampicillin-resistant Haemophilus influenzae type B infection. JAMA 1974;229:295–7.

38. Bush K. Top 10 Beta-lactamase papers for 2015. ASM Microbe 2016, Boston, MA, June 16–20, 2016.

39. Bush K, Jacoby GA. Updated functional classification of beta-lactamases. Antimicrob Agents Chemother 2010;54:969–76.

40. Poirel L, Naas T, Nordmann P. Diversity, epidemiology, and genetics of class D beta-lactamases. Antimicrob Agents Chemother 2010;54:24–38.

41. Poirel L, Bonnin RA, Nordmann P. Genetic features of the widespread plasmid coding for the carbapenemase OXA-48. Antimicrob Agents Chemother 2012;56:559–62.

42. Paterson DL, Bonomo RA. Extended-spectrum beta-lactamases: a clinical update. Clin Microbiol Rev 2005;18:657–86.

43. Lukac PJ, Bonomo RA, Logan LK. Extended-spectrum β-lactamase-producing Enterobacteriaceae in children: old foe, emerging threat. Clin Infect Dis 2015;60:1389–97.

44. Logan LK, Hujer AM, Marshall SH, et al. Analysis of beta-lactamase resistance determinants in enterobacteriaceae from Chicago children: a multicenter survey. Antimicrob Agents Chemother 2016;60(6):3462–9.

45. Ambler RP. The structure of beta-lactamases. Philos Trans R Soc Lond B Biol Sci 1980;289:321–31.

46. Patel G, Bonomo RA. "Stormy waters ahead": global emergence of carbapenemases. Front Microbiol 2013;4:48.

47. Nordmann P, Cuzon G, Naas T. The real threat of Klebsiella pneumoniae carbapenemase-producing bacteria. Lancet Infect Dis 2009;9:228–36.

48. Logan LK, Weinstein RA. The epidemiology of carbapenem-resistant Enterobacteriaceae: the impact and evolution of a global menace. J Infect Dis 2017;215:S28–36.

49. Mojica MF, Bonomo RA, Fast W. B1-Metallo-β-Lactamases: where do we stand? Curr Drug Targets 2016;17:1029–50.

50. Dortet L, Poirel L, Nordmann P. Worldwide dissemination of the NDM-type carbapenemases in Gram-negative bacteria. Biomed Res Int 2014;2014:249856.

51. Wendt C, Dietze B, Dietz E, et al. Survival of Acinetobacter baumannii on dry surfaces. J Clin Microbiol 1997;35:1394–7.

52. Bonomo RA, Szabo D. Mechanisms of multidrug resistance in *Acinetobacter* species and *Pseudomonas aeruginosa*. Clin Infect Dis 2006;43(Suppl 2):S49–56.

53. Segal SC, Zaoutis TE, Kagen J, et al. Epidemiology of and risk factors for Acinetobacter species bloodstream infection in children. Pediatr Infect Dis J 2007;26: 920–6.
54. Logan LK, Gandra S, Mandal S, et al. Multidrug- and carbapenem-resistant Pseudomonas aeruginosa in children, United States, 1999-2012. J Pediatr Infect Dis Soc 2017;6:352–9.
55. Crivaro V, Bagattini M, Salza MF, et al. Risk factors for extended-spectrum beta-lactamase-producing Serratia marcescens and Klebsiella pneumoniae acquisition in a neonatal intensive care unit. J Hosp Infect 2007;67:135–41.
56. Logan LK, Braykov NP, Weinstein RA, et al, CDC Epicenters Prevention Program. Extended-spectrum β-lactamase-producing and third-generation cephalosporin-resistant Enterobacteriaceae in children: trends in the United States, 1999-2011. J Pediatr Infect Dis Soc 2014;3:320–8.
57. Zerr DM, Miles-Jay A, Kronman MP, et al. Previous antibiotic exposure increases risk of infection with extended-spectrum-β-lactamase- and AmpC-producing Escherichia coli and Klebsiella pneumoniae in pediatric patients. Antimicrob Agents Chemother 2016;60:4237–43.
58. Zerr DM, Weissman SJ, Zhou C, et al. The molecular and clinical epidemiology of extended-spectrum cephalosporin- and carbapenem-resistant Enterobacteriaceae at 4 US pediatric hospitals. J Pediatr Infect Dis Soc 2017;6:366–75.
59. Stillwell T, Green M, Barbadora K, et al. Outbreak of KPC-3 producing carbapenem-resistant Klebsiella pneumoniae in a US pediatric hospital. J Pediatr Infect Dis Soc 2015;4:330–8.
60. Rispens JR, Medernach RL, Hujer AM, et al. A Multicenter Study of the Clinical and Molecular Epidemiology of TEM- and SHV-type Extended- Spectrum Beta-Lactamase producing (ESBL) Enterobacteriaceae (Ent) Infections in Children. IDWeek 2017, San Diego, CA, October 4–8, 2017.
61. Logan LK. Carbapenem-resistant enterobacteriaceae: an emerging problem in children. Clin Infect Dis 2012;55:852–9.
62. Suwantarat N, Logan LK, Carroll KC, et al. The prevalence and molecular epidemiology of multidrug-resistant Enterobacteriaceae colonization in a pediatric intensive care unit. Infect Control Hosp Epidemiol 2016;37:1–9.
63. Nguyen DC, Scaggs FA, Charnot-Katsikas A, et al. A Multicenter Case-Case-Control Study of Factors Associated with Klebsiella pneumoniae Carbapenemase (KPC)-Producing Enterobacteriaceae (KPC-CRE) Infections in Children. IDWeek 2017, San Diego, CA, October 4–8. 2017.
64. Logan L, Renschler J, Gandra S, et al. Carbapenem-resistant Enterobacteriaceae in children, United States, 1999-2012. Emerg Infect Dis 2015;21:2014–21.
65. Logan LK, Bonomo RA. Metallo-β-lactamase (MBL)-producing Enterobacteriaceae in United States children. Open Forum Infect Dis 2016;3:ofw090.
66. Zerr DM, Qin X, Oron AP, et al. Pediatric infection and intestinal carriage due to extended-spectrum-cephalosporin-resistant Enterobacteriaceae. Antimicrob Agents Chemother 2014;58:3997–4004.
67. Herra C, Falkiner FR. Serratia marcescens. In: Antimicrobe Microbes. Available at: http://www.antimicrobe.org/b26.asp. Accessed July 27, 2017.
68. Klompas M, Branson R, Eichenwald EC, et al. Strategies to prevent ventilator associated pneumonia in acute care hospitals: 2014 update. Infect Control Hosp Epidemiol 2014;35:915–36.
69. Priebe GP, Larsen G, Logan LK, et al. Etiologies for pediatric ventilator associated conditions – the need for a broad VAC prevention bundle. Crit Care Med 2015;43:80.

70. Viale P, Giannella M, Bartoletti M, et al. Considerations about antimicrobial stewardship in settings with epidemic extend-spectrum β-lactamase-producing or carbapenem-resistant Enterobacteriaceae. Infect Dis Ther 2015;4(Suppl 1): 65–83.

71. Perez F, Pultz MJ, Endimiani A, et al. Effect of antibiotic treatment on establishment and elimination of intestinal colonization by KPC-producing Klebsiella pneumoniae in mice. Antimicrob Agents Chemother 2011;55:2585–9.

72. Trick WE, Lin MY, Cheng-Leidig R, et al. Electronic public health registry of extensively drug-resistant organisms, Illinois, USA. Emerg Infect Dis 2015;21:1725–32.

73. Tamma PD, Newland JG, Pannaraj PS, et al. The use of intravenous colistin among children in the U.S.: results from a multicenter, case series. Pediatr Infect Dis J 2013;32:17–22.

74. Olaitan AO, Morand S, Rolain JM. Mechanisms of polymyxin resistance: acquired and intrinsic resistance in bacteria. Front Microbiol 2014;5:643.

75. Liu YY, Wang Y, Walsh TR, et al. Emergence of plasmid-mediated colistin resistance mechanism MCR-1 in animals and human beings in China: a microbiological and molecular biological study. Lancet Infect Dis 2016;16:161–8.

76. Yin W, Li H, Shen Y, et al. Novel plasmid-mediated colistin resistance gene *mcr-3* in *Escherichia coli*. MBio 2017;8:e00543–7.

77. Gu DX, Huang YL, Ma JG, et al. Detection of colistin resistance gene mcr-1 in hypervirulent Klebsiella pneumoniae and Escherichia coli isolates from an infant with diarrhea in China. Antimicrob Agents Chemother 2016;60:5099–100.

New Developments in Rapid Diagnostic Testing for Children

Mark D. Gonzalez, PhD, D(ABMM)[a], Erin McElvania, PhD, D(ABMM)[b],*

KEYWORDS

- Rapid diagnostic assays • Group A streptococcus • Influenza • RSV
- Syndromic multiplex panels • Gastrointestinal panel • Respiratory panel
- Meningitis encephalitis panel

KEY POINTS

- Compared with traditional rapid antigen testing, new diagnostics assays for Group A Streptococcus, influenza, and respiratory syncytial virus combine rapid turnaround time with high sensitivity and specificity.
- There has been a surge in the availability of multiplex syndromic panels that test for a broad range of pathogens associated with a single clinical presentation.
- Molecular infectious disease testing that was previously performed in microbiology laboratories is now being developed in easy-to-use platforms, which are available at point of care.

It is an exciting time in the field of microbiology because of the expansion of rapid diagnostic tests. Pathogen testing previously was performed by traditional laboratory methods such as bacterial, fungal, and viral culture or ova and parasite (O&P) examination. Testing could have a slow time to results; some testing lacked sensitivity, and most testing was centralized in the laboratory. Newer advances in pathogen detection assays are now providing rapid results and have greater sensitivity and specificity, and many assays are moving out of the centralized laboratory and to the patient as point-of-care tests. In this review, the authors chose to highlight the currently available US Food and Drug Administration (FDA)–cleared molecular assays for various infectious syndromes relevant to the pediatric population. Although outcome studies in this area are sparse, rapid results may result in decreased time to optimal antimicrobial treatment and improved patient outcomes.

Disclosure Statement: E. McElvania is a consultant for Luminex Corporation. M.D. Gonzalez has no disclosures.
[a] Department of Pathology, Children's Healthcare of Atlanta, 1405 Clifton Road, Northeast, Atlanta, GA 30322, USA; [b] Department of Pathology, NorthShore University Health System, 2650 Ridge Avenue, Evanston, IL 60201, USA
* Corresponding author.
E-mail address: emcelvania@northshore.org

Infect Dis Clin N Am 32 (2018) 19–34
https://doi.org/10.1016/j.idc.2017.11.006
0891-5520/18/© 2017 Elsevier Inc. All rights reserved.

id.theclinics.com

RAPID DIAGNOSTIC TESTING FOR GROUP A STREPTOCOCCUS

Group A streptococcus (GAS), *Streptococcus pyogenes*, is the most common bacterial cause of pharyngitis, which infrequently can result in serious conditions such as bacteremia, post–streptococcal glomerulonephritis, and rheumatic fever. Strep throat is most common in children 5 to 15 years of age, which is complicated by the fact that approximately 15% of children in this group are asymptomatic carriers of GAS.[1] Throat culture is the gold standard for diagnosis of GAS pharyngitis, but due to the 24- to 48-hour turnaround time, rapid antigen testing has been the standard of practice in emergency departments (EDs) and outpatient clinics for many years. Because rapid antigen assays have low sensitivity compared with culture, throat swabs that test negative by the GAS rapid antigen assay must be cultured when collected from children less than 18 years of age. Rapid antigen testing when combined with reflex throat culture brings the sensitivity of GAS detection to an acceptable level of greater than 95%.

To increase the sensitivity of GAS detection, second-generation antigen assays have been recently developed. These assays use a reading device to interpret the assay rather than the naked eye, which increases the sensitivity of antigen detection and reduces the subjective nature of reading low positive test results. In a study of 48 pediatric patients with pharyngitis, the Sofia Strep A + FID (Quidel Corp, San Diego, CA, USA) was 88.9% sensitive and 93.3% specific for detection of GAS compared with culture.[2]

Illumigene group A Streptococcus assay (Meridian Bioscience Inc, Cincinnati, OH, USA) uses isothermal amplification for detection of GAS and was found to be 100% sensitive and 95.9% specific compared with culture in a study of 437 throat swabs collected from primarily pediatric patients (98% of patients <18 years of age).[3] A second study of 361 pediatric patients reported the Illumigene assay to be 98.6% sensitive and 96.5% specific.[4] For comparison, traditional GAS rapid antigen tests were also run on all specimens in both studies and had a sensitivity of 73.3% and 55.2%, respectively, and specificity of 89.1% and 99.1%, respectively. The Simplexa Group A Strep Direct Assay (DiaSorin Molecular LLC, Cypress, CA, USA) was found to be 97.4% sensitive and 95.2% specific compared with culture in a study of 1352 specimens across 4 pediatric testing sites.[5]

Molecular tests have also been developed that allow rapid, point-of-care detection of GAS. These assays are highly sensitive and specific and may not require reflex to culture if testing is negative. Many of these tests are also Clinical Laboratory Improvement Amendments (CLIA) waived, which allows molecular testing to be performed by nonlaboratory personnel, such as physicians and nurses in an outpatient or ED setting. The Cobas Liat Strep A Assay (Roche Diagnostics, Indianapolis, IN, USA) is a waived, polymerase chain reaction (PCR)-based assay found to be 100% sensitive and 98.3% specific for GAS detection compared with an in-house developed molecular assay using 198 throat swabs from adults and children.[6] Another point-of-care molecular test is the Alere i strep A (Alere Inc, Waltham, MA, USA). In a study conducted across 10 US medical centers, 481 primarily pediatric specimens were tested by nonlaboratory personnel and found the Alere i strep A assay to be 98.7% sensitive and 98.5% specific compared with bacterial culture.[7]

In the past few years, there has been an explosion in the field of GAS assays. These new assays are rapid, have increased sensitivity over traditional rapid antigen tests, and in many cases, can be performed at point of care. Because molecular testing is more sensitive than culture, clinicians must be cognizant to only test patients with signs and symptoms of pharyngitis to prevent detecting GAS colonization. Molecular testing does not distinguish between live or dead organisms, so molecular tests cannot be used to determine clearance of GAS following treatment. Testing for GAS by molecular methods can result in the missed opportunity to detect less common causes of bacterial pharyngitis such as Lancefield groups C and G β-hemolytic streptococci, which are identified by throat culture. In an effort to identify additional bacterial causes of pharyngitis, some assays such as the Simplexa Group A Strep Assay detect Lancefield groups C and G β-hemolytic streptococci in addition to GAS. A summary of FDA-cleared rapid second-generation and molecular GAS assays can be found in **Table 1**.

RAPID DIAGNOSTIC TESTING FOR RESPIRATORY VIRUSES

Millions of children are infected each year with influenza and respiratory syncytial virus (RSV), with even more falling ill with a variety of other respiratory viruses. Respiratory viral infections can span the clinical spectrum from no symptoms to death in rare cases. Children under the age of 5, and especially those under 2 years of age, are at high risk for complications from influenza, resulting in thousands of hospitalizations and approximately 100 to 150 deaths per year.[8] RSV is the leading cause of bronchiolitis and pneumonia in children under 1 year of age, causing 60,000 hospitalizations in children each year.[9]

Traditionally, viral culture was the gold standard for respiratory virus detection, but because of the long turnaround time, rapid antigen testing became the mainstay for influenza and RSV testing in the ED and outpatient settings. Just like rapid antigen testing for GAS, testing for influenza and RSV is rapid and inexpensive, but lacks sensitivity at 50% to 70%. For this reason, the Centers for Disease Control and Prevention (CDC) has discouraged the use of rapid antigen testing for influenza and RSV and promoted the use of molecular detection of these viruses. If rapid antigen testing must be used, the CDC recommends using these assays only when the prevalence of influenza or RSV in the community is greater than 10%, which raises the positive predictive value of the assay. Even when the prevalence is high, clinicians must interpret rapid antigen test results with caution, because a negative result does not exclude infection in a symptomatic patient.[10]

Like GAS testing, second-generation rapid antigen assays using a reading device have been developed to increase the sensitivity of influenza and RSV detection. A study of 240 pediatric specimens tested on 3 second-generation influenza platforms, the Veritor System Flu A + B (BD Diagnostics, Sparks, MD, USA), Sofia Influenza A + B FIA (Quidel Corp, San Diego, CA, USA), and BinaxNOW Influenza A&B (Alere Scarborough, Inc, Scarborough, ME, USA), found testing to be in agreement 93.8%, 94.2%, and 95.8% of the time for influenza A and 98.1%, 79.2%, and 80.8% of the time for influenza B, respectively, compared with real-time PCR.[11]

Assays using molecular methods of influenza and RSV detection have drastically increased the sensitivity of viral detection over previous methods, including rapid antigen testing and viral culture. The increased speed of detection is partially due to removal of an external extraction step before molecular testing, allowing testing platforms such as the Simplexa Flu A/B & RSV Direct (DiaSorin Molecular LLC, Cypress, CA, USA), Solana Influenza A + B (Quidel Corp, San Diego, CA, USA), and Xpert Xpress Flu/RSV (Cepheid, Sunnyvale, CA, USA) assays to provide results in 30 to 60 minutes. Because the sensitivity and specificity of molecular tests are high, testing can be performed year round regardless of the prevalence of influenza or RSV.

An exciting new development in the field of influenza and RSV detection has been the development of rapid, point-of-care molecular testing. These assays combine the quick

Table 1
Second-generation and molecular group A streptococcus testing, US Food and Drug Administration approved

Assay	Targets	Methodology	Turnaround Time, min	CLIA Waived	Pediatric References
BD Veritor System	Group A streptococci	Immunochromatographic assay	5	Yes	—
Quidel Sofia Strep A + FIA	Group A streptococci	Immunofluorescence-based lateral flow	5	Yes	Roper et al,[2] 2017
Alere i Strep A	Group A streptococci	Isothermal nucleic acid amplification	8	Yes	Cohen et al,[7] 2015
Roche cobas LiatStrep A Assay	Group A streptococci	Real-time PCR	15	Yes	Uhl & Patel,[6] 2016
Cepheid Xpert Xpress Strep A Assay	Group A streptococci	Real-time PCR	30	No	—
Quidel Solana Strep Complete Assay	Group A, C, and G streptococci	Isothermal helicase-dependent amplification	25	No	—
Meridian illumigene Group A Strep	Group A streptococci	Loop-mediated isothermal amplification	<60	No	Henson et al,[3] 2013; Felsenstein et al,[4] 2014
DiaSorin Simplexa Group A Strep	Group A, C, and G streptococci	Real-time PCR	60	No	Tabb & Batterman,[5] 2016

turnaround time of rapid antigen testing with the high sensitivity and specificity associated with molecular testing. Several of these assays are CLIA waived and can be performed at point of care by non-laboratory-trained individuals. Although molecular assays cost more than traditional rapid antigen assays, they provide accurate test results while patients are being seen in clinic or in the ED, allowing treatment decisions to be made while the patient is in house. A study of 545 specimens (85% collected from children) found the Alere i Influenza A&B assay to be 99.3% sensitive and 98.1% specific for influenza A, and 97.6% sensitive and 100% specific for influenza B, compared with viral culture and real-time reverse transcription (RT)-PCR used for discrepant analysis.[12]

A study of 2 CLIA-waived, point-of-care, molecular assays, Cobas Liat Influenza A/B (Roche Diagnostics, Indianapolis, IN, USA) and Alere i Influenza A&B (Alere Scarborough, Inc, Scarborough, ME, USA), tested 129 respiratory specimens (41% pediatric specimens). They found the Alere i to be 71.3% sensitive for influenza A and 93.3% sensitive for influenza B with 100% specificity for both viruses.[13] The Cobas Liat had 100% sensitivity and specificity for influenza A and B. The low sensitivity of the Alere i was thought to be due to specimens below the limit of detection (LOD) for the assay, and since this study, the assay has been revised to address this issue. A summary of FDA-cleared rapid second-generation and molecular influenza and combined influenza and RSV assays can be found in **Table 2**.

SYNDROMIC MULTIPLEX RESPIRATORY PANELS

Although influenza and RSV are the most common respiratory pathogens, there are many other respiratory viruses that cause significant disease, especially in immunosuppressed patients. The advent of syndromic multiplex assays allows for rapid identification of a large number of respiratory pathogens, both bacterial and viral, from respiratory specimens (**Table 3**). A study of 300 respiratory specimens (49% from pediatric patients) were tested on 4 multiplex respiratory panels, FilmArray RP, GenMark Dx eSensor (GenMark Diagnostics, Inc, Carlsbad, CA, USA), Luminex xTAG RVPv1 (Luminex, Austin, TX, USA), and the Luminex xTAG (bioMérieux, Durham, NC, USA) RVP fast.[14] The overall sensitivity was 84.5% for the FilmArray RP, 98.3% for the eSensor RVP (Luminex, Austin, TX, USA), 92.7% for the xTAG RVPv1, and 84.4% for the RVP fast. The specificity was greater than 99% for all assays. It should be noted that all assays used have been updated since the time of this study. Recently, the first CLIA-waived respiratory panel, FilmArray Respiratory Panel EZ (bioMérieux, Durham, NC, USA), has come to the market, allowing respiratory panels to be performed in outpatient settings. More information on rapid influenza and respiratory panel testing can be found in recent *Clinics in Laboratory Medicine* articles by Peaper and Landry[15] and Buller.[16]

Rapid influenza testing is valuable for more than just convenience—it can affect patient outcomes. A study of influenza testing for pediatric patients presenting to the ED found that the use of rapid, multiplex PCR was the most cost-effective testing method (based on quality-adjusted life-years) compared with traditional PCR, direct-fluorescent antibody, and rapid antigen testing.[17] A meta-analysis of greater than 1500 pediatric patients found that rapid influenza detection in the ED decreased antibiotic usage, but the trend was not statistically significant.[18] The study did find that having rapid viral testing available did significantly decrease the rate of chest radiographs performed in the ED. Another pediatric study by Rogers and colleagues[19] found that implementation of the BioFire RP reduced antibiotic duration when test results were obtained in less than 4 hours. Also, if test results were positive for a respiratory virus, inpatient length of stay and time in isolation were decreased compared with before the BioFire RP was in use.

Table 2
Second-generation and molecular influenza and respiratory syncytial virus testing, US Food and Drug Administration approved

Assay	Targets Detected	Methodology	Turnaround Time, min	CLIA Waived	Pediatric References
BD Veritor System Flu A + B	Influenza A & B	Immunochromatographic assay	5–10	Yes	Dunn et al,[11] 2014
Quidel Sofia Influenza A + B FIA	Influenza A & B	Immunofluorescence-based lateral flow with reader	3–15	Yes	Dunn et al,[11] 2014
Alere i Influenza A & B 2	Influenza A & B	Isothermal nucleic acid amplification	<15	Yes	Bell et al,[12] 2014; Nolte et al,[13] 2016
Roche cobas Liat Influenza A/B and RSV	Influenza A & B and RSV	Real-time PCR	20	Yes	Nolte et al,[13] 2016
Cepheid Xpert Xpress Flu/RSV Assay	Influenza A & B and RSV	Real-time RT-PCR	30	No	—
DiaSorin Simplexa Flu A/B & RSV Direct	Influenza A & B and RSV	Real-time RT-PCR	60	No	—
Quidel Solana Influenza A + B Assay	Influenza A & B	RT-PCR followed by isothermal helicase-dependent amplification	45	No	—

Table 3
Multiplex respiratory panels, US Food and Drug Administration approved

Assay	Turnaround Time, h	Bacterial Targets	Viral Targets	Pediatric References
bioMérieux FilmArray Respiratory Panel	1	*Bordetella pertussis* *Chlamydophila pneumoniae* *Mycoplasma pneumoniae*	Influenza A, A/H1, A/H3, A/H1-2009 Influenza B RSV Parainfluenza virus 1, 2, 3, and 4 Human metapneumovirus Human rhinovirus/enterovirus[a] Adenovirus Coronavirus HKU1, NL63, 229E, and OC43	Popowitch et al,[14] 2013
bioMérieux FilmArray Respiratory Panel EZ (CLIA waived)	1	*B pertussis* *C pneumoniae* *M pneumoniae*	Influenza A, A/H1, A/H3, A/H1-2009 Influenza B RSV Parainfluenza virus Human metapneumovirus Human rhinovirus/enterovirus[a] Adenovirus Coronavirus	—
GenMark ePlex Respiratory Pathogen Panel (RP)	1.5	*C pneumoniae* *M pneumoniae*	Influenza A, A/H1, A/H3, A/H1-2009 Influenza B Respiratory syncytial virus A and B Parainfluenza virus 1, 2, 3, and 4 Human metapneumovirus, Human rhinovirus/enterovirus Adenovirus Coronavirus HKU1, NL63, 229E, and OC43	Popowitch et al,[14] 2013
Luminex Verigene Respiratory Pathogens Flex Test (RP Flex)	<2	*B pertussis* *Bordetella parapertussis/B bronchiseptica* *Bordetella holmesii*	Influenza A, A/H1, A/H3 Influenza B Respiratory syncytial virus A and B Human rhinovirus Parainfluenza virus 1, 2, 3, and 4 Human metapneumovirus, Adenovirus	—
Luminex NxTAG Respiratory Pathogen Panel	5	*C pneumoniae* *M pneumoniae*	Influenza A, A/H1, A/H3 Influenza B Respiratory syncytial virus A and B Human rhinovirus/enterovirus Parainfluenza virus 1, 2, 3, and 4 Human metapneumovirus, Adenovirus Coronavirus HKU1, NL63, 229E, and OC43 Human bocavirus	Popowitch et al,[14] 2013

[a] Unable to differentiate human rhinovirus and enterovirus.

DETECTION OF GASTROINTESTINAL PATHOGENS

Traditional testing for the array of the gastrointestinal pathogens, which includes bacteria, viruses, and parasites, has relied on a range of testing methodologies. The decision of the appropriate tests to order is complicated by the lack of symptoms/biomarkers to reliably differentiate between pathogen groups.[20] The identification of bacterial pathogens relies on stool culture, which can take days to result and has reduced sensitivity because of the fastidious nature of some pathogens, such as *Campylobacter* and *Shigella*. In an effort to increase the sensitivity of *Campylobacter* detection in stool specimens, antigen tests are available for rapid *Campylobacter* spp testing. Unfortunately, a large multicenter study evaluated 4 *Campylobacter* antigen assays and found that despite relatively high specificity (>95%), the positive predictive value was only 36% to 51%.[21] Based on these results, the use of *Campylobacter* antigen assays as stand-alone tests is not recommended.

Antigen testing has also been used for detection of viral and parasitic causes of gastroenteritis, including adenovirus 40/41, rotavirus, *Giardia lamblia*, and *Cryptosporidium*. Antigen testing offers a more rapid and relatively sensitive method for viral and parasitic pathogen detection relative to viral culture and O&P examination. Rapid antigen testing for parasites does not require multiple specimens to rule out infections, which is the practice for O&P examination. Readers are referred to a review of protozoal diagnostics for additional information.[22]

Detection of norovirus has always been difficult, because it cannot be cultured. For years, laboratory-developed molecular tests were the only method for norovirus testing. Recently, the first FDA-cleared molecular assay, Xpert Norovirus (Cepheid, Sunnyvale, CA, USA) became available for detection of norovirus genogroups GI and GII from stool specimens. In a multicenter study of approximately 1400 fresh and frozen stool specimens, this assay demonstrated high sensitivity (>98%) and specificity (>98%) for both norovirus genogroups.[23]

There is much overlap in symptoms of bacterial and viral causes of gastroenteritis, making them unable to be differentiated clinically. Often clinicians are not aware of which bacteria are included in their institution's standard stool culture, because this varies among laboratories. To solve these problems, multiplexed syndromic panels are now available for detection of numerous gastrointestinal pathogens. The FilmArray Gastrointestinal (bioMérieux, Durham, NC, USA) and xTAG Gastrointestinal (Luminex, Austin, TX, USA) panels detect bacterial, viral, and parasitic targets, whereas the Verigene Enteric Pathogens Panel (Luminex, Austin, TX, USA) detects both bacterial and viral pathogens. The ProGastro SSCS (Hologic Inc, Marlborough, MA, USA) only detects bacterial pathogens, whereas the BDMax Enteric system (BD, Franklin Lakes, NJ, USA) has a bacterial panel, extended bacterial panel, and a parasite panel. All assay targets are summarized in **Table 4**. Studies on each of these assays has been published, and all assays show high sensitivity and specificity for their respective targets.[24–31] In fact, these multiplex panels result in increased and unexpected detections that would not be identified by the ordering preference of the clinician. For example, in a study by Stockmann and colleagues,[32] they noted that for patients with only *Clostridium difficile* testing, the FilmArray Gastrointestinal pathogen panel identified an alternative pathogen in 29% of those patients.

Currently, there are few studies directly comparing these multiplex panels. Huang and colleagues[29] evaluated the performance for the shared analytes of the Verigene Enteric, FilmArray Gastrointestinal, and xTAG Gastrointestinal panels and found that the FilmArray and xTAG panels performed similarly except for reduced *Salmonella* detection with the later assay (79.2%) relative to the former assay (95.8%). The

Table 4
Multiplex gastrointestinal panels, US Food and Drug Administration approved

Assay	Turnaround Time, h	Bacterial Targets	Viral Targets	Parasitic Targets	References
BDMax Enteric Bacterial Panel[a]	3	Campylobacter spp Salmonella spp Shigella/EIEC STEC	—	—	Harrington et al,[24] 2015
BDMax Extended Enteric Bacterial Panel[b]	3.5	ETEC Plesiomonas shigelloides Vibrio spp Yersinia enterocolitica	—	—	Simner et al,[26] 2017
BDMax Enteric Parasite Panel	4.5	—	—	Cryptosporidium Entamoeba histolytica Giardia	Madison-Antenucci et al,[25] 2016
bioMérieux FilmArray Gastrointestinal Panel[c]	1	Campylobacter spp C difficile P shigelloides Salmonella spp Vibrio spp (cholerae) EAEC EPEC ETEC STEC (Escherichia coli O157) Shigella/EIEC	Adenovirus 40/41 Astrovirus Norovirus Rotavirus Sapovirus	Cryptosporidium Cyclospora cayetanensis E histolytica Giardia	27,29,32,34,36

(continued on next page)

Table 4
(continued)

Assay	Turnaround Time, h	Bacterial Targets	Viral Targets	Parasitic Targets	References
Hologic Prodesse ProGastro SSCS Assay	4	Campylobacter spp Salmonella spp Shiga toxin 1 and 2 Shigella spp	—	—	Buchan et al,[28] 2013
Luminex Verigene Enteric Pathogens Test[d]	2	Campylobacter spp Salmonella spp Shigella spp Vibrio spp Y enterocolitica Shiga toxin 1 and 2 (stx1 and stx2)	Norovirus Rotavirus	—	Huang et al,[29] 2016
Luminex xTAG Gastrointestinal Pathogen Panel[e]	5	Campylobacter spp C difficile E coli O157 ETEC STEC Salmonella spp Shigella spp Vibrio cholera	Adenovirus 40/41 Norovirus Rotavirus	Cryptosporidium E histolytica Giardia	29–31,34

Abbreviations: EAEC, enteroaggregative *E coli*; EPEC, enteropathogenic *E coli*; ETEC, enterotoxigenic *E coli*; STEC, shiga-toxin–like producing *E coli*.

[a] BDMax Enteric Bacterial Panel detects specific *Campylobacter* (*coli* and *jejuni*) species but only reports as a group.

[b] BDMax Extended Enteric Bacterial Panel detects specific *Vibrio* (*cholerae*, *parahaemolyticus*, and *vulnificus*) species but only reports as a group.

[c] FilmArray Gastrointestinal panel detects specific *Campylobacter* (*coli*, *jejuni*, and *upsaliensis*) and *Vibrio* (*cholerae*, *parahaemolyticus*, and *vulnificus*) species but only reports as a group. When STEC is detected, the assay then determines if it is an *E coli* O157 serotype.

[d] Verigene Enteric Pathogen Test detects specific *Campylobacter* (*coli*, *jejuni*, and *lari*) and *Vibrio* (*cholera* and *parahaemolyticus*) species but only reports as a group.

[e] xTAG Gastrointestinal Pathogen Panel detects specific *Campylobacter* (*coli*, *jejuni*, and *lari*) species but only reports as a group.

Verigene Enteric panel demonstrated similar specificity to the other assays but reduced sensitivity for detection of *Campylobacter* (83.3%), *Salmonella* (83.3%), norovirus (89%), and rotavirus (71.4%). In another study, the investigators evaluated the FilmArray Gastrointestinal and xTAG Gastrointestinal panels and found similar performance between both tests for shared analytes except the xTAG panel demonstrated lower specificity for norovirus in prospective and retrospective specimens.[33] Finally, in the study by Chhabra and colleagues,[34] the investigators specifically examined the analytical performance of the FilmArray Gastrointestinal and xTAG Gastrointestinal panels for detection of gastrointestinal viruses. The investigators noted that the FilmArray Gastrointestinal Panel demonstrated overall better analytical performance for viral detection relative to the xTAG panel.[34]

Although multiplex gastrointestinal panels offer more rapid results to clinicians, they can present a potential problem for public health surveillance efforts if bacterial pathogens are not cultured.[35] In addition, the lack of bacterial isolates could complicate treatment without antimicrobial susceptibility results. Another caveat to these molecular panel tests is that multiple pathogens can be present, as observed with 31.5% of specimens in a multicenter study of the FilmArray,[27] and 30.3% for the xTAG Gastrointestinal panel.[33] The clinical significance of multiple positive targets is currently unclear and can cause frustration for clinicians unsure which target or targets detected are responsible for their patient's symptoms. Finally, limited information is available on repeat multiplex testing. Park and colleagues[36] retrospectively evaluated patients with initially negative FilmArray Gastrointestinal results and found that 92.5% remained negative upon retesting within 4 weeks. Conversely, of patients with initially positive results, 53.8% remained positive for the same target within 4 weeks.[36] Continued asymptomatic shedding has been observed for gastrointestinal pathogens.[37,38] Taken together, these results show that molecular testing is not appropriate as a test of cure and that continued detection of targets can occur for an indeterminate amount of time regardless of patient symptoms. It is absolutely necessary to restrict testing to symptomatic individuals and carefully interpret any repeat positive results.

Several of the multiplex syndromic panels contain a target for *C difficile*. For pediatric patients, the American Academy of Pediatrics guidelines for *Clostridium difficile* infection (CDI) diagnosis discourages testing in those less than 1 years of age due to the high percentage of children in this age group who are asymptomatically colonized with *C difficile*.[39] In children aged 1 to 3 years, causes such as viruses should be considered before testing for *C difficile* for the same reason. As a discussion of *C difficile* testing is outside the scope of this article, the authors refer readers to a review of *C difficile* testing in pediatrics.[40]

RAPID DETECTION OF CENTRAL NERVOUS SYSTEM INFECTIONS

Traditional rapid diagnostic testing of cerebrospinal fluid (CSF) specimens uses cell count, protein, glucose, and Gram stain. However, this testing has limited analytical sensitivity and specificity in differentiating infectious versus noninfectious causes or in differentiating the bacterial versus viral versus fungal pathogens. The gold standard for identification of bacterial pathogens is CSF culture, whereas fungal causes are identified by culture and antigen testing (eg, Cyptococcal antigen testing). Bacterial and fungal cultures can take days to grow, test, and obtain a result. In addition, treatment with antimicrobial therapy before obtaining CSF can reduce microbial viability, leaving clinicians without a target for therapy. There exist bacterial antigen tests for CSF specimens that can provide rapid results, but such testing is not recommended by the Infectious Diseases Society of America.[41] Viral testing is now performed using molecular-based methods, which surpass viral culture in sensitivity and turn-around time.

Molecular testing of CSF specimens for viral pathogens is frequently performed using laboratory developed tests (LDTs), which uses various methods for nucleic acid extraction, purification, oligonucleotide primer sets, and detection methods. Taken together, this can create interlaboratory variability of test performance, requiring clinicians to be aware of the relative performance of their institutional assays. Currently, there are 2 stand-alone FDA-cleared assays for detection of viral pathogens from CSF specimens, the Cepheid Xpert EV (Enterovirus) (Cepheid, Sunnyvale, CA, USA) and Simplexa HSV 1 and 2 Direct (**Table 5**). Both are qualitative assays performed directly off of CSF specimens. The Xpert EV (DiaSorin Molecular LLC, Cypress, CA, USA) detects an array of enterovirus serotypes, but not parechoviruses, and overall demonstrates high sensitivity (>97%) and specificity (100%).[42,43] Similarly, the Simplexa HSV 1 and 2 Direct has shown high sensitivity (96%) and specificity (97%), although depending on the comparator LDT, the LOD may be slightly higher than the evaluated LDT.[44,45]

There is only one FDA-cleared syndromic multiplex panel, the FilmArray Meningitis/Encephalitis panel (bioMérieux, Durham, NC, USA) (**Table 6**). It detects bacterial (n = 6), viral (n = 7), and fungal pathogens (n = 1) from CSF specimens. One large prospective study examined 1560 CSF specimens from adults and children using the FilmArray Meningitis/Encephalitis panel and found an 84.4% positive and greater than 99.9% negative agreement with the comparator methods.[46] Although it was noted that an additional 21 pathogens were detected using the FilmArray Meningitis/Encephalitis panel, there was also 22 unconfirmed/false positive detections. *Streptococcus pneumoniae* (n = 7) was the most frequent unconfirmed/false positive target, which the investigators proposed could be oral flora contamination during testing, necessitating the need for adherence to strict molecular testing procedures. In 2 pediatric specific studies examining the FilmArray Meningitis/Encephalitis panel, strong agreement was seen with conventional methods.[47,48] Although in 1 study, 2 herpes simplex virus (HSV)-1 detections were missed by the FilmArray Meningitis/Encephalitis panel that were likely near the LOD of the assay, HSV-1 was detected in both specimens by the standard-of-care LDT.[48] It should be noted that 2 studies found that this panel demonstrated reduced sensitivity for *Cryptococcus* detection relative to antigen testing.[49,50] Finally, to date, there is no clinical report of the performance of this assay for detecting relatively low incident pathogen *Listeria monocytogenes* and only 1 report for *Neisseria meningitidis*,[49] which was detected by the panel.

Molecular testing for bacterial and fungal CSF pathogens does not replace traditional culture, because culture provides isolates for antimicrobial susceptibility testing and can detect pathogens not on the panel. Careful interpretation of the results from CSF multiplex panels needs to take into account the patient's clinical picture because false positive results can occur from contamination events. In particular, positive results for herpes viruses (eg, cytomegalovirus, HSV, human herpesvirus 6, and varicella zoster virus) could represent detection of latent or actively replicating virus.

Table 5			
Singleplex detection of viral pathogens directly from cerebrospinal fluid specimens			
Assay	**Turnaround Time (h)**	**Targets Detected**	**Methodology**
Cepheid Xpert EV	1	Enterovirus	Real-time PCR
DiaSorin Simplexa HSV 1 and 2 direct	1	HSV 1 and HSV 2[a]	Real-time PCR

[a] Simplexa HSV 1 and 2 Direct detects and differentiates between HSV1 and/or HSV2.

Table 6				
Multiplex meningitis encephalitis panel, US Food and Drug Administration approved				
Assay	Turnaround Time, h	Bacterial Targets	Viral Targets	Fungal Targets
bioMérieux FilmArray Meningitis/ Encephalitis Panel	1 h	*Escherichia coli* K1[a] *Haemophilus influenzae* *L monocytogenes* *N meningitidis* *Streptococcus agalactiae* (Group B) *S pneumoniae*	CMV Enterovirus HSV-1 HSV-2 HHV-6 Human parechovirus VZV	*Cryptococcus neoformans/gattii*[b]

Abbreviations: CMV, cytomegalovirus; HSV-1, herpes simplex virus 1; HSV-2, herpes simplex virus 2; HHV-6, human herpesvirus 6; VZV, varicella zoster virus.
[a] The FilmArray Meningitis/Encephalitis panel only detects *E coli* K1, which accounts for up to 80% of *E coli* causes of neonatal meningitis.
[b] *C neoformans* and *C gattii* are not differentiated by this assay.

DETECTION OF *KINGELLA KINGAE* FROM SEPTIC JOINTS

K kingae is a frequent colonizer of the oropharynx in young children 2 to 36 months of age, and its prevalence is increased in children who attend daycare.[51] In children colonized with *K kingae*, bacteria can translocate to the bloodstream, causing bacteremia and seeding of distal body sites, primarily joints and bones, where it causes infection. *K kingae* is a fastidious bacterium that rarely grows in culture from septic joints. To improve sensitivity of pathogen detection, excess joint fluid can be inoculated into blood culture bottles and incubated for increased recovery of *K kingae*.[52] Although there are no FDA-cleared molecular assays for detection of *K kingae*, testing is offered at reference laboratories and some hospitals have LDT PCR assays that are used clinically. Some pediatric orthopedic practices routinely test for *K kingae* in patients ≤4 years of age using either a *K kingae*–specific PCR assays or 16S ribosomal DNA sequencing directly from joint specimens.[53,54] Both inoculation of joint fluid into blood culture bottles and molecular detection assays have markedly improved the rate of *K kingae* detection from joint specimens compared with bacterial culture alone.

SUMMARY

New diagnostic assays for GAS, influenza, and RSV are pressing the boundaries of maintaining a rapid turnaround time and providing increased sensitivity and specificity of pathogen detection. Molecular testing is no longer confined to the walls of the laboratory but has been reimagined into easy-to-use platforms which can be used by nonlaboratory personnel at point of care. In addition, multiplex syndromic panels are allowing broad testing of pathogens associated with a single clinical presentation in a single assay. Together with clinicians, rapid and accurate pathogen detection in children may result in decreased time to optimal antimicrobial treatment and improved patient outcomes.

REFERENCES

1. Martin JM, Green M, Barbadora KA, et al. Group A streptococci among school-aged children: clinical characteristics and the carrier state. Pediatrics 2004; 114(5):1212–9.

2. Roper SM, Edwards R, Mpwo M, et al. Reducing errors in an emergency center setting using an automated fluorescence immunoassay for group A streptococcus identification. Clin Pediatr (Phila) 2017;56(7):675–7.
3. Henson AM, Carter D, Todd K, et al. Detection of Streptococcus pyogenes by use of Illumigene group A Streptococcus assay. J Clin Microbiol 2013;51(12):4207–9.
4. Felsenstein S, Faddoul D, Sposto R, et al. Molecular and clinical diagnosis of group A streptococcal pharyngitis in children. J Clin Microbiol 2014;52(11):3884–9.
5. Tabb MM, Batterman HJ. The Simplexa™ group A strep direct assay: a sample-to-answer molecular assay for the diagnosis of group A streptococcal pharyngitis. Expert Rev Mol Diagn 2016;16(3):269–76.
6. Uhl JR, Patel R. Fifteen-minute detection of Streptococcus pyogenes in throat swabs by use of a commercially available point-of-care PCR assay. J Clin Microbiol 2016;54(3):815.
7. Cohen DM, Russo ME, Jaggi P, et al. Multicenter clinical evaluation of the novel Alere i strep a isothermal nucleic acid amplification test. J Clin Microbiol 2015; 53(7):2258–61.
8. Available at: https://www.cdc.gov/flu/protect/children.htm. Accessed October 25, 2017.
9. Available at: https://www.cdc.gov/rsv. Accessed October 27, 2017.
10. Available at: https://www.cdc.gov/flu/professionals/diagnosis/rapidlab.htm. Accessed October 25, 2017.
11. Dunn J, Obuekwe J, Baun T, et al. Prompt detection of influenza A and B viruses using the BD Veritor™ system flu A+B, Quidel® Sofia® influenza A+B FIA, and Alere binaxNOW® influenza A&B compared to real-time reverse transcription-polymerase chain reaction (RT-PCR). Diagn Microbiol Infect Dis 2014;79(1):10–3.
12. Bell J, Bonner A, Cohen DM, et al. Multicenter clinical evaluation of the novel Alere™ i Influenza A&B isothermal nucleic acid amplification test. J Clin Virol 2014;61(1):81–6.
13. Nolte FS, Gauld L, Barrett SB. Direct comparison of Alere i and Cobas Liat influenza A and B tests for rapid detection of influenza virus infection. J Clin Microbiol 2016;54(11):2763–6.
14. Popowitch EB, O'Neill SS, Miller MB. Comparison of the Biofire FilmArray RP, Genmark eSensor RVP, Luminex xTAG RVPv1, and Luminex xTAG RVP fast multiplex assays for detection of respiratory viruses. J Clin Microbiol 2013;51(5):1528–33.
15. Peaper DR, Landry ML. Rapid diagnosis of influenza: state of the art. Clin Lab Med 2014;34(2):365–85.
16. Buller RS. Molecular detection of respiratory viruses. Clin Lab Med 2013;33(3): 439–60.
17. Nelson RE, Stockmann C, Hersh AL, et al. Economic analysis of rapid and sensitive polymerase chain reaction testing in the emergency department for influenza infections in children. Pediatr Infect Dis J 2015;34(6):577–82.
18. Doan Q, Enarson P, Kissoon N, et al. Rapid viral diagnosis for acute febrile respiratory illness in children in the emergency department. Cochrane Database Syst Rev 2014;(9):CD006452.
19. Rogers BB, Shankar P, Jerris RC, et al. Impact of a rapid respiratory panel test on patient outcomes. Arch Pathol Lab Med 2015;139(5):636–41.
20. Gonzalez MD, Wilen CB, Burnham CA. Markers of intestinal inflammation for the diagnosis of infectious gastroenteritis. Clin Lab Med 2015;35(2):333–44.
21. Fitzgerald C, Patrick M, Gonzalez A, et al. Multicenter evaluation of clinical diagnostic methods for detection and isolation of campylobacter spp. from stool. J Clin Microbiol 2016;54(5):1209–15.

22. McHardy IH, Wu M, Shimizu-Cohen R, et al. Detection of intestinal protozoa in the clinical laboratory. J Clin Microbiol 2014;52(3):712–20.
23. Gonzalez MD, Langley LC, Buchan BW, et al. Multicenter evaluation of the xpert norovirus assay for detection of norovirus genogroups I and II in fecal specimens. J Clin Microbiol 2016;54(1):142–7.
24. Harrington S, MBuchan BW, Doern C, et al. Multicenter evaluation of the BD max enteric bacterial panel PCR assay for rapid detection of Salmonella spp., Shigella spp., Campylobacter spp. (C. jejuni and C. coli), and Shiga toxin 1 and 2 genes. J Clin Microbiol 2015;53(5):1639–47.
25. Madison-Antenucci S, Relich RF, Doyle L, et al. Multicenter evaluation of BD max enteric parasite real-time PCR assay for detection of Giardia duodenalis, Cryptosporidium hominis, Cryptosporidium parvum, and Entamoeba histolytica. J Clin Microbiol 2016;54(11):2681–8.
26. Simner PJ, Oethinger M, Stellrecht KA, et al. Multisite evaluation of the BD Max extended enteric bacterial panel for detection of yersinia enterocolitica, enterotoxigenic escherichia coli, vibrio, and plesiomonas shigelloides from stool specimens. J Clin Microbiol 2017;55(11):3258–66.
27. Buss SN, Leber A, Chapin K, et al. Multicenter evaluation of the BioFire FilmArray gastrointestinal panel for etiologic diagnosis of infectious gastroenteritis. J Clin Microbiol 2015;53(3):915–25.
28. Buchan BW, Olson WJ, Pezewski M, et al. Clinical evaluation of a real-time PCR assay for identification of Salmonella, Shigella, Campylobacter (Campylobacter jejuni and C. coli), and shiga toxin-producing Escherichia coli isolates in stool specimens. J Clin Microbiol 2013;51(12):4001–7.
29. Huang RS, Johnson CL, Pritchard L, et al. Performance of the Verigene® enteric pathogens test, Biofire FilmArray™ gastrointestinal panel and Luminex xTAG® gastrointestinal pathogen panel for detection of common enteric pathogens. Diagn Microbiol Infect Dis 2016;86(4):336–9.
30. Claas EC, Burnham CA, Mazzulli T, et al. Performance of the xTAG® gastrointestinal pathogen panel, a multiplex molecular assay for simultaneous detection of bacterial, viral, and parasitic causes of infectious gastroenteritis. J Microbiol Biotechnol 2013;23(7):1041–5.
31. Mengelle C, Mansuy JM, Prere MF, et al. Simultaneous detection of gastrointestinal pathogens with a multiplex Luminex-based molecular assay in stool samples from diarrhoeic patients. Clin Microbiol Infect 2013;19(10):E458–65.
32. Stockmann C, Rogatcheva M, Harrel B, et al. How well does physician selection of microbiologic tests identify Clostridium difficile and other pathogens in paediatric diarrhoea? Insights using multiplex PCR-based detection. Clin Microbiol Infect 2015;21(2):179.e9-15.
33. Khare R, Espy MJ, Cebelinski E, et al. Comparative evaluation of two commercial multiplex panels for detection of gastrointestinal pathogens by use of clinical stool specimens. J Clin Microbiol 2014;52(10):3667–73.
34. Chhabra P, Gregoricus N, Weinberg GA, et al. Comparison of three multiplex gastrointestinal platforms for the detection of gastroenteritis viruses. J Clin Virol 2017;95:66–71.
35. Shea S, Kubota KA, Maguire H, et al. Clinical microbiology laboratories' adoption of culture-independent diagnostic tests is a threat to foodborne-disease surveillance in the United States. J Clin Microbiol 2017;55(1):10–9.
36. Park S, Hitchcock MM, Gomez CA, et al. Is follow-up testing with the film array gastrointestinal multiplex PCR panel necessary? J Clin Microbiol 2017;55(4):1154–61.

37. Humphries RM, Linscott AJ. Laboratory diagnosis of bacterial gastroenteritis. Clin Microbiol Rev 2015;28(1):3–31.
38. Robilotti E, Deresinski S, Pinsky BA. Norovirus. Clin Microbiol Rev 2015;28(1):134–64.
39. Schutze GE, Willoughby RE, Committee on Infectious Diseases, et al. Clostridium difficile infection in infants and children. Pediatrics 2013;131(1):196–200.
40. Antonara S, Leber AL. Diagnosis of Clostridium difficile infections in children. J Clin Microbiol 2016;54(6):1425–33.
41. Baron EJ, Miller JM, Weinstein MP, et al. A guide to utilization of the microbiology laboratory for diagnosis of infectious diseases: 2013 recommendations by the Infectious Diseases Society of America (IDSA) and the American Society for Microbiology (ASM)(a). Clin Infect Dis 2013;57(4):e22–121.
42. Kost CB, Rogers B, Oberste MS, et al. Multicenter beta trial of the GeneXpert enterovirus assay. J Clin Microbiol 2007;45(4):1081–6.
43. Marlowe EM, Novak SM, Dunn JJ, et al. Performance of the GeneXpert enterovirus assay for detection of enteroviral RNA in cerebrospinal fluid. J Clin Virol 2008;43(1):110–3.
44. Binnicker MJ, Espy MJ, Irish CL. Rapid and direct detection of herpes simplex virus in cerebrospinal fluid by use of a commercial real-time PCR assay. J Clin Microbiol 2014;52(12):4361–2.
45. Kuypers J, Boughton G, Chung J, et al. Comparison of the Simplexa HSV1 & 2 direct kit and laboratory-developed real-time PCR assays for herpes simplex virus detection. J Clin Virol 2015;62:103–5.
46. Leber AL, Everhart K, Balada-Llasat JM, et al. Multicenter evaluation of BioFire filmarray meningitis/encephalitis panel for detection of bacteria, viruses, and yeast in cerebrospinal fluid specimens. J Clin Microbiol 2016;54(9):2251–61.
47. Messacar K, Breazeale G, Robinson CC, et al. Potential clinical impact of the film array meningitis encephalitis panel in children with suspected central nervous system infections. Diagn Microbiol Infect Dis 2016;86(1):118–20.
48. Graf EH, Farquharson MV, Cárdenas AM. Comparative evaluation of the FilmArray meningitis/encephalitis molecular panel in a pediatric population. Diagn Microbiol Infect Dis 2017;87(1):92–4.
49. Hanson KE, Slechta ES, Killpack JA, et al. Preclinical assessment of a fully automated multiplex PCR panel for detection of central nervous system pathogens. J Clin Microbiol 2016;54(3):785–7.
50. Rhein J, Bahr NC, Hemmert AC, et al. Diagnostic performance of a multiplex PCR assay for meningitis in an HIV-infected population in Uganda. Diagn Microbiol Infect Dis 2016;84(3):268–73.
51. Yagupsky P. Kingella kingae: carriage, transmission, and disease. Clin Microbiol Rev 2015;28(1):54–79.
52. Yagupsky P, Dagan R, Howard CW, et al. High prevalence of Kingella kingae in joint fluid from children with septic arthritis revealed by the BACTEC blood culture system. J Clin Microbiol 1992;30(5):1278–81.
53. Chometon S, Benito Y, Chaker M, et al. Specific real-time polymerase chain reaction places Kingella kingae as the most common cause of osteoarticular infections in young children. Pediatr Infect Dis J 2007;26(5):377–81.
54. Carter K, Doern C, Jo CH, et al. The clinical usefulness of polymerase chain reaction as a supplemental diagnostic tool in the evaluation and the treatment of children with septic arthritis. J Pediatr Orthop 2016;36(2):167–72.

Current Concepts in the Evaluation and Management of Bronchiolitis

Kathryn E. Kyler, MD[a], Russell J. McCulloh, MD[b,c],*

KEYWORDS

- Bronchiolitis • Respiratory syncytial virus • Viral infection • Pediatrics • Evaluation
- Management

KEY POINTS

- Bronchiolitis is a lower respiratory tract illness caused by viral infection in children 2 years of age and younger, frequently associated with wheezing.
- It is a common cause of hospitalization, particularly in patients with risk factors for serious disease.
- Care is generally supportive with a focus on safely doing less.
- Many therapies have been shown to have no significant effect on hospitalization rates, length of stay, or duration of symptoms.

OVERVIEW

Bronchiolitis is a common lower respiratory tract illness caused by viral infection in children 2 years of age and younger. Bronchiolitis is characterized by inflammation and increased mucus production, leading to a spectrum of respiratory symptoms including rhinitis, tachypnea, and increased work of breathing. Diagnostic criteria vary across countries.[1] In North America, the American Academy of Pediatrics (AAP) defined bronchiolitis as "a constellation of clinical symptoms and signs including a viral upper respiratory prodrome followed by increased respiratory effort and wheezing."[2] Older children can have wheezing induced by viral infection but not fit the classic picture of bronchiolitis, making differentiating bronchiolitis from viral-induced wheeze in these patients challenging.[2]

Disclosure Statement: The authors have no conflicts of interest to disclose.
[a] Pediatric Hospital Medicine, Department of Pediatrics, Children's Mercy Kansas City, University of Missouri-Kansas City, 2401 Gillham Road, Kansas City, MO 64108, USA; [b] Department of Pediatrics, Children's Mercy Kansas City, University of Missouri-Kansas City, 2401 Gillham Road, Kansas City, MO 64108, USA; [c] Department of Internal Medicine, University of Missouri-Kansas City, 2411 Holmes Street, Kansas City, MO 64108, USA
* Corresponding author. Children's Mercy Hospital, 2401 Gillham Road, Kansas City, MO 64108.
E-mail address: rmcculloh@cmh.edu

Infect Dis Clin N Am 32 (2018) 35–45
https://doi.org/10.1016/j.idc.2017.10.002
0891-5520/18/© 2017 Elsevier Inc. All rights reserved.
id.theclinics.com

Bronchiolitis is the most common cause of hospital admission in children 12 months old and younger, accounting for 16% to 18% of hospitalizations yearly and costing approximately $1.73 billion.[3,4] It most commonly affects infants and young children, with a peak incidence in infants less than 6 months of age.[4,5] Approximately 2% to 3% of children with bronchiolitis require hospitalization.[6] The most commonly identified causative viral pathogen is respiratory syncytial virus (RSV), which is found in 50% to 80% of cases.[3,7] Other common viral etiologies include human enterovirus/rhinovirus (16%–18%), influenza (10%–15%), human metapneumovirus (3%–19%), and parainfluenza virus (1%–7%).[7–10] Up to 10% to 30% of bronchiolitis cases result from coinfection with multiple viruses.[10] The peak season for RSV and most other viruses is during the winter months in the United States (December to March), with some regional variation in areas with a warmer climate.[3]

Several risk factors can predispose children to more severe disease from bronchiolitis (**Box 1**). Infants with a history of preterm birth (<37 weeks gestation) and infants less than 12 weeks of age are at increased risk for severe disease. Infants and young children who are immunocompromised, have congenital cardiac disease, or chronic lung disease of prematurity are also at increased risk. Other congenital/genetic abnormalities may put infants at risk, including: cystic fibrosis, Down syndrome, cerebral palsy, or other congenital abnormalities.[5,11] Other potential risk factors for disease severity include in utero and postnatal cigarette smoke exposure or duration of exclusive breast feeding.[12–14]

PATHOPHYSIOLOGY

Viruses commonly causing bronchiolitis usually affect only the upper respiratory tract or nasal mucus membranes, leading to nasal congestion and upper respiratory symptoms. However, in 30% to 40% of infected infants, the lower respiratory tract will become affected.[15] This lower airway inflammation leads to shedding of the epithelial layers in the small airways, airway edema, and ciliary dysfunction. The resulting collection of necrotic cells and mucus in the airways can lead to varying degrees of obstruction, atelectasis, and pulmonary ventilation/perfusion mismatch, causing hypoxemia.[2]

Bronchospasm through smooth muscle constriction is a minor pathophysiological component of bronchiolitis, which may explain the limited effects of bronchodilators in symptomatic treatment.[2] Additionally, tissue inflammation is minimal; the primary driver of symptoms is debris accumulation in the smaller airways, which likely explains why corticosteroids and epinephrine provide little benefit for children with bronchiolitis.[16,17]

Box 1
Risk factors for severe bronchiolitis

- Age less than 12 weeks
- History of prematurity (birth <37 weeks gestation)
- Hemodynamically significant cardiac disease
- Chronic lung disease of prematurity
- Immunodeficiency (eg, hypogammaglobulinemia)
- Genetic/chromosomal abnormalities (eg, Down syndrome, cystic fibrosis)
- Other congenital anomalies (eg, spina bifida, anencephaly)
- Other high-risk chronic conditions (eg, cancer, chronic kidney disease)
- In-utero smoke exposure

CLINICAL MANIFESTATIONS

Bronchiolitis starts with upper airway manifestations such as rhinorrhea, nasal congestion, and sneezing. After a few days, symptoms shift to the lower airway, causing increased cough and respiratory distress. Patients may exhibit crackles, rhonchi, and/or wheezing on lung examination, and may have mild-to-severe retractions, nasal flaring, and/or head bobbing in cases of more severe respiratory distress. Apnea may occur, especially in infants 6 months of age and younger with RSV infections.[18] Poor oral intake can result from nasal obstruction, respiratory distress, and tachypnea.[19] Generalized symptoms including fever or malaise are also common.

Bronchiolitis is a self-limited viral disease, but symptom severity of can vary greatly, ranging from mild congestion and cough without difficulty breathing to severe respiratory distress, apnea, or hypoxemia that may ultimately require mechanical ventilation. Symptoms are typically mild for the first few days and peak at approximately days 3 to 5 of illness. Symptoms may begin to improve by days 5 to 6 of illness, with a median duration of approximately 12 days.[20] Once a child begins improving, it is uncommon for his or her disease to worsen again.[21] Some symptoms (primarily cough) may linger for several weeks.[22]

DIAGNOSIS

Diagnosis and assessment of bronchiolitis severity should be made clinically, using the history and physical examination.[3] Important history elements to review include the effect of symptoms on the child's oral intake in order to maintain adequate hydration and effects on mental status.[3] Clinicians should assess the ability of families to recognize concerning symptoms that should prompt a return for evaluation. Assessing past medical history to identify potential risk factors for disease progression is also important.

Diagnosis based on physical examination may require serial examinations over time due to frequent fluctuations in symptom severity. Clinicians should be aware of the normal values for respiratory rate and heart rate for different age groups, as normal ranges change considerably over the first few years of life. Using specific physical examination findings to predict disease severity is difficult; severe adverse events in children with bronchiolitis are rare (<1% of children will require intensive care unit [ICU] admission), making detection of clinically important associations difficult.[3,23] Several respiratory symptom scores have been developed to assess respiratory distress severity in bronchiolitis, but none has achieved widespread acceptance.[24]

There is a growing consensus over the past 20 years for safely doing less when diagnosing and managing bronchiolitis.[25] Based on available evidence, the following laboratory and radiological work ups are generally not recommended for bronchiolitis, except in cases where the diagnosis is uncertain or when a concomitant diagnosis is suspected: complete blood cell (CBC) count, blood cultures, or routine virologic testing. Current evidence does not support obtaining routine chest radiographs in children with bronchiolitis.[3] Most infants will have some abnormalities on chest radiography, but studies have failed to correlate radiographic findings with risk for severe disease. Radiography should be considered if symptoms warrant ICU admission or with clinical concerns for another complication (eg, pneumothorax or bacterial pneumonia).

Routine virologic testing is generally not recommended in bronchiolitis, as test results will not alter clinical management. An exception is children receiving palivizumab prophylaxis who present with symptoms concerning for bronchiolitis; prophylaxis should be discontinued if RSV is identified (see Prevention, below). Rapid viral testing for influenza during peak season should also be considered, as antiviral therapy is recommended by the AAP for influenza-infected children:

Hospitalized with influenza
With severe, complicated, or progressive symptoms
At high risk for complications
Otherwise healthy but for whom a decrease in symptoms duration is deemed necessary by their provider[26]

A systematic review found that infants less than 60 to 90 days of age with bronchiolitis were unlikely to have concomitant serious bacterial infection (SBI); 3.3% had urinary tract infections (UTIs), and incidence of bacteremia or meningitis were extremely rare, with studies reporting an incidence of less than 0.1%.[27] This information could argue for a more selective approach to SBI screening in infants younger than 60 to 90 days who present with fever and symptoms consistent with bronchiolitis or who have been found to have a documented RSV infection.

MANAGEMENT
Determining Disposition

When caring for a child with bronchiolitis in any clinical setting, the initial evaluation should assess illness severity to help determine if hospitalization is warranted (**Table 1**). Indications for hospital admission include hypoxemia (oxygen saturation of <90% in room air), significantly increased work of breathing/retractions, dehydration, or an inability to maintain hydration with oral intake because of respiratory distress. Careful consideration of a child's risk factors for progression to serious disease and the natural history of bronchiolitis may further aid clinicians in determining proper disposition.[5] If a patient does not require admission, families should be carefully counseled on signs and symptoms that would necessitate return for evaluation.

Supportive Care

Care for children with bronchiolitis is supportive, including hydration, respiratory support, and supplemental oxygen if needed. As mentioned previously, caring for infants and children with bronchiolitis should focus on safely doing less, and a significant amount of research over the last few decades has shed light on the efficacy of particular therapies in bronchiolitis.[25]

Suctioning

Oral and nasal suctioning are often beneficial for infants and children with bronchiolitis with tachypnea and respiratory distress.[28] Suctioning helps temporarily clear nasal and airway secretions, thereby improving respiratory symptoms. Nasal suctioning may be performed by health care providers or at home by parents. Nasopharyngeal suctioning (ie, deep suctioning) may not provide any additional benefit over nasal suctioning, and 1 study identified a longer length of stay for infants receiving deep suctioning, possibly because of increased airway trauma from the procedure.[28]

Oxygen therapy and pulse oximetry monitoring

Supplemental oxygen should be provided to all infants and children with bronchiolitis with hypoxemia (oxygen saturations of <90%).[3] Oxygen saturations of 89% or higher are generally adequate for tissue perfusion, and the risk to the patient from mild hypoxemia is minimal. Additionally, mild, transient episodes of hypoxemia are common

Table 1
Indications for therapy in bronchiolitis

Intervention	Indications	Limitations
Nebulized hypertonic saline (3%)	Increased work of breathing in inpatient setting only	Not indicated for use in the emergency room: does not change need for admission; does not decrease length of stay when stay expected to be <3 d
Oxygen	Hypoxemia with O_2 saturation <90%	O_2 saturation of 89% or greater are adequate for tissue perfusion and the risk from hypoxemia is minimal
Fluid resuscitation	Dehydration, poor oral intake, or respiratory distress increasing the risk of aspiration	Intravenous hydration may result in iatrogenic hyponatremia
Albuterol	Not indicated; albuterol trial no longer recommended	May transiently improve symptom scores, but no change in need for hospitalization, resolution of symptoms, or length of stay
Epinephrine	Not indicated	Provides no improvement in length of stay or other inpatient outcomes
Systemic corticosteroids	Not indicated	Provides no improvement in length of stay or other inpatient outcomes
Antibiotics	Use only if suspicion for concomitant bacterial infection is high	Will not provide benefit for viral bronchiolitis
Chest physiotherapy	Not indicated	Studies have shown no benefit
Continuous pulse oximetry	Use only in patients requiring oxygen for hypoxemia; otherwise not indicated	Intermittent pulse oximetry is adequate for patients who do not require O_2; studies show this decreases length of stay

Data from Ralston SL, Lieberthal AS, Meissner HC, et al. Clinical practice guideline: the diagnosis, management, and prevention of bronchiolitis. Pediatrics 2014;134(5):e1474–502.

even in well infants.[29] Supplemental oxygen can be delivered using conventional nasal cannula or via minimally invasive positive pressure support.

Continuous pulse oximetry may be monitored in patients requiring supplemental oxygen. However, because oxygen saturations are a poor indicator of respiratory distress, it is unnecessary to continuously monitor pulse oximetry of infants not requiring supplemental oxygen.[3] One study evaluating the role of continuous pulse oximetry in infants hospitalized with bronchiolitis found that 1 in 4 patients had unnecessarily prolonged hospital stays because of a perceived need for oxygen therapy.[30] Thus, the AAP recommends only intermittent pulse oximetry checks for children admitted with bronchiolitis who do not require supplemental oxygen.[3]

Minimally invasive positive pressure ventilation
Varying degrees of respiratory support may be provided to admitted infants and children with significant respiratory distress, hypoxemia, or respiratory failure. Increased air flow (with or without supplemental oxygen) may be provided by simple nasal

cannula, high flow nasal cannula, or if necessary, positive pressure ventilation or intubation and mechanical ventilation. Although the mechanisms behind providing high flow nasal cannula or positive pressure ventilation are not well understood, and data regarding their efficacy are lacking, they are thought to improve respiratory distress and oxygenation by increasing the end expiratory lung volumes and decreasing airway resistance.[31,32] The use of minimally invasive respiratory supports may help decrease the need for intubation in children with bronchiolitis, but more studies are necessary to determine their effectiveness.[32]

Hydration therapy

Infants who are unable to meet their hydration needs orally because of bronchiolitis symptoms should receive hydration therapy.[3] Hydration and nutrition may be provided orally, via a nasogastric tube, or intravenously. Enteral hydration may be appropriate for patients who do not have vomiting and are not at significant risk of clinical decompensation that would potentially require positive pressure ventilation support or intubation.

Recommendations Regarding Specific Therapies

Nebulized hypertonic saline

The use of nebulized hypertonic (3%) saline (HTS) may be considered for inpatients with bronchiolitis, but should not be administered in the emergency department.[3] HTS may improve mucociliary clearance, resulting in reduced respiratory distress and improved oxygenation.[33] Data regarding HTS efficacy in decreasing length of stay and disease severity are mixed; however, the most recent systematic review concluded that HTS may help decrease the length of stay of patients admitted with bronchiolitis.[33,34] HTS should be scheduled every 6 to 8 hours. The risk of adverse events from HTS is low, and treatments are generally well tolerated.[33]

Albuterol

Using albuterol or other bronchodilators is not recommended for infants and children with bronchiolitis.[3] Despite the fact that many patients with bronchiolitis will have wheezing on examination and administration of albuterol may transiently improve clinical respiratory scores, albuterol has no meaningful effect on disease resolution, oxygen requirement, need for hospitalization, or length of hospital stay.[18,35,36]

Epinephrine

Racemic epinephrine for infants and children with bronchiolitis is not recommended.[3] A systematic review of evidence regarding epinephrine use in bronchiolitis found no difference in need for hospital admission or length of stay, and no difference in symptom resolution.[17]

Systemic corticosteroids

The administration of systemic corticosteroids to patients with bronchiolitis is not recommended.[3] Corticosteroid use does not result in any improvement in clinical respiratory scores, hospitalization rates, or lengths of stay.[16,18]

Antibiotics

Given that the risk of SBI in children with bronchiolitis is less than 1%, administration of antibiotics in patients diagnosed with bronchiolitis is generally not recommended.[3,27,37] However, other bacterial infections such as pneumonia or acute otitis media are possible, and appropriate treatment should be considered if a clinician has a high degree of suspicion for a concomitant bacterial illness.[3,37]

Chest physiotherapy

Chest physiotherapy (vibration, percussion, passive forced exhalation) is not recommended in the treatment of bronchiolitis.[3] Chest physiotherapy provided no improvement in bronchiolitis severity or clinical symptom scores, time to recovery, or length of hospital stay.[38]

COMPLICATIONS

Potential complications secondary to bronchiolitis include apnea, aspiration, respiratory failure, and secondary bacterial pneumonia. Neonates and infants younger than 6 months are at highest risk of apnea episodes. Any infant or child with tachypnea or respiratory distress is at increased risk of aspirating orally ingested liquids or solids. Children with risk factors for severe disease are at higher risk of respiratory failure (see **Box 1**). Approximately 2% of infants and children hospitalized with bronchiolitis will require intubation and mechanical ventilation, but the risk of mortality is low (<0.05%).[4] The prevalence of secondary bacterial pneumonia in children with bronchiolitis has been estimated to be low (<2%), although the prevalence in patients who require ICU care is higher (up to 40%).[37,39,40]

PREVENTION
Palivizumab

Palivizumab is a monoclonal antibody vaccine that is highly active against RSV and has been shown to decrease RSV infections in at-risk infants.[41] A 2011 meta-analysis showed that palivizumab prophylaxis in at-risk infants did not modify the mortality rate from RSV disease (which was low among vaccinated and unvaccinated groups), but did lower rates of hospitalization due to RSV disease in the vaccinated group.[42] The use of palivizumab for certain populations of at-risk children is indicated for the prevention of serious lower respiratory tract disease from RSV during peak season (**Table 2**).

Table 2
Recommendations for administration of palivizumab in first year of life

Should Receive Immunization	Immunization not Recommended	May Consider Immunization
All preterm infants delivered at <29.0 weeks gestation	Preterm infants delivered at ≥29.0 weeks gestation without chronic lung disease	Children <1 y with pulmonary abnormalities impairing ability to clear secretions
Any infant delivered at <32.0 weeks gestation with chronic lung disease of prematurity	Infants with hemodynamically insignificant heart disease	Children <1 y with neuromuscular disease
Any infant with hemodynamically significant heart disease	Infants with heart disease adequately corrected by surgery (do not require medication for heart failure)	Severely immunocompromised children <2 y
	For prophylaxis of health care-associated RSV disease	Children undergoing cardiac transplant in second year of life during RSV season
	Infants 12–24 months with any heart disease, including hemodynamically significant disease	Preterm infants <32.0 weeks gestation with chronic lung disease of prematurity who continue to require oxygen/corticosteroids/diuretics in the 6-month period leading up to their second RSV season

Data from Refs.[41–43]

Clinicians should not administer palivizumab to otherwise healthy infants delivered beyond gestational age of 28 weeks, 6 days. Infants who qualify for palivizumab can receive up to 5 doses during the first year of life (or second, if appropriate) during peak RSV season (November to March). If an at-risk patient is born during RSV season, he or she may require fewer than 5 doses, as every infant should receive their final dose in March. Insufficient data exist to recommend palivizumab prophylaxis to infants with cystic fibrosis or Down syndrome. As the likelihood of repeat RSV hospitalization in the same season is extremely low (<0.5%), further palivizumab doses should be halted for infants who have a breakthrough RSV hospitalization during the winter season they are receiving prophylaxis.[43]

Other Preventive Measures and Counseling

An important way for clinicians to prevent the spread of respiratory viruses during peak season is to provide proper counseling on preventive measures to families. Chief among these recommendations is good hand hygiene.[3] All clinicians should disinfect their hands by washing with soap and water, or using alcohol-based hand sanitizer, both before and after direct contact with or in the vicinity of an infected person. Hand hygiene is of obvious clinical importance, especially because viral shedding of RSV in immunocompetent hosts can persist for up to 3 weeks.[19]

Clinicians should assess smoke exposure of children at risk for bronchiolitis, as tobacco smoke exposure has been shown to increase the risk and severity of bronchiolitis.[3,44] Appropriate counseling to families with children exposed to tobacco smoke should be provided, including risks of smoking outside the home and dangers of smoke lingering on clothing/in rooms for long periods of time.[45]

Clinicians may also recommend exclusive breastfeeding for at least 6 months, as breastfeeding has shown proven benefits for infants, including decreased incidence of respiratory infections.[3] A meta-analysis from the Agency for Healthcare Research (AHRQ) found a 72% reduction in the risk of hospitalization due to respiratory infection in infants exclusively breastfed for at least 4 months compared with formula-fed infants.[46] Other studies have found decreased illness severity in breastfed infants, with breastfed infants possibly having shorter lengths of stay and fewer days requiring supplemental oxygen.[47,48] Clinicians should foster continued breastfeeding by providing counseling and other additional support to mothers, such as lactation consultation.

The AAP also recommends clinicians educate family members and personnel on evidence-based diagnosis, treatment, and prevention of bronchiolitis.[3] Family expectations and experience should be elicited and addressed. Infants and children with bronchiolitis are often symptomatic for 2 to 3 weeks; providing anticipatory guidance at the first instance of a family seeking care may prevent repeat visits due to lingering symptoms. Efforts to prevent spread of disease at home should be recommended, including good hand hygiene and possible restriction of visitors to homes with newborns during the respiratory virus season. With education and open discussion about the nature of the disease, and use of a shared decision-making model with families, clinicians may avoid promoting inappropriate antibiotic or other therapy use and prevent unnecessary health care visits because of lingering symptoms.[22,49]

SUMMARY

Bronchiolitis is a viral infection of the lower respiratory tract in children 2 years of age and younger, frequently associated with wheezing on physical examination. It is a common cause of respiratory distress and hospitalization, particularly in patients with risk factors for more serious disease. The diagnosis can be made based on clinical signs and symptoms alone, and care is generally supportive, with a focus on safely doing less for symptomatic children. Bronchodilators, systemic corticosteroids, and other therapies have no significant effect on hospitalization rates, length of stay, or symptom duration.

REFERENCES

1. Bronchiolitis in children: diagnosis and management. Guidance and guidelines. NICE. Available at: https://www.nice.org.uk/guidance/ng9/chapter/1-Recommendations#assessment-and-diagnosis. Accessed May 16, 2017.
2. American Academy of Pediatrics Subcommittee on Diagnosis and Management of Bronchiolitis. Diagnosis and Management of Bronchiolitis. Pediatrics 2006; 118(4):1774–93.
3. Ralston SL, Lieberthal AS, Meissner HC, et al. Clinical practice guideline: the diagnosis, management, and prevention of bronchiolitis. Pediatrics 2014; 134(5):e1474–502.
4. Hasegawa K, Tsugawa Y, Brown DFM, et al. Trends in bronchiolitis hospitalizations in the United States, 2000–2009. Pediatrics 2013;132(1):28–36.
5. Murray J, Bottle A, Sharland M, et al. Risk factors for hospital admission with RSV bronchiolitis in England: a population-based birth cohort study. PLoS One 2014; 9(2):e89186.
6. Boyce TG, Mellen BG, Mitchel EF Jr, et al. Rates of hospitalization for respiratory syncytial virus infection among children in Medicaid. J Pediatr 2000;137(6): 865–70.
7. Miller EK, Gebretsadik T, Carroll KN, et al. Viral etiologies of infant bronchiolitis, croup, and upper respiratory illness during four consecutive years. Pediatr Infect Dis J 2013;32(9):950–5.
8. Wolf DG, Greenberg D, Kalkstein D, et al. Comparison of human metapneumovirus, respiratory syncytial virus and influenza A virus lower respiratory tract infections in hospitalized young children. Pediatr Infect Dis J 2006;25(4): 320–4.
9. Mansbach JM, McAdam AJ, Clark S, et al. Prospective multicenter study of the viral etiology of bronchiolitis in the emergency department. Acad Emerg Med 2008;15(2):111–8.
10. Paranhos-Baccalà G, Komurian-Pradel F, Richard N, et al. Mixed respiratory virus infections. J Clin Virol 2008;43(4):407–10.
11. Ricart S, Marcos MA, Sarda M, et al. Clinical risk factors are more relevant than respiratory viruses in predicting bronchiolitis severity. Pediatr Pulmonol 2013; 48(5):456–63.
12. Brand HK, de Groot R, Galama JMD, et al. Infection with multiple viruses is not associated with increased disease severity in children with bronchiolitis. Pediatr Pulmonol 2012;47(4):393–400.
13. Richard N, Komurian-Pradel F, Javouhey E, et al. The impact of dual viral infection in infants admitted to a pediatric intensive care unit associated with severe bronchiolitis. Pediatr Infect Dis J 2008;27(3):213–7.
14. Hall CB, Weinberg GA, Iwane MK, et al. The burden of respiratory syncytial virus infection in young children. N Engl J Med 2009;360(6):588–98.
15. Bope ET, Conn HF, Kellerman RD. Conn's Current Therapy 2017. 2017. Available at: https://www-clinicalkey-com.ezproxy.cmh.edu/#!/browse/book/3-s2.0-C20130194974. Accessed August 8, 2017.

16. Fernandes RM, Bialy LM, Vandermeer B, et al. Glucocorticoids for acute viral bronchiolitis in infants and young children. Cochrane Database Syst Rev 2013;(6):CD004878.

17. Hartling L, Bialy LM, Vandermeer B, et al. Epinephrine for bronchiolitis. Cochrane Database Syst Rev 2011;(6):CD003123.

18. Zorc JJ, Hall CB. Bronchiolitis: recent evidence on diagnosis and management. Pediatrics 2010;125(2):342–9.

19. Piedimonte G, Perez MK. Respiratory syncytial virus infection and bronchiolitis. Pediatr Rev 2014;35(12):519–30.

20. Swingler GH, Hussey GD, Zwarenstein M. Duration of illness in ambulatory children diagnosed with bronchiolitis. Arch Pediatr Adolesc Med 2000;154(10): 997–1000.

21. Mansbach JM, Clark S, Piedra PA, et al. Hospital course and discharge criteria for children hospitalized with bronchiolitis. J Hosp Med 2015;10(4):205–11.

22. Petruzella FD, Gorelick MH. Duration of illness in infants with bronchiolitis evaluated in the emergency department. Pediatrics 2010;126(2):285–90.

23. Shay DK, Holman RC, Newman RD, et al. Bronchiolitis-associated hospitalizations among US children, 1980-1996. JAMA 1999;282(15):1440–6.

24. Destino L, Weisgerber MC, Soung P, et al. Validity of respiratory scores in bronchiolitis. Hosp Pediatr 2012;2(4):202–9.

25. Society of Hospital Medicine – Pediatric Hospital Medicine. Choosing wisely. Available at: http://www.choosingwisely.org/societies/society-of-hospital-medicine-pediatric/. Accessed July 14, 2017.

26. AAP Committee on Infectious Diseases. Recommendations for prevention and control of influenza in children, 2016-2017. Pediatrics 2016;138(4):e20162527.

27. Ralston S, Hill V, Waters A. Occult serious bacterial infection in infants younger than 60 to 90 days with bronchiolitis: a systematic review. Arch Pediatr Adolesc Med 2011;165(10):951–6.

28. Mussman GM, Parker MW, Statile A, et al. Suctioning and length of stay in infants hospitalized with bronchiolitis. JAMA Pediatr 2013;167(5):414–21.

29. Hunt CE, Corwin MJ, Lister G, et al. Longitudinal assessment of hemoglobin oxygen saturation in healthy infants during the first 6 months of age. Collaborative Home Infant Monitoring Evaluation (CHIME) Study Group. J Pediatr 1999;135(5): 580–6.

30. Schroeder AR, Marmor AK, Pantell RH, et al. Impact of pulse oximetry and oxygen therapy on length of stay in bronchiolitis hospitalizations. Arch Pediatr Adolesc Med 2004;158(6):527–30.

31. Hough JL, Pham TMT, Schibler A. Physiologic effect of high-flow nasal cannula in infants with bronchiolitis. Pediatr Crit Care Med 2014;15(5):e214–9.

32. Beggs S, Wong ZH, Kaul S, et al. High-flow nasal cannula therapy for infants with bronchiolitis. Cochrane Database Syst Rev 2014. https://doi.org/10.1002/14651858.CD009609.pub2. John Wiley & Sons, Ltd.

33. Zhang L, Mendoza-Sassi RA, Klassen TP, et al. Nebulized hypertonic saline for acute bronchiolitis: a systematic review. Pediatrics 2015;136(4):687–701.

34. Zhang L, Mendoza-Sassi RA, Wainwright C, et al. Nebulised hypertonic saline solution for acute bronchiolitis in infants. Cochrane Database Syst Rev 2013;(7):CD006458.

35. Gadomski AM, Scribani MB. Bronchodilators for bronchiolitis. Cochrane Database Syst Rev 2014;(6):CD001266.

36. King VJ, Viswanathan M, Bordley WC, et al. Pharmacologic treatment of bronchiolitis in infants and children: a systematic review. Arch Pediatr Adolesc Med 2004;158(2):127–37.
37. Farley R, Spurling GKP, Eriksson L, et al. Antibiotics for bronchiolitis in children under two years of age. Cochrane Database Syst Rev 2014;(10):CD005189.
38. Roqué i Figuls M, Giné-Garriga M, Granados Rugeles C, et al. Chest physiotherapy for acute bronchiolitis in paediatric patients between 0 and 24 months old. Cochrane Database Syst Rev 2016. https://doi.org/10.1002/14651858. CD004873.pub5. John Wiley & Sons, Ltd.
39. Hall CB, Powell KR, Schnabel KC, et al. Risk of secondary bacterial infection in infants hospitalized with respiratory syncytial viral infection. J Pediatr 1988; 113(2):266–71.
40. Thorburn K, Harigopal S, Reddy V, et al. High incidence of pulmonary bacterial co-infection in children with severe respiratory syncytial virus (RSV) bronchiolitis. Thorax 2006;61(7):611–5.
41. Palivizumab, a humanized respiratory syncytial virus monoclonal antibody, reduces hospitalization from respiratory syncytial virus infection in high-risk infants. The IMpact-RSV Study. Pediatrics 1998;102(3):531–7.
42. Checchia PA, Nalysnyk L, Fernandes AW, et al. Mortality and morbidity among infants at high risk for severe respiratory syncytial virus infection receiving prophylaxis with palivizumab: a systematic literature review and meta-analysis. Pediatr Crit Care Med 2011;12(5):580–8.
43. American Academy of Pediatrics Committee on Infectious Diseases, American Academy of Pediatrics Bronchiolitis Guidelines Committee. Updated guidance for palivizumab prophylaxis among infants and young children at increased risk of hospitalization for respiratory syncytial virus infection. Pediatrics 2014; 134(2):415–20.
44. Jones LL, Hashim A, McKeever T, et al. Parental and household smoking and the increased risk of bronchitis, bronchiolitis and other lower respiratory infections in infancy: systematic review and meta-analysis. Respir Res 2011;12:5.
45. Matt GE, Quintana PJE, Destaillats H, et al. Thirdhand tobacco smoke: emerging evidence and arguments for a multidisciplinary research agenda. Environ Health Perspect 2011;119(9):1218–26.
46. Ip S, Chung M, Raman G, et al. Breastfeeding and maternal and infant health outcomes in developed countries. Evid Rep Technol Assess (Full Rep) 2007;(153): 1–186.
47. Oddy WH, Sly PD, de Klerk NH, et al. Breast feeding and respiratory morbidity in infancy: a birth cohort study. Arch Dis Child 2003;88(3):224–8.
48. Nishimura T, Suzue J, Kaji H. Breastfeeding reduces the severity of respiratory syncytial virus infection among young infants: a multi-center prospective study. Pediatr Int 2009;51(6):812–6.
49. Taylor JA, Kwan-Gett TSC, McMahon EM. Effectiveness of an educational intervention in modifying parental attitudes about antibiotic usage in children. Pediatrics 2003;111(5 Pt 1):e548–54.

Pediatric Community-Acquired Pneumonia in the United States

Changing Epidemiology, Diagnostic and Therapeutic Challenges, and Areas for Future Research

Sophie E. Katz, MD[a], Derek J. Williams, MD, MPH[b],*

KEYWORDS

• Community-acquired pneumonia • Pediatric • Epidemiology

KEY POINTS

• Pediatric community-acquired pneumonia (CAP) continues to cause significant morbidity and remains one of the most common serious infections of childhood.

• Routine childhood vaccination against *Streptococcus pneumoniae* has greatly reduced invasive disease rates caused by this pathogen.

• Although molecular diagnostics have helped highlight the important role that respiratory viruses play in pediatric CAP, bacterial diagnostics remain suboptimal.

• Biomarkers and molecular host responses to infection are current areas of intense study that may facilitate a deeper understanding of pneumonia etiology and disease outcomes.

INTRODUCTION

Pneumonia is an infection of the lower airways (distal bronchi and alveoli) caused by both viruses and bacteria. Community-acquired pneumonia (CAP) specifically refers to clinical signs and symptoms of pneumonia acquired outside a hospital setting.[1] It is one of the most common serious infections in childhood, accounting for more than 900,000 deaths among children younger than 5 years of age in 2015.[2] Although

Disclosures: The authors have no relevant financial disclosures.
[a] Division of Infectious Diseases, Monroe Carell Jr. Children's Hospital at Vanderbilt, Vanderbilt University Medical Center, D-7235 Medical Center North, 1161 21st Avenue South, Nashville, TN 37232-2581, USA; [b] Division of Hospital Medicine, Monroe Carell Jr. Children's Hospital at Vanderbilt, Vanderbilt University Medical Center, CCC 5324 Medical Center North, 1161 21st Avenue South, Nashville, TN 37232, USA
* Corresponding author.
E-mail address: Derek.Williams@Vanderbilt.edu

Infect Dis Clin N Am 32 (2018) 47–63
https://doi.org/10.1016/j.idc.2017.11.002
0891-5520/18/© 2017 Elsevier Inc. All rights reserved.

the rate of mortality due to CAP is much lower in the developed world compared with the developing world, CAP continues to account for a significant proportion of health care visits and hospitalizations in high-income countries. This review focuses on pediatric CAP in the United States and other industrialized nations, specifically highlighting the changing epidemiology of CAP, diagnostic and therapeutic challenges, and areas for further research.

EPIDEMIOLOGY

In the United States, CAP accounts for approximately 2 million outpatient visits annually[3] and is among the most common causes for hospitalization, with approximately 124,000 pediatric hospitalizations annually (annual incidence of 15.7–22.5 hospitalizations per 100,000 children).[4–6] The highest rate of health care utilization occurs in children younger than 2 years of age and decreases with increasing age in the pediatric population.[4]

DIAGNOSIS

Children with pneumonia most often present with fever, tachypnea, and other signs of respiratory distress (**Table 1**). Signs and symptoms may include tachypnea, cough, dyspnea, retractions, grunting, hypoxemia, abdominal pain, or lethargy, and physical examination findings of decreased breath sounds, crackles, rales, or wheezing on auscultation of lung fields. Many of these findings overlap with other acute lower respiratory tract diseases (eg, asthma and viral bronchiolitis), and identifying children with pneumonia based only on clinical signs and symptoms is sometimes difficult. As a result, chest radiographs are commonly used to confirm the diagnosis. Even when a chest radiograph reveals an infiltrate, however, it is sometimes difficult to differentiate between consolidation representing pneumonia and atelectasis commonly seen in children with asthma or bronchiolitis. As a result, variation in chest radiograph interpretation is common and may contribute to antibiotic overuse.[7,8] For this reason, the guideline developed by the Pediatric Infectious Diseases Society (PIDS) and Infectious Diseases Society of America (IDSA) discourages use of chest radiographs in children with suspected uncomplicated pneumonia in an outpatient setting.[7] Chest

Table 1	
Manifestations of community-acquired pneumonia requiring hospitalization among those enrolled in the Centers for Disease Control Etiology of Pneumonia in the Community study	
Characteristic	**Frequency in Children with Radiographic Evidence of Pneumonia (N = 2358) no. (%)**
Symptom	
Cough	2230 (95)
Abnormal temperature	2155 (91)
Anorexia	1766 (75)
Dyspnea	1657 (70)
Chest indrawing	1278 (55)
Radiographic finding	
Consolidation	1376 (58)
Alveolar or interstitial infiltrate	1195 (51)
Pleural effusion	314 (13)

Adapted from Jain S, Williams DJ, Arnold SR, et al. Community-acquired pneumonia requiring hospitalization among U.S. children. NEJM 2015;372(9):839. Table 1; with permission.

radiographs are recommended in children who are hospitalized with hypoxemia or respiratory distress and in those with suspected complications, such as parapneumonic effusions, necrotizing pneumonia, or pneumothorax (**Fig. 1**).

Chest ultrasound is most often used for evaluating local complications, such as parapneumonic effusion and empyema, but recent studies have demonstrated high sensitivity (92%–98%) and specificity (92%–100%) for detecting lung consolidation compared with chest radiography.[9–13] Additional benefits of chest ultrasound include a lack of ionizing radiation and availability in most emergency department settings. An important limitation of ultrasound is that evaluation and interpretation are highly operator dependent. Thus, despite these promising early studies, large-scale, pragmatic studies are needed to better evaluate the effectiveness of this imaging technique versus standard chest radiography.

ETIOLOGY

Pneumonia is a heterogeneous disease caused by a variety of pathogens, including viruses and bacteria. Historically, CAP was largely considered a bacterial process, most often due to *Streptococcus pneumoniae, Haemophilus influenzae, Streptococcus pyogenes*, and *Staphylococcus aureus*.[14–18] The introduction of routine childhood vaccination against both *Streptococcus pneumoniae* and *H influenzae*, however, has dramatically reduced disease caused by these pathogens. At the same time,

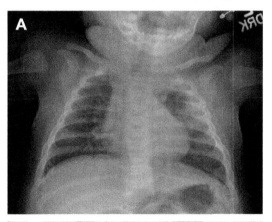

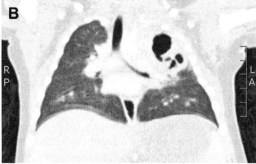

Fig. 1. Radiographic imaging in cavitating pneumonia. (*A*) Chest radiograph demonstrating a complex air space opacity in the left upper lobe with central lucency consistent with cavitating pneumonia. (*B*) CT of the same lesion demonstrates a large cavity with central necrosis and multiple air fluid levels occupying most of the left upper lobe.

highly sensitive molecular diagnostics for viral respiratory pathogens have heightened awareness of the impact of viruses as a cause of CAP.

Pneumonia Etiology Prior to Introduction of Pneumococcal Conjugate Vaccine

A 2004 study by Michelow and colleagues[15] exemplifies pre–pneumococcal conjugate vaccine (PCV) era etiology studies. That study used traditional culture methods, pneumolysin-based polymerase chain reaction (PCR) assays, viral direct fluorescent antibody tests, and serologic tests for viruses, *Mycoplasma* spp, and *Chlamydia* spp to identify pathogens in 154 hospitalized children with radiographically confirmed lower respiratory infections at a single institution. A majority of patients (60%) were noted to have infection with typical respiratory bacteria (most commonly, *Streptococcus pneumoniae*, detected in 73% of children with documented bacterial disease), with viruses identified in 45% of children.

Impact of Pneumococcal Conjugate Vaccines

A 7-valent PCV (PCV7) targeting the most common clinically important pneumococcal serotypes was introduced into the United States childhood immunization schedule in 2000. Rates of invasive pneumococcal disease caused by PCV7 serotypes in children less than 5 years of age plummeted from an average of 95.2 cases to 22.6 cases per 100,000 population within 4 years after the introduction of PCV7.[19] By 2006, hospitalization rates for CAP and pneumonia-associated complications among young children decreased by 39% and 36%, respectively.[5,20] Despite these declines, disease caused by nonvaccine serotypes soon emerged, and rates of complicated pneumonia increased, prompting introduction of an expanded, 13-valent PCT (PCV13) into the US childhood immunization program in 2010.[21] Since that time, hospitalization rates decreased from 53.6 per 100,000 admissions in the pre-PCV13 era to 23.3 per 100,000 admissions in the post-PCV13 era, and rates of complicated pneumococcal pneumonia decreased significantly.[22]

Pneumonia Etiology in the Post–Pneumococcal Conjugate Vaccine Era

The multicenter Centers for Disease Control and Prevention (CDC) Etiology of Pneumonia in the Community (EPIC) Study was a prospective, population-based surveillance study of greater than 2300 pediatric CAP hospitalizations in the United States conducted from 2010 to 2012.[4] This study used serology and nasopharyngeal PCR to identify 8 different viruses, culture-based methods and whole-blood PCR (pneumococcal *lyt-A*) to identify typical bacteria, and nasopharyngeal PCR to identify atypical bacterial pathogens.

Viruses were identified in greater than 70% of children, whereas bacteria were identified in only 15% of children (**Fig. 2**).[4] The most common viral pathogens included respiratory syncytial virus (RSV), human rhinovirus, human metapneumovirus, and adenovirus, all detected in greater than 10% of children. RSV, adenovirus, and human metapneumovirus were more commonly identified in children younger than 5 years of age compared with older children.

Bacteria were identified in approximately 15% of children in the CDC EPIC study, although *Streptococcus pneumoniae* was only identified in 4% of children, further underscoring the impact that PCV has had on the epidemiology of pediatric CAP.[4] *Mycoplasma pneumoniae* was the most frequently identified bacterial pathogen, detected in 8% of children, including 19% of school-aged children, but only 3% of children younger than 5 years of age. Other bacteria were identified in 1% or less of children. Importantly, 19% of children in the CDC EPIC study had no pathogen identified, highlighting the continued need for enhanced diagnostics and novel pathogen discovery techniques.

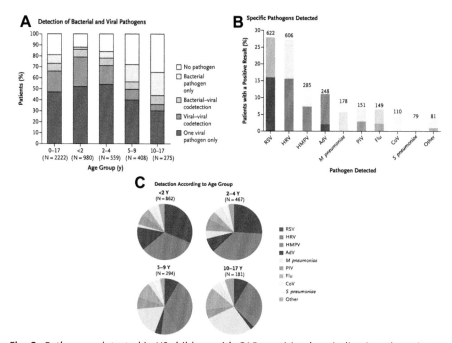

Fig. 2. Pathogens detected in US children with CAP requiring hospitalization, detection according to age group. Darker shading in the bar graph in panel B indicates that only the single pathogen was detected, and lighter shading indicates the pathogen was detected in combination with at least one other pathogen. Panel A shows the proportion of pathogen types among 2222 hospitalized children in the CDC EPIC study. A total of 4 patients had more than one bacterial pathogen without a virus detected. Panel C shows the proportions of pathogens detected, according to age group. AdV, denotes adenovirus; CoV, coronavirus; Flu, influenza A or B virus; HMPV, human metapneumovirus; HRV, human rhinovirus; PIV, parainfluenza virus. (*Data from* Jain S, Williams DJ, Arnold SR, et al. Community-acquired pneumonia requiring hospitalization among U.S. children. NEJM 2015;372(9):840. Fig. 2; with permission.)

Uncommon Causes of Community-acquired Pneumonia

Other pathogens that are less commonly seen among US children include *Mycobacterium tuberculosis*, fungi, *Burkholderia cepacia*, *Aspergillus fumigatus*, and *Pseudomonas aeruginosa* and usually occur in patients with underlying risk factors, such as immunocompromising conditions; chronic conditions, such as cystic fibrosis and spinal muscular atrophy; or history of international travel (**Table 2**). These pathogens should also be suspected in patients who experience treatment failure for more common etiologic agents.

CHALLENGES AND AREAS FOR FUTURE RESEARCH
Bacterial Diagnostics

Blood cultures
The 2011 PIDS/IDSA CAP guideline recommends obtaining blood cultures in children hospitalized with CAP.[7,23,24] In this setting, however, blood cultures identify a pathogen in only 2% to 7% of children with CAP.[24–27] Blood cultures are more often positive in children with parapneumonic effusion, ranging from 10% to 35%.[25,26,28] In the outpatient setting, blood cultures are not routinely recommended, because positivity rates are low and results are unlikely to change management. Regardless, despite

Table 2
Rare microorganisms causing pediatric community-acquired pneumonia or occurring in specialized populations

Microorganism	Comment
Viruses	
Varicella zoster virus	Potential complication after primary varicella infection. Often severe and associated with secondary bacterial infection.
Measles virus	Rubeola. Pneumonia is a frequent complication.
Hantavirus	Hantavirus pulmonary syndrome. Rodent exposure.
Bacteria	
Bordatella pertussis	Pneumonia uncommon manifestation. Bacterial coinfection may be severe, especially in infants.
Group B streptococci	Neonatal pneumonia and sepsis.
Listeria monocytogenes	Neonatal pneumonia and sepsis.
Gram-negative enterics	Neonatal pneumonia and sepsis. Potential pathogens in aspiration pneumonia.
Chlamydia trachomatis	Cause of afebrile pneumonia in young infants <3 mo of age.
Anaerobes (oral flora)	Potential pathogens in aspiration pneumonia.
Legionella pneumophila	Legionnaires' disease. Rare in children but associated with community outbreaks. Exposure to contaminated artificial freshwater systems.
Coxiella burnetti	Q fever. Exposure to wild and domesticated herbivores or unpasteurized dairy (eg, cattle, sheep, and goats). Also potential bioterrorism agent.
Chlamydia psittaci	Psittacosis. Bird (eg, pet birds and pigeons) exposure.
Francisella tularensis	Tularemia. Rabbit exposure.
Yersinia pestis	Pneummonic plague. Rodent flea exposure.
Bacillus anthracis	Anthrax. Woolsorter's disease. Wild and domesticated herbivore (eg, cattle, sheep, goats) exposure. Also potential bioterrorism agent.
Leptospira interrogans	Leptospirosis. Exposure to urine of wild and domestic animals carrying the bacterium.
Mycobacterium tuberculosis	Rare in US children. Usually associated with high-risk exposures.
Brucella abortus	Brucellosis. Exposure to wild and domesticated animals or unpasteurized dairy (eg, cattle, sheep, pigs, goats, deer, and dogs).
Fungi	
Histoplasma capsulatum	Histoplasmosis. Exposure to bird or bat droppings (eg, poultry/bird roosts and caves). Endemic to eastern and central United States.
Blastomyces dermaitidis	Blastomycosis. Environmental exposure to fungal spores (wooded areas). Endemic to Southeastern and Midwestern United States.
Cryptococcus neoformans	Cryptococcosis. Exposure to soil contaminated with bird droppings. Significant pathogen nearly exclusively among immunocompromised.
Coccidioides immitis	Coccidiomycosis. Valley fever. Environmental exposure to fungal spores (dry, dusty environments). Endemic to Southwestern United States.

Adapted from Williams DJ, Shah SS. Community-acquired pneumonia in the conjugate vaccine era. J Pediatric Infect Dis Soc 2012;1(4):320. Table 2; with permission.

their low yield, blood cultures currently provide the best opportunity to identify typical bacterial pathogens in most children with CAP.

Diagnostic yield of blood cultures can be optimized by restricting their use to those patients with increased pretest probability of having a positive culture, such as those who are severely ill or have parapneumonic effusion.[29–31] Isolation of pathologic organisms occurs significantly less frequently in patients exposed to antibiotics before specimen collection.[32,33] Studies have also demonstrated increased yield of blood cultures with each additional milliliter of blood drawn.[34–36] Obtaining adequate weight-based blood volumes is also associated with lower rates of blood culture contamination, for reasons yet unknown.[35,37] Contamination rates can also be minimized by adhering to proper sterile collection methods.[32,35,37]

Cultures of the lower respiratory tract

Pleural fluid cultures are positive in up to 35% of cases and should be performed whenever pleural fluid is obtained.[7,25,26,38–40] The invasive methods associated with sampling the pleural space, however, make it impractical to obtain pleural fluid specimens except when dictated for clinical care. Bronchoalveolar lavage is rarely indicated in CAP, except in instances of lack of response to therapy, very severe pneumonia, or immunocompromised hosts in whom opportunistic pathogens are suspected.[41] Sputum cultures are of low diagnostic yield in children, due to the inability of most young children with pneumonia to produce an adequate sputum sample. Pretreatment with antibiotics further hinders diagnostic yield. Induced sputum has been explored as an opportunity to collect sputum samples in young children, although utility is limited by frequent detection of upper respiratory tract bacteria and similar rates of recovery of pathogens in pneumonia cases compared with children without pneumonia.[42,43]

Molecular Diagnostics

Bacterial diagnostics

Pneumococcal urinary antigen testing is often used in the evaluation of pneumonia in adults. In children, however, detection of *Streptococcus pneumoniae* urinary antigen is associated with false-positive results due to high rates of nasopharyngeal colonization.[44,45] More recently, a serotype-specific urinary antigen detection method has been developed and validated in adults with pneumonia[46]; whether or not this test could prove useful in children remains to be determined.

Although not widely used in clinical settings, whole-blood pneumococcal PCR (*lyt-A*) has been used in epidemiologic studies, including EPIC and Pneumonia Etiology Research for Child Health (PERCH). Potential benefits include improved sensitivity, rapid turnaround time, and less influence of antibiotic pretreatment compared with culture-based methods.[47,48] In the EPIC study, 2.5% of children tested were PCR-positive for *Streptococcus pneumoniae*, whereas blood cultures were positive for pneumococcus in only 1% of children ($P<.001$).[4] In the PERCH study, 291 children with pneumonia (7.3%) were pneumococcal PCR-positive, whereas only 44 children (denominator not provided) had a positive blood culture for *Streptococcus pneumoniae*.[49] Moreover, although prior studies demonstrated 100% specificity of *lyt-A* pneumococcal PCR from the blood,[50] the PERCH study also identified pneumococcal DNA in the blood of 273 control children (5.5%).[49] Thus, although pneumococcal PCR may increase rate of detection over blood culture, suboptimal test specificity hampers interpretation.

PCR also increases yield for pleural fluid specimens. In a study evaluating archived pleural fluid specimens from 63 pediatric patients with CAP, a pathogen was detected in 84% of samples using PCR compared with only 35% of samples when using conventional culture methods ($P<.001$).[28] The most frequent pathogen detected using both methods was *Streptococcus pneumoniae*, 71% using PCR and 24% using conventional culture. The next most frequent pathogens identified were *Streptococcus pyogenes* (11% using PCR and 5% using conventional culture) and *S aureus* (8% using PCR and 6% using conventional culture). This study also highlighted the potential for bias with respect to pathogen identification introduced when relying on culture alone for epidemiologic studies, because penicillin-resistant pneumococcal isolates and *S aureus* were more likely to be positive in culture, whereas other serotypes of *Streptococcus pneumoniae* and bacterial pathogens commonly susceptible to penicillins were more commonly identified by PCR.

Up to two-thirds of children younger than 5 years are colonized in the upper respiratory tract with common bacterial pathogens known to cause pneumonia,[51] and PCR from the upper respiratory tract is not a reliable method for ascertaining bacterial etiologies of pneumonia. A possible exception is *M pneumoniae*, which has not previously been considered a frequent colonizer of the upper respiratory tract. Consistent with this theory, the CDC EPIC study demonstrated that although *M pneumoniae* was detected in 8% of children with pneumonia, fewer than 1% of controls had evidence of *M pneumoniae*.[4] In contrast, a cross-sectional, observational study in the Netherlands of asymptomatic children and children with symptoms of upper and lower respiratory tract infection detected *M pneumoniae* DNA not only in 16% of symptomatic children but also in 21% of asymptomatic children.[52] Given the conflicting results of these 2 studies and the increasing commercial availability of *M pneumoniae* PCR tests, caution is warranted when interpreting test results in the clinical setting.

Viral diagnostics

In contrast to bacteria, PCR testing for viruses from upper respiratory samples has largely replaced culture and serology-based methods to investigate pneumonia etiology, owing to superior sensitivity, rapid turnaround time, and ability to identify viruses that are difficult to grow in culture. A major concern, however, is whether lower respiratory tract disease can be attributed to a viral pathogen detected in the upper airway. The scope of the problem is well illustrated in a study conducted by Self and colleagues[53] that compared PCR detections of 13 viruses from the upper respiratory tract among 1024 children with CAP and 759 healthy, asymptomatic children enrolled in the CDC EPIC study. Overall, approximately 25% of asymptomatic children had 1 or more viruses detected compared with approximately 65% of children with CAP. Detection of most viruses was higher among children with CAP compared with asymptomatic controls, including influenza (3% vs 0%), RSV (27% vs 2%), and human metapneumovirus (15% vs 2%), with attributable fractions greater than 90% for all. Conversely, rhinovirus was detected at a similar frequency in both children with CAP and asymptomatic children (22% vs 17%; attributable fraction 12%; 95% CI, 18% to 34%). Attributable fractions for other viruses studied ranged from 44% to 68%. Thus, although some viruses detected in the upper airway likely reflect lower airway disease (eg, RSV, influenza, and human metapneumovirus), detection of other viruses must be interpreted with caution. As proposed for adults, investigating viral loads may further help to differentiate disease versus asymptomatic colonization.[54]

Because sensitive methods of diagnosing viral infections have become more widely available, the recognition of viral and bacterial coinfection has also increased. It is well known that upper tract disease with respiratory viruses often precedes the development of bacterial pneumonia.[55–57] Although it is not always clear if a virus detected in the upper airway represents prior or concurrent infection in a subject with bacterial pneumonia, studies suggest that viral-bacterial codetections are associated with a more severe clinical course compared with single viral or bacterial detections.[58–60] The association between influenza and coinfection with pneumococcal or staphylococcal pneumonia is perhaps the best described of these viral and bacterial coinfections.[61,62]

Acute-Phase Reactants and Biomarkers

Elevated leukocyte count was traditionally considered to be associated with serious bacterial infection, but the specificity of leukocyte count in making the diagnosis of bacterial pneumonia in children is poor, and the degree of elevation does not reliably distinguish between viral and bacterial pneumonia.[7,63–65] As such, routine measurement of leukocyte count is likely not beneficial.

More recent biomarkers used in the detection of pneumonia include C-reactive protein (CRP) and procalcitonin (PCT). These biomarkers may perform better than leukocyte count for identifying bacterial infections,[64,66,67] although identifying relevant clinical cutpoints remains a challenge. To evaluate the impact of CRP in the etiologic diagnosis of pneumonia, a meta-analysis of 8 studies with more than 1200 children with viral or bacterial causes of CAP demonstrated that CRP levels greater than or equal to 40 mg/L to 60 mg/L were associated with only a 64% positive predictive value for identifying children with bacterial pneumonia.[68]

PCT is a peptide precursor of calcitonin and is produced by C cells in the thyroid gland and by neuroendocrine cells in the lung and intestine. Levels are usually undetectable in healthy individuals but increase in response to systemic inflammation. Cytokines typically associated with bacterial infection enhance PCT release, whereas interferons, which are more often associated with viral infections, inhibit PCT release.[69,70] Thus, much interest has been directed at PCT as a potential biomarker for bacterial disease.

Among 532 hospitalized children enrolled in the CDC EPIC study, a PCT cutoff value of 0.25 ng/mL demonstrated a sensitivity of 85% and specificity of 45% for CAP caused by typical bacterial pathogens.[71] The study also found that higher PCT levels were associated with more severe disease. Multiple studies have shown utility in using PCT levels to guide antibiotic initiation and duration.[71–76]

Biomarker studies using transcriptomics show promise for enhancing diagnostic capabilities by using host responses to identify possible pathogens and study disease severity.[77–80] Transcriptomics uses gene expression profiling to measure the activity or expression of thousands of genes at once, thereby creating a global picture of cellular activity. Profiles of peripheral blood leukocytes in patients with lower respiratory tract infection can accurately distinguish influenza viral infection from bacterial infection and predict disease severity.[81] Host transcriptional profiling has also been shown useful in distinguishing symptomatic rhinovirus infection from incidental detection in children.[80] These promising studies will likely add much to the understanding of pneumonia etiology and outcomes, although much work remains prior to translating these new technologies to the bedside.

Prediction of Outcomes

Several prognostic models are available for adults with pneumonia,[82,83] and their application has been shown to contribute to improved outcomes. Unfortunately, no analogous models have been validated in children, a recognized key knowledge gap.[7] Recently, Williams and colleagues[84] derived 3 prognostic models to identify risk for severe outcomes among children with CAP; each model demonstrated good predictive accuracy (concordance index 0.78–0.81). In that study, extremes of age, vital signs, chest indrawing, and radiographic infiltrate pattern ranked among the most important predictors of disease outcomes. Although these models require further validation, their use could reduce variability and improve care for children with pneumonia.

TREATMENT

Although viruses are a major cause of childhood pneumonia, a majority of children with pneumonia receive antibiotics. Pneumonia is associated with more antibiotic use in US pediatric hospitals than any other condition.[85] When antibiotics are indicated, amoxicillin or ampicillin is recommended as first-line therapy in most children[7] (**Table 3**). Prior

Table 3
Empiric antimicrobial strategies for pediatric community-acquired pneumonia

Population		Bacterial Pneumonia	Atypical Pneumonia
Outpatient			
Neonates — 3 mo			
Preschool (<5 y)	Preferred	Amoxicillin	Azithromycin
	Alternative(s)	Amoxiciilin/clavulanate	Clarithromycin or erythromycin
5–17 y	Preferred	Amoxicillin	Azithromycin
	Alternative(s)	Amoxicillin/clavulanate	Clarithromycin or erythromycin Doxycycline if >7 y
Inpatient			
Neonates	Preferred	Ampicillin + gentamicin	N/A
	Alternative(s)	Ampicillin + cefotaxime	
1–3 mo	Preferred	Cefotaxime	N/A
	Alternative(s)	Azithromycin if suspect *C trachomatis* or *B pertussis*	
3 mo–17 y, fully immunized, local epidemiology indicates low prevalence of penicillin nonsusceptible *Streptococcus pneumoniae*	Preferred	Ampicillin or penicillin G	Azithromycin
	Alternative(s)	Ceftriaxone or cefotaxime Antistaphylococcal coverage for suspected *S aureus*, including clindamycin or vancomycin in methicillin-resistant *S aureus*–prevalent regions	Clarithromycin or erythromycin Doxycycline if >7 y Levofloxacin for those who have reached skeletal maturity
3 mo–17 y, not fully immunized, or local epidemiology indicates moderate to high prevalence of penicillin nonsusceptible *Streptococcus pneumoniae*	Preferred	Ceftriaxone or cefotaxime	Azithromycin
	Alternative(s)	Levofloxacin Antistaphylococcal coverage for suspected *S aureus*, including clindamycin or vancomycin in methicillin-resistant *S aureus*–prevalent regions	Clarithromycin or erythromycin Doxycycline if >7 y Levofloxacin for those who have reached skeletal maturity

Adapted from Bradley JS, Byington CL, Shah SS, et al. Empiric therapy for pediatric community-acquired pneumonia (CAP). The management of community-acquired pneumonia in infants and children older than 3 months of age: clinical practice guidelines by the Pediatric Infectious Diseases Society and the Infectious Diseases Society of America. Clin Infect Dis 2011;53:e34. Table 7; with permission.

to release of the national guideline, however, broader-spectrum third-generation cephalosporins and macrolides were commonly used.

To date, the impact of the national guideline on prescribing has been mixed. Approximately 4 years after guideline publication, penicillin use increased approximately 27.6% and cephalosporin use decreased approximately 27.8% across 48 tertiary care children's hospitals in the United States, although substantial variability was noted across institutions.[86] Similar variability persists in the outpatient setting.[87] Antimicrobial stewardship programs, local clinical practice guidelines, and quality improvement methods all play important roles in raising awareness of these recommendations and reducing unnecessary and inappropriate antibiotic use.[86,88,89]

Current practices for treatment of uncomplicated CAP generally use 7-day to 10-day antibiotic courses, although 2 large pediatric randomized controlled studies are currently evaluating the safety and efficacy of shorter courses of antibiotics, a United Kingdom community-acquired pneumonia study (CAP-IT) and the US phase IV double-blind, placebo-controlled, randomized trial Short Course Outpatient Therapy of Community Acquired Pneumonia (SCOUT-CAP).[90,91]

Consideration of alternative etiologies, such as S aureus, is warranted in children with severe or rapidly progressive disease, extensive local complications, or poor treatment response. S aureus is an uncommon cause of CAP, detected in only 1% of children hospitalized with pneumonia.[4] Thus, to preserve the effectiveness of antistaphylococcal antibiotics, care must be taken when considering when to use these agents empirically, and efforts to de-escalate therapy whenever possible should be emphasized.

Although M pneumoniae is a frequent cause of CAP in children, it is impossible to reliably distinguish this pathogen from other common causes of pneumonia. Questions regarding the utility of currently available PCR tests for M pneumoniae, as outlined previously, further complicate treatment considerations. Moreover, azithromycin use is associated with the development of multidrug resistance.[92,93] Perhaps the most important consideration governing when to use macrolide therapy, however, is that currently available studies have failed to consistently demonstrate their benefit in children with pneumonia.[94]

SUMMARY

Despite advances in recent years, CAP continues to cause significant morbidity and mortality and poses diagnostic and therapeutic challenges. Vaccination against Haemophilus influenzae type b and Streptococcus pneumoniae has greatly reduced invasive disease rates caused by these pathogens, and the introduction of molecular diagnostics has highlighted the important role that respiratory viruses play in disease pathogenesis while also introducing new challenges. This updated understanding brings into question whether all children with CAP would benefit from antibiotic therapy, and if so, which therapies might be most effective. Limitations of current diagnostics, however, impede advances toward addressing these important questions. Biomarkers and host responses to infection are current areas of intense study that may facilitate a deeper understanding of pneumonia etiology and disease outcomes. As this important work progresses, future epidemiologic studies using state-of-the-art diagnostics will continue to serve an important role in informing understanding of the changing epidemiology of CAP.

ACKNOWLEDGMENTS

The authors thank Kathryn Edwards, MD, and Ritu Banerjee, MD, PhD, Vanderbilt University Medical Center, for their critical review and input during article preparation.

REFERENCES

1. Harris M, Clark J, Coote N, et al. British thoracic society guidelines for the management of community acquired pneumonia in children: update 2011. Thorax 2011;66(Suppl 2):ii1–23.
2. World Health Organization, 2016. Fact Sheet – Pneumonia. Available at: http://www.who.int/mediacentre/factsheets/fs331/en/. Accessed November 22, 2017.
3. Kronman MP, Hersh AL, Feng R, et al. Ambulatory visit rates and antibiotic prescribing for children with pneumonia, 1994-2007. Pediatrics 2011;127(3):411–8.
4. Jain S, Williams DJ, Arnold SR, et al. Community-acquired pneumonia requiring hospitalization among U.S. children. N Engl J Med 2015;372(9):835–45.
5. Lee GE, Lorch SA, Sheffler-Collins S, et al. National hospitalization trends for pediatric pneumonia and associated complications. Pediatrics 2010;126(2):204–13.
6. Healthcare Cost and Utilization Project (HCUP). HCUP Kids' Inpatient Database (KID) 2009; Available at: http://hcup-us.ahrq.gov/kidsoverview.jsp. Accessed June 28, 2017.
7. Bradley JS, Byington CL, Shah SS, et al. The management of community-acquired pneumonia in infants and children older than 3 months of age: clinical practice guidelines by the pediatric infectious diseases society and the infectious diseases society of America. Clin Infect Dis 2011;53(7):e25–76.
8. Novack V, Avnon LS, Smolyakov A, et al. Disagreement in the interpretation of chest radiographs among specialists and clinical outcomes of patients hospitalized with suspected pneumonia. Eur J Intern Med 2006;17(1):43–7.
9. Shah VP, Tunik MG, Tsung JW. Prospective evaluation of point-of-care ultrasonography for the diagnosis of pneumonia in children and young adults. JAMA Pediatr 2013;167(2):119–25.
10. Copetti R, Cattarossi L. Ultrasound diagnosis of pneumonia in children. Radiol Med 2008;113(2):190–8.
11. Pereda MA, Chavez MA, Hooper-Miele CC, et al. Lung ultrasound for the diagnosis of pneumonia in children: a meta-analysis. Pediatrics 2015;135(4):714–22.
12. Boursiani C, Tsolia M, Koumanidou C, et al. Lung ultrasound as first-line examination for the diagnosis of community-acquired pneumonia in children. Pediatr Emerg Care 2017;33(1):62–6.
13. Claes AS, Clapuyt P, Menten R, et al. Performance of chest ultrasound in pediatric pneumonia. Eur J Radiol 2017;88:82–7.
14. Juven T, Mertsola J, Waris M, et al. Etiology of community-acquired pneumonia in 254 hospitalized children. Pediatr Infect Dis J 2000;19(4):293–8.
15. Michelow IC, Olsen K, Lozano J, et al. Epidemiology and clinical characteristics of community-acquired pneumonia in hospitalized children. Pediatrics 2004; 113(4):701–7.
16. Wubbel L, Muniz L, Ahmed A, et al. Etiology and treatment of community-acquired pneumonia in ambulatory children. Pediatr Infect Dis J 1999;18(2):98–104.
17. Claesson BA, Trollfors B, Brolin I, et al. Etiology of community-acquired pneumonia in children based on antibody responses to bacterial and viral antigens. Pediatr Infect Dis J 1989;8(12):856–62.
18. Heiskanen-Kosma T, Korppi M, Jokinen C, et al. Etiology of childhood pneumonia: serologic results of a prospective, population-based study. Pediatr Infect Dis J 1998;17(11):986–91.
19. Hicks LA, Harrison LH, Flannery B, et al. Incidence of pneumococcal disease due to non-pneumococcal conjugate vaccine (PCV7) serotypes in the United States

during the era of widespread PCV7 vaccination, 1998-2004. J Infect Dis 2007; 196(9):1346–54.

20. Grijalva CG, Nuorti JP, Arbogast PG, et al. Decline in pneumonia admissions after routine childhood immunisation with pneumococcal conjugate vaccine in the USA: a time-series analysis. Lancet 2007;369(9568):1179–86.

21. Moore MR, Gertz RE Jr, Woodbury RL, et al. Population snapshot of emergent Streptococcus pneumoniae serotype 19A in the United States, 2005. J Infect Dis 2008;197(7):1016–27.

22. Olarte L, Barson WJ, Barson RM, et al. Pneumococcal pneumonia requiring hospitalization in us children in the 13-valent pneumococcal conjugate vaccine era. Clin Infect Dis 2017;64(12):1699–704.

23. Campbell SG, Marrie TJ, Anstey R, et al. The contribution of blood cultures to the clinical management of adult patients admitted to the hospital with community-acquired pneumonia: a prospective observational study. Chest 2003;123(4): 1142–50.

24. Hickey RW, Bowman MJ, Smith GA. Utility of blood cultures in pediatric patients found to have pneumonia in the emergency department. Ann Emerg Med 1996; 27(6):721–5.

25. Myers AL, Hall M, Williams DJ, et al. Prevalence of bacteremia in hospitalized pediatric patients with community-acquired pneumonia. Pediatr Infect Dis J 2013; 32(7):736–40.

26. Shah SS, Dugan MH, Bell LM, et al. Blood cultures in the emergency department evaluation of childhood pneumonia. Pediatr Infect Dis J 2011;30(6):475–9.

27. Iroh Tam PY, Bernstein E, Ma X, et al. Blood culture in evaluation of pediatric community-acquired pneumonia: a systematic review and meta-analysis. Hosp Pediatr 2015;5(6):324–36.

28. Blaschke AJ, Heyrend C, Byington CL, et al. Molecular analysis improves pathogen identification and epidemiologic study of pediatric parapneumonic empyema. Pediatr Infect Dis J 2011;30(4):289–94.

29. Dien Bard J, McElvania TeKippe E. Diagnosis of bloodstream infections in children. J Clin Microbiol 2016;54(6):1418–24.

30. Self WH, Speroff T, Grijalva CG, et al. Reducing blood culture contamination in the emergency department: an interrupted time series quality improvement study. Acad Emerg Med 2013;20(1):89–97.

31. Hall RT, Domenico HJ, Self WH, et al. Reducing the blood culture contamination rate in a pediatric emergency department and subsequent cost savings. Pediatrics 2013;131(1):e292–7.

32. Driscoll AJ, Deloria Knoll M, Hammitt LL, et al. The effect of antibiotic exposure and specimen volume on the detection of bacterial pathogens in children with pneumonia. Clin Infect Dis 2017;64(suppl_3):S368–77.

33. Harris AM, Bramley AM, Jain S, et al. Influence of antibiotics on the detection of bacteria by culture-based and culture-independent diagnostic tests in patients hospitalized with community-acquired pneumonia. Open Forum Infect Dis 2017;4(1):ofx014.

34. Isaacman DJ, Karasic RB, Reynolds EA, et al. Effect of number of blood cultures and volume of blood on detection of bacteremia in children. J Pediatr 1996; 128(2):190–5.

35. Gonsalves WI, Cornish N, Moore M, et al. Effects of volume and site of blood draw on blood culture results. J Clin Microbiol 2009;47(11):3482–5.

36. Berkley JA, Lowe BS, Mwangi I, et al. Bacteremia among children admitted to a rural hospital in Kenya. N Engl J Med 2005;352(1):39–47.

37. Connell TG, Rele M, Cowley D, et al. How reliable is a negative blood culture result? Volume of blood submitted for culture in routine practice in a children's hospital. Pediatrics 2007;119(5):891–6.

38. Byington CL, Spencer LY, Johnson TA, et al. An epidemiological investigation of a sustained high rate of pediatric parapneumonic empyema: risk factors and microbiological associations. Clin Infect Dis 2002;34(4):434–40.

39. Hoff SJ, Neblett WW, Edwards KM, et al. Parapneumonic empyema in children: decortication hastens recovery in patients with severe pleural infections. Pediatr Infect Dis J 1991;10(3):194–9.

40. Picard E, Joseph L, Goldberg S, et al. Predictive factors of morbidity in childhood parapneumonic effusion-associated pneumonia: a retrospective study. Pediatr Infect Dis J 2010;29(9):840–3.

41. Brownback KR, Thomas LA, Simpson SQ. Role of bronchoalveolar lavage in the diagnosis of pulmonary infiltrates in immunocompromised patients. Curr Opin Infect Dis 2014;27(4):322–8.

42. Thea DM, Seidenberg P, Park DE, et al. Limited utility of polymerase chain reaction in induced sputum specimens for determining the causes of childhood pneumonia in resource-poor settings: findings from the Pneumonia Etiology Research for Child Health (PERCH) Study. Clin Infect Dis 2017;64(suppl_3):S289–300.

43. Murdoch DR, Morpeth SC, Hammitt LL, et al. The diagnostic utility of induced sputum microscopy and culture in childhood pneumonia. Clin Infect Dis 2017; 64(suppl_3):S280–8.

44. Murdoch DR, Laing RT, Mills GD, et al. Evaluation of a rapid immunochromatographic test for detection of Streptococcus pneumoniae antigen in urine samples from adults with community-acquired pneumonia. J Clin Microbiol 2001;39(10): 3495–8.

45. Dowell SF, Garman RL, Liu G, et al. Evaluation of Binax NOW, an assay for the detection of pneumococcal antigen in urine samples, performed among pediatric patients. Clin Infect Dis 2001;32(5):824–5.

46. Pride MW, Huijts SM, Wu K, et al. Validation of an immunodiagnostic assay for detection of 13 Streptococcus pneumoniae serotype-specific polysaccharides in human urine. Clin Vaccine Immunol 2012;19(8):1131–41.

47. Resti M, Micheli A, Moriondo M, et al. Comparison of the effect of antibiotic treatment on the possibility of diagnosing invasive pneumococcal disease by culture or molecular methods: a prospective, observational study of children and adolescents with proven pneumococcal infection. Clin Ther 2009;31(6):1266–73.

48. Clark JE. Determining the microbiological cause of a chest infection. Arch Dis Child 2015;100(2):193–7.

49. Morpeth SC, Deloria Knoll M, Scott JAG, et al. Detection of pneumococcal DNA in blood by polymerase chain reaction for diagnosing pneumococcal pneumonia in young children from low- and middle-income countries. Clin Infect Dis 2017; 64(suppl_3):S347–56.

50. Azzari C, Cortimiglia M, Moriondo M, et al. Pneumococcal DNA is not detectable in the blood of healthy carrier children by real-time PCR targeting the lytA gene. J Med Microbiol 2011;60(Pt 6):710–4.

51. Abdullahi O, Nyiro J, Lewa P, et al. The descriptive epidemiology of Streptococcus pneumoniae and Haemophilus influenzae nasopharyngeal carriage in children and adults in Kilifi district, Kenya. Pediatr Infect Dis J 2008;27(1):59–64.

52. Spuesens EB, Fraaij PL, Visser EG, et al. Carriage of Mycoplasma pneumoniae in the upper respiratory tract of symptomatic and asymptomatic children: an observational study. PLoS Med 2013;10(5):e1001444.

53. Self WH, Williams DJ, Zhu Y, et al. Respiratory viral detection in children and adults: comparing asymptomatic controls and patients with community-acquired pneumonia. J Infect Dis 2016;213(4):584–91.

54. Jansen RR, Wieringa J, Koekkoek SM, et al. Frequent detection of respiratory viruses without symptoms: toward defining clinically relevant cutoff values. J Clin Microbiol 2011;49(7):2631–6.

55. Ampofo K, Bender J, Sheng X, et al. Seasonal invasive pneumococcal disease in children: role of preceding respiratory viral infection. Pediatrics 2008;122(2):229–37.

56. Peltola VT, McCullers JA. Respiratory viruses predisposing to bacterial infections: role of neuraminidase. Pediatr Infect Dis J 2004;23(1 Suppl):S87–97.

57. Fiore AE, Iverson C, Messmer T, et al. Outbreak of pneumonia in a long-term care facility: antecedent human parainfluenza virus 1 infection may predispose to bacterial pneumonia. J Am Geriatr Soc 1998;46(9):1112–7.

58. Randolph AG, Vaughn F, Sullivan R, et al. Critically ill children during the 2009-2010 influenza pandemic in the United States. Pediatrics 2011;128(6):e1450–8.

59. Nguyen T, Kyle UG, Jaimon N, et al. Coinfection with Staphylococcus aureus increases risk of severe coagulopathy in critically ill children with influenza A (H1N1) virus infection. Crit Care Med 2012;40(12):3246–50.

60. Voiriot G, Visseaux B, Cohen J, et al. Viral-bacterial coinfection affects the presentation and alters the prognosis of severe community-acquired pneumonia. Crit Care 2016;20(1):375.

61. McCullers JA. Insights into the interaction between influenza virus and pneumococcus. Clin Microbiol Rev 2006;19(3):571–82.

62. Dawood FS, Chaves SS, Perez A, et al. Complications and associated bacterial coinfections among children hospitalized with seasonal or pandemic influenza, United States, 2003-2010. J Infect Dis 2014;209(5):686–94.

63. Nohynek H, Valkeila E, Leinonen M, et al. Erythrocyte sedimentation rate, white blood cell count and serum C-reactive protein in assessing etiologic diagnosis of acute lower respiratory infections in children. Pediatr Infect Dis J 1995;14(6):484–90.

64. Berg AS, Inchley CS, Fjaerli HO, et al. Clinical features and inflammatory markers in pediatric pneumonia: a prospective study. Eur J Pediatr 2017;176(5):629–38.

65. Hoshina T, Nanishi E, Kanno S, et al. The utility of biomarkers in differentiating bacterial from non-bacterial lower respiratory tract infection in hospitalized children: difference of the diagnostic performance between acute pneumonia and bronchitis. J Infect Chemother 2014;20(10):616–20.

66. Van den Bruel A, Thompson MJ, Haj-Hassan T, et al. Diagnostic value of laboratory tests in identifying serious infections in febrile children: systematic review. BMJ 2011;342:d3082.

67. Higdon MM, Le T, O'Brien KL, et al. Association of C-reactive protein with bacterial and respiratory syncytial virus-associated pneumonia among children aged <5 years in the PERCH study. Clin Infect Dis 2017;64(suppl_3):S378–86.

68. Flood RG, Badik J, Aronoff SC. The utility of serum C-reactive protein in differentiating bacterial from nonbacterial pneumonia in children: a meta-analysis of 1230 children. Pediatr Infect Dis J 2008;27(2):95–9.

69. Gilbert DN. Procalcitonin as a biomarker in respiratory tract infection. Clin Infect Dis 2011;52(Suppl 4):S346–50.

70. Linscheid P, Seboek D, Nylen ES, et al. In vitro and in vivo calcitonin I gene expression in parenchymal cells: a novel product of human adipose tissue. Endocrinology 2003;144(12):5578–84.

71. Stockmann C, Ampofo K, Killpack J, et al. Procalcitonin accurately identifies hospitalized children with low risk of bacterial community-acquired pneumonia. J Pediatric Infect Dis Soc 2017. [Epub ahead of print].

72. Christ-Crain M, Jaccard-Stolz D, Bingisser R, et al. Effect of procalcitonin-guided treatment on antibiotic use and outcome in lower respiratory tract infections: cluster-randomised, single-blinded intervention trial. Lancet 2004;363(9409): 600–7.

73. Bouadma L, Luyt CE, Tubach F, et al. Use of procalcitonin to reduce patients' exposure to antibiotics in intensive care units (PRORATA trial): a multicentre randomised controlled trial. Lancet 2010;375(9713):463–74.

74. Schuetz P, Briel M, Christ-Crain M, et al. Procalcitonin to guide initiation and duration of antibiotic treatment in acute respiratory infections: an individual patient data meta-analysis. Clin Infect Dis 2012;55(5):651–62.

75. Baer G, Baumann P, Buettcher M, et al. Procalcitonin guidance to reduce antibiotic treatment of lower respiratory tract infection in children and adolescents (ProPAED): a randomized controlled trial. PLoS One 2013;8(8):e68419.

76. Esposito S, Tagliabue C, Picciolli I, et al. Procalcitonin measurements for guiding antibiotic treatment in pediatric pneumonia. Respir Med 2011;105(12):1939–45.

77. Mejias A, Dimo B, Suarez NM, et al. Whole blood gene expression profiles to assess pathogenesis and disease severity in infants with respiratory syncytial virus infection. Plos Med 2013;10(11):e1001549.

78. Suarez NM, Bunsow E, Falsey AR, et al. Superiority of transcriptional profiling over procalcitonin for distinguishing bacterial from viral lower respiratory tract infections in hospitalized adults. J Infect Dis 2015;212(2):213–22.

79. Mahajan P, Kuppermann N, Mejias A, et al. Association of RNA biosignatures with bacterial infections in febrile infants aged 60 days or younger. JAMA 2016;316(8): 846–57.

80. Heinonen S, Jartti T, Garcia C, et al. Rhinovirus detection in symptomatic and asymptomatic children: value of host transcriptome analysis. Am J Respir Crit Care Med 2016;193(7):772–82.

81. Ramilo O, Allman W, Chung W, et al. Gene expression patterns in blood leukocytes discriminate patients with acute infections. Blood 2007;109(5):2066–77.

82. Fine MJ, Auble TE, Yealy DM, et al. A prediction rule to identify low-risk patients with community-acquired pneumonia. N Engl J Med 1997;336(4):243–50.

83. Charles PG, Wolfe R, Whitby M, et al. SMART-COP: a tool for predicting the need for intensive respiratory or vasopressor support in community-acquired pneumonia. Clin Infect Dis 2008;47(3):375–84.

84. Williams DJ, Zhu Y, Grijalva CG, et al. Predicting severe pneumonia outcomes in children. Pediatrics 2016;138(4) [pii:e20161019].

85. Gerber JS, Kronman MP, Ross RK, et al. Identifying targets for antimicrobial stewardship in children's hospitals. Infect Control Hosp Epidemiol 2013;34(12): 1252–8.

86. Williams DJ, Hall M, Gerber JS, et al. Impact of a national guideline on antibiotic selection for hospitalized pneumonia. Pediatrics 2017;139(4) [pii:e20163231].

87. Handy LK, Bryan M, Gerber JS, et al. Variability in antibiotic prescribing for community-acquired pneumonia. Pediatrics 2017;139(4) [pii:e20162331].

88. Smith MJ, Kong M, Cambon A, et al. Effectiveness of antimicrobial guidelines for community-acquired pneumonia in children. Pediatrics 2012;129(5):e1326–33.

89. Ambroggio L, Thomson J, Murtagh Kurowski E, et al. Quality improvement methods increase appropriate antibiotic prescribing for childhood pneumonia. Pediatrics 2013;131(5):e1623–31.

90. CAP-IT: Efficacy, safety and impact on antimicrobial resistance of duration and dose of amoxicillin treatment for young children with Community-Acquired Pneumonia (CAP): A randomised controlled trial. 2017; Available at: https://www.capitstudy.org.uk/. Accessed June 28, 2017.

91. A Phase IV Double-Blind, Placebo-Controlled, Randomized Trial to Evaluate Short Course vs. Standard Course Outpatient Therapy of Community Acquired Pneumonia in Children (SCOUT-CAP). 2017; https://clinicaltrials.gov/ct2/show/NCT02891915. Accessed June 28, 2017.

92. Hicks LA, Chien YW, Taylor TH Jr, et al, Active Bacterial Core Surveillance Team. Outpatient antibiotic prescribing and nonsusceptible Streptococcus pneumoniae in the United States, 1996-2003. Clin Infect Dis 2011;53(7):631–9.

93. Spuesens EB, Meyer Sauteur PM, Vink C, et al. Mycoplasma pneumoniae infections–does treatment help? J Infect 2014;69(Suppl 1):S42–6.

94. Biondi E, McCulloh R, Alverson B, et al. Treatment of mycoplasma pneumonia: a systematic review. Pediatrics 2014;133(6):1081–90.

Emerging Respiratory Viruses in Children

Jennifer E. Schuster, MD, MSCI[a],*, John V. Williams, MD[b]

KEYWORDS

- Novel influenza A • Influenza C • Middle East respiratory syndrome virus
- Rhinovirus C

KEY POINTS

- Molecular diagnostics have led to the increased identification and recognition of existing and new viruses.
- Mutations and gene reassortment have caused transmission of animal viruses to humans.
- Emerging respiratory viruses can circulate seasonally or year-round as intermittent epidemics, or as outbreaks with subsequent resolution.

INTRODUCTION

Respiratory viruses are a leading cause of pediatric morbidity and mortality worldwide. In the last 15 years, molecular detection and sequencing have led to increased pathogen identification in common respiratory illnesses as well as identification of pathogens during outbreak scenarios. Heightened awareness for these and other emerging viruses is necessary to provide the best care for pediatric patients and to alert public health officials of novel diseases.

NOVEL INFLUENZA A

Background

Seasonal influenza A generally causes a yearly epidemic with variable prevalence based on vaccine efficacy and antigenic drift. Antigenic drift occurs in seasonal influenza due to minor mutations in the viral hemagglutinin (H) and neuraminidase (NA) genes. Antigenic shift occurs because of the ability of the virus to infect multiple

Disclosure Statement: J.E. Schuster has nothing to disclose. J.V. Williams serves on the Scientific Advisory Board of Quidel and an Independent Data Monitoring Committee for GlaxoSmithKline.

[a] Department of Pediatrics, Children's Mercy Kansas City, 2401 Gillham Road, Kansas City, MO 64108, USA; [b] Department of Pediatrics, Children's Hospital of Pittsburgh of UPMC, University of Pittsburgh School of Medicine, 9122 Rangos Research Building, 4400 Penn Avenue, Pittsburgh, PA 15224, USA
* Corresponding author.
E-mail address: jeschuster@cmh.edu

Infect Dis Clin N Am 32 (2018) 65–74
https://doi.org/10.1016/j.idc.2017.10.001
id.theclinics.com

animals, especially birds, and the ability of the segmented genome to undergo reassortment, mixing different proteins from different viral strains (**Table 1**). Novel influenza strains are antigenically distinct because of complete exchange of gene segments encoding the H or NA proteins, introducing H and NA variants that have not previously circulated in humans; thus, reassortant viruses have the ability to cause pandemics because of minimal preexisting population immunity. Avian influenza viruses can be passed to humans directly through close contact, or indirectly through another animal host. Because these viruses are adapted to birds, they usually have limited ability to replicate in humans, restricting person-to-person transmission. However, this can be circumvented by either mutation or reassortment with a human virus, as in the pandemic 2009 H1N1, which was a reassortment between avian, human, and swine influenza viruses.[1,2] Initially, reports of novel influenza A viruses centered on cases of H5N1. H5N1 human cases have occurred predominantly in Southeast Asia, the Indian subcontinent, and the Middle East; however, H5N1 has been detected in birds across Eurasia, Indonesia, and North Africa. Newly emerging avian influenza strains, including H7N9 and H10N8, have been identified in patients with poultry exposure in China. Seasonal outbreaks of H7N9 in humans have occurred since 2013, with a recent spike in cases in China.[3] Most cases have been reported in adults.[4] Influenza A H5N1 causes more severe disease and higher mortality in children, whereas person-to-person transmission is more common with H7N9, with nearly half of pediatric cases occurring in secondary clusters.[5] These novel influenza strains retain their preference for avian receptors and are not well adapted for human-to-human transmission.[6] Thus, pediatric cases are less common, likely because of lower rates of poultry exposure in children. Nonetheless, these viruses have been adapted in a controlled setting to be transmissible among mammals[7]; therefore, sustained human-to-human transmission could be possible, placing children at risk.

Clinical Symptoms

The clinical symptoms associated with novel influenza A strains are similar to yearly epidemic strains; however, symptoms are often more severe due to lack of preexisting immunity. Since its reemergence in 2003, fatal reports of H5N1 pediatric cases have been described, including symptoms consistent with acute encephalitis.[8] Compared with seasonal H3N2 and H1N1, H5N1-infected patients had a higher viral load and

Table 1
Differences among the influenza virus species

	Influenza A	Influenza B	Influenza C
Outer membrane proteins (total proteins)	Hemagglutinin and neuraminidase (10)	Hemagglutinin and neuraminidase (11)	Hemagglutinin-esterase fusion (9)
Host	Humans, swine, poultry, other animals	Humans and seals	Humans and swine
Variation	Antigenic shift and drift	Antigenic drift	Antigenic drift
Epidemiology	Able to cause pandemics due to reassortment with associated severe disease	Epidemics, but not pandemics, and severe disease can occur	Rare epidemics with generally mild disease

Adapted from Bennett JE, Dolin R, Blaser MJ. Mandell, Douglas, and Bennett's principles and practice of infectious diseases. 8th edition. Philadelphia: Elsevier/Saunders; 2015; with permission.

more exuberant cytokine response,[9] and mortalities are approximately 60%.[10] Any cytopenia and/or liver involvement is associated with more severe disease.[11,12] H7N9 infection in humans was first reported in China in 2013. Three patients suffered from rapidly progressive, fatal acute respiratory distress syndrome with multiorgan system failure; 2 were known to have recent poultry exposure. Fever and cough are common symptoms,[13] and similar to H5N1, laboratory findings included cytopenia, elevated liver function tests, and elevated creatinine kinase.[13,14] In 2013, a fatal case of novel H10N8 was reported in a patient with recent poultry market exposure in China.[15] Retrospective testing demonstrated that this was a newly emerged virus with no prior evidence of infection in poultry workers.[16]

Diagnosis

Travel history is important for persons with acute respiratory illnesses, because most novel influenza A viruses occur in Southeast Asia. Although influenza can be detected in cell culture, molecular diagnostics are crucial for the rapid identification of novel influenza viruses. Reverse transcriptase polymerase chain reaction (RT-PCR) can identify a broad range of influenza A strains with subsequent genome sequencing for complete identification of novel strains. Alternatively, RT-PCR primers and probes specific for avian H and NA genes are available.[17]

Prevention and Treatment

A whole-virus influenza H5N1 vaccine was found to be safe in a pediatric population with good antibody responses to both H and NA components.[18] Inactivated H7N9 vaccines are undergoing clinical trials,[19] and viruslike particle vaccine candidates are effective in small animal models.[20] Oseltamivir is recommended for persons infected with novel influenza A viruses, although reports of resistance have been described.[21] Chemoprophylaxis with oseltamivir can be considered based on exposure risk. Oseltamivir chemoprophylaxis is recommended in the highest-risk exposure groups (ie, household or close family member contacts of a confirmed or probable case of novel influenza A) and can be considered in moderate-risk exposure groups (ie, health care personnel with unprotected close contact with a confirmed or probable case).[22] Institution of appropriate isolation precautions is important (**Table 2**).[23]

INFLUENZA C
Background

Although initially identified in 1950, influenza C, a member of the *Orthomyxoviridae* family, is less well described than influenza A and B viruses. Influenza C has 9 viral proteins in contrast with the 10 and 11 viral proteins of influenza A and B, respectively. Unlike influenza A and B, it does not contain the NA outer membrane protein. This difference contributes to unique disease characteristics and important considerations

Table 2
Isolation for emerging respiratory viruses

	Standard	Contact	Droplet	Airborne
Novel influenza A	✓	✓	—	✓
Influenza C	✓	—	✓	—
MERS	✓	✓	—	✓
Rhinovirus C	✓	Consider	✓	—

Data from Refs.[23,50,69]

with respect to antiviral treatment. Similar to influenza B, influenza C does not undergo reassortment and antigenic shift, which is in contrast to influenza A. Influenza C does exhibit antigenic drift, and multiple variants can co-circulate (see **Table 1**). Data suggest that the virus circulates globally, and like other respiratory viruses, infection occurs early in life.[1] Most children infected are less than 6 years old.[24] Influenza C has been rarely identified as a cause of medically attended illness in adults.[25] The prevalence of influenza C is typically less than influenza A, but it can approach influenza B for some years.[26] Although overall rates are low, less than 1% of all respiratory specimens in one study,[24] epidemics do occur in conjunction with replacement of the dominant antigenic group.[27,28] Influenza C circulates primarily during the winter to early summer.[24] Recent studies using molecular detection have suggested that influenza C is more frequent in children than previously recognized.[24,26,28–31]

Clinical Symptoms

Influenza C symptoms are indistinguishable from influenza A and B. In one cohort, almost one-fifth of children with influenza C, predominantly those less than 2 years old, were hospitalized primarily due to pneumonia and bronchiolitis. In the ambulatory setting, upper respiratory tract infections were common. Fever and cough were common symptoms in both groups,[24] and influenza C has been identified as a cause of hospitalized pediatric community-acquired pneumonia.[31] Influenza C has been associated with fewer febrile days and less health care utilization than influenza A or B, suggesting a milder pathogen.[29] Like other influenza types, influenza C has been associated with encephalopathy.[32]

Diagnosis

RT-PCR methods have been used to identify influenza C.[30,33] Viral culture is difficult because of limited cell culture methods. Furthermore, the virus does not display an easily distinguishable strong cytopathic effect like influenza A and B.

Prevention and Treatment

Treatment of influenza C is not well described. Neuraminidase inhibitors are ineffective because of the lack of NA glycoprotein on the outer membrane of the virus. In vitro data suggest that amantadine has activity against influenza C[34]; however, the adamantanes have broad toxicities and are not routinely recommended because of high rates of resistance by influenza A.[35] Currently licensed seasonal influenza vaccines do not contain antigens to influenza C and are not protective. Supportive care is recommended. Droplet isolation should be used for children hospitalized with influenza C infection (see **Table 2**).

MIDDLE EAST RESPIRATORY SYNDROME VIRUS
Background

Coronaviruses (CoV) are a common cause of pediatric respiratory tract disease, accounting for about 15% of common colds. Viruses are classified into different genera (*Alpha-*, *Beta-*, *Gamma-*, and *Deltacoronavirus*). CoVs can infect multiple species, and crossover from animals to humans can lead to outbreaks.[1] Epidemic CoVs have been reported, most notably severe acute respiratory syndrome–associated coronavirus (SARS-CoV) in 2002 to 2003.[36] In 2012, a ≥60-year-old Saudi Arabian presented with pneumonia and respiratory failure. A novel *Betacoronavirus*, subsequently termed Middle East respiratory syndrome (MERS-CoV), was identified. Although most of the cases were detected in Saudi Arabia and United Arab Emirates, imported cases to the United States were described.[37] The virus was closely related to bat CoVs.[38]

However, camels were later identified as an intermediary host when zoonotic transmissions occurred,[39] and MERS-CoV seroprevalence was significantly higher among persons with camel exposure.[40] Person-to-person transmission did occur, which led to secondary hospital outbreaks.[41] Although initial reports primarily occurred in adults, likely related to zoonotic and occupational exposures, pediatric cases developed in household contacts.[42]

Clinical Symptoms

Case descriptions of patients with MERS-CoV are primarily in adults and in patients hospitalized with SARS-CoV. In one case series, fever was present in 62% of symptomatic patients, and cough was present in 50%. Upper respiratory tract symptoms were less common with only 19% of subjects having rhinorrhea.[43] Gastrointestinal symptoms, including diarrhea, have been reported. Although initial case fatality rates exceeded 50%,[44] a large number (25%) of patients with laboratory-confirmed infection were asymptomatic in other studies.[43] Data are sparse in children. In one case series of 11 Saudi children with confirmed MERS-CoV, the median age was 13 years (range 2–16 years), older than most respiratory viruses. Only 2 patients had symptoms, and both had underlying medical diseases, a 2-year-old with cystic fibrosis and a 14-year-old with Down syndrome and cardiopulmonary disease. Although the younger child died of respiratory failure, the older child had a relatively uncomplicated hospital course. Pulmonary imaging for both children demonstrated bilateral diffuse infiltrates.[45] In one cohort of household contacts of MERS-CoV-infected subjects, the secondary attack rate was relatively low at 5%. The virus did not have an increased predilection for children, and none of the infected children developed symptoms, suggesting that disease may be worse with primary transmission and/or in adults.[42]

Diagnosis

As with novel influenza A viruses, travel and exposure history are important. Real-time RT-PCR is available for the diagnosis of MERS-CoV, and serologic testing also exists.[46] Viral culture can be performed but requires proper specimen handling and biosafety at level-3 facilities.[47]

Prevention and Treatment

No MERS-CoV-specific treatment exists. In a small retrospective study of adults with severe MERS-CoV, patients treated with oral ribavirin and subcutaneous pegylated interferon alpha-2a had improved survival at 14 days (70% vs 29%). However, 28-day survival was not significantly different (30% vs 17%).[48] Candidate vaccines are being studied; however, most are in the preclinical stage.[49] Airborne and contact precautions are recommended to prevent person-to-person transmission (see **Table 2**).[50]

RHINOVIRUS C
Background

Human rhinoviruses (RV), members of the Picornaviridae family, are leading causes of respiratory illness in children. A new RV species, distinct from species A and B, was identified in 2004.[51,52] Sequencing of the viral protein 4 (VP4) region from specimens of children hospitalized with respiratory illness corroborated the discovery of this new species, rhinovirus C (RV-C). Most children in whom the isolate was identified were hospitalized with asthma or febrile wheeze.[53] Sixty genotypes of RV-C have been identified. The global burden of RV-C is significant with approximately one-quarter of RV infections attributed to RV-C. Rates of RV-C are generally higher than RV-B and comparable to RV-A in some studies.[54] RV-C is detected year-round.[55,56]

Clinical Symptoms

Although RVs are detected in both symptomatic and asymptomatic children, RV-C is more commonly associated with episodes of clinical illness.[57] Only 3% of RV-C is detected in healthy children.[58] RV-C can cause severe respiratory disease, particularly in asthmatics, and was associated with asthma exacerbations in children in a case-control study.[59] Children with RV-C are more likely to require supplemental oxygen and to have wheezing than children with RV-A.[60] However, in other studies, RV-A and RV-C produce similar clinical symptoms.[55,56] In one case series, 40% of RV-C-infected hospitalized children required supplemental oxygen and 95% wheezed.[56] RV-C-infected children in the outpatient and emergency department settings were more likely to have radiographically confirmed/clinically diagnosed lower respiratory tract illness (eg, bronchiolitis, pneumonia, croup, and asthma) compared with children with other RVs.[61,62] In addition, children with RV-C-related wheezing were more likely to be hospitalized for respiratory problems compared with non-RV respiratory viruses.[63]

Diagnosis

RV is typically detected from nasopharyngeal specimens using RT-PCR. Broad range PCR allows for detection of a variety of RVs by using primers targeting a conserved region. A subsequent step, including seminested PCR or sequencing, can identify the specific species and serotype. RV-C has also been detected in stool[64] as well as in blood, in which higher rates of viremia occurred with RV-C compared with other RV types.[65] RV can be detected using cell culture; however, this method is highly variable and depends on optimal temperatures (33°C–34°C), motion, and time (10–14 days to see cytopathic effect).[1] Furthermore, RV-C is extremely difficult to culture and requires highly specialized methods.[66] Antigen and antibody detection is hampered by the presence of numerous RV serotypes.

Prevention and Treatment

No licensed treatment of RV-C exists. Experimental antivirals have had some in vitro efficacy against RV-C, although notably, pleconaril did not have activity.[67] RV vaccine development has been complicated by the numerous viral serotypes and lack of cross-serotype protection.[68] Droplet isolation should be used for children hospitalized with clinically apparent RV-C infection.

SUMMARY

Respiratory viruses remain a leading cause of childhood disease. The identification and emergence of novel respiratory viruses are important for pediatricians and infectious diseases clinicians. Viruses that were previously difficult to culture can now be rapidly identified using molecular diagnostics and sequencing, and these techniques are highly useful for detecting outbreaks. In addition, the ongoing evolution of viruses and ability to mutate allows for species-to-species transmission of novel viruses. Practitioners should remain on high alert for emerging viruses in cases whereby a cause cannot be identified for a clinical syndrome or if the clinical syndrome is more severe than expected for the identified pathogen. Travel and animal exposure history are important to maintain a high index of suspicion, and rapid institution of appropriate isolation precautions is crucial to prevent person-to-person transmission (see **Table 2**).

REFERENCES

1. Bennett JE, Dolin R, Blaser MJ. Mandell, Douglas, and Bennett's principles and practice of infectious diseases. 8th edition. Philadelphia: Elsevier/Saunders; 2015.
2. Garten RJ, Davis CT, Russell CA, et al. Antigenic and genetic characteristics of swine-origin 2009 A(H1N1) influenza viruses circulating in humans. Science 2009;325(5937):197–201.
3. Zhou L, Ren R, Yang L, et al. Sudden increase in human infection with avian influenza A(H7N9) virus in China, September-December 2016. Western Pac Surveill Response J 2017;8(1):6–14.
4. Qi X, Qian YH, Bao CJ, et al. Probable person to person transmission of novel avian influenza A (H7N9) virus in Eastern China, 2013: epidemiological investigation. BMJ 2013;347:f4752.
5. Sha J, Dong W, Liu S, et al. Differences in the epidemiology of childhood infections with avian influenza A H7N9 and H5N1 viruses. PLoS One 2016;11(10): e0161925.
6. Zhang H, de Vries RP, Tzarum N, et al. A human-infecting H10N8 influenza virus retains a strong preference for avian-type receptors. Cell Host Microbe 2015; 17(3):377–84.
7. Imai M, Watanabe T, Hatta M, et al. Experimental adaptation of an influenza H5 HA confers respiratory droplet transmission to a reassortant H5 HA/H1N1 virus in ferrets. Nature 2012;486(7403):420–8.
8. de Jong MD, Bach VC, Phan TQ, et al. Fatal avian influenza A (H5N1) in a child presenting with diarrhea followed by coma. N Engl J Med 2005;352(7):686–91.
9. de Jong MD, Simmons CP, Thanh TT, et al. Fatal outcome of human influenza A (H5N1) is associated with high viral load and hypercytokinemia. Nat Med 2006; 12(10):1203–7.
10. Centers for Disease Control and Prevention. Highly pathogenic asian avian influenza A (H5N1) in people. Available at: https://www.cdc.gov/flu/avianflu/h5n1-people.htm. Accessed July 12, 2017.
11. Kawachi S, Luong ST, Shigematsu M, et al. Risk parameters of fulminant acute respiratory distress syndrome and avian influenza (H5N1) infection in Vietnamese children. J Infect Dis 2009;200(4):510–5.
12. Furuya H, Kawachi S, Shigematsu M, et al. Clinical factors associated with severity in hospitalized children infected with avian influenza (H5N1). Environ Health Prev Med 2011;16(1):64–8.
13. Liu S, Sun J, Cai J, et al. Epidemiological, clinical and viral characteristics of fatal cases of human avian influenza A (H7N9) virus in Zhejiang Province, China. J Infect 2013;67(6):595–605.
14. Gao R, Cao B, Hu Y, et al. Human infection with a novel avian-origin influenza A (H7N9) virus. N Engl J Med 2013;368(20):1888–97.
15. Chen H, Yuan H, Gao R, et al. Clinical and epidemiological characteristics of a fatal case of avian influenza A H10N8 virus infection: a descriptive study. Lancet 2014;383(9918):714–21.
16. Jia K, Jiao G, Hong ML, et al. No evidence H10N8 avian influenza virus infections among poultry workers in Guangdong province before 2013. J Clin Virol 2015;62: 6–7.
17. Monne I, Ormelli S, Salviato A, et al. Development and validation of a one-step real-time PCR assay for simultaneous detection of subtype H5, H7, and H9 avian influenza viruses. J Clin Microbiol 2008;46(5):1769–73.

18. van der Velden MV, Geisberger A, Dvorak T, et al. Safety and immunogenicity of a vero cell culture-derived whole-virus H5N1 influenza vaccine in chronically ill and immunocompromised patients. Clin Vaccine Immunol 2014;21(6):867–76.

19. Mulligan MJ, Bernstein DI, Winokur P, et al. Serological responses to an avian influenza A/H7N9 vaccine mixed at the point-of-use with MF59 adjuvant: a randomized clinical trial. JAMA 2014;312(14):1409–19.

20. Liu YV, Massare MJ, Pearce MB, et al. Recombinant virus-like particles elicit protective immunity against avian influenza A(H7N9) virus infection in ferrets. Vaccine 2015;33(18):2152–8.

21. Centers for Disease Control and Prevention. Prevention and treatment of avian influenza A viruses in people. 2017. Available at: https://www.cdc.gov/flu/avianflu/prevention.htm. Accessed July 12, 2017.

22. Centers for Disease Control and Prevention. Interim guidance on follow-up of close contacts of persons infected with novel influenza A viruses associated with severe human disease and on the use of antiviral medications for chemoprophylaxis. 2015. Available at: https://www.cdc.gov/flu/avianflu/novel-av-chemoprophylaxis-guidance.htm. Accessed October 12, 2017.

23. Centers for Disease Control and Prevention. Interim guidance for infection control within healthcare settings when caring for confirmed cases, probable cases, and cases under investigation for infection with novel influenza A viruses associated with severe disease. 2016. Available at: https://www.cdc.gov/flu/avianflu/novel-flu-infection-control.htm. Accessed August 9, 2017.

24. Matsuzaki Y, Katsushima N, Nagai Y, et al. Clinical features of influenza C virus infection in children. J Infect Dis 2006;193(9):1229–35.

25. Nesmith N, Williams JV, Johnson M, et al. Sensitive diagnostics confirm that influenza C is an uncommon cause of medically attended respiratory illness in adults. Clin Infect Dis 2017;65(6):1037–9.

26. Calvo C, Garcia-Garcia ML, Borrell B, et al. Prospective study of influenza C in hospitalized children. Pediatr Infect Dis J 2013;32(8):916–9.

27. Matsuzaki Y, Sugawara K, Abiko C, et al. Epidemiological information regarding the periodic epidemics of influenza C virus in Japan (1996-2013) and the seroprevalence of antibodies to different antigenic groups. J Clin Virol 2014;61(1): 87–93.

28. Matsuzaki Y, Abiko C, Mizuta K, et al. A nationwide epidemic of influenza C virus infection in Japan in 2004. J Clin Microbiol 2007;45(3):783–8.

29. Budge PJ, Griffin MR, Edwards KM, et al. Impact of home environment interventions on the risk of influenza-associated ARI in Andean children: observations from a prospective household-based cohort study. PLoS One 2014;9(3):e91247.

30. Matsuzaki Y, Ikeda T, Abiko C, et al. Detection and quantification of influenza C virus in pediatric respiratory specimens by real-time PCR and comparison with infectious viral counts. J Clin Virol 2012;54(2):130–4.

31. Principi N, Scala A, Daleno C, et al. Influenza C virus-associated community-acquired pneumonia in children. Influenza Other Respir Viruses 2013;7(6): 999–1003.

32. Takayanagi M, Umehara N, Watanabe H, et al. Acute encephalopathy associated with influenza C virus infection. Pediatr Infect Dis J 2009;28(6):554.

33. Howard LM, Johnson M, Gil AI, et al. A novel real-time RT-PCR assay for influenza C tested in Peruvian children. J Clin Virol 2017;96:12–6.

34. Neumayer EM, Haff RF, Hoffman CE. Antiviral activity of amantadine hydrochloride in tissue culture and in ovo. Proc Soc Exp Biol Med 1965;119:393–6.

35. Centers for Disease Control and Prevention. Antiviral dosage. Guidance on the use of influenza antiviral agents. 2015. Available at: https://www.cdc.gov/flu/professionals/antivirals/antiviral-dosage.htm. Accessed October 12, 2017.

36. Ksiazek TG, Erdman D, Goldsmith CS, et al. A novel coronavirus associated with severe acute respiratory syndrome. N Engl J Med 2003;348(20):1953–66.

37. Bialek SR, Allen D, Alvarado-Ramy F, et al. First confirmed cases of Middle East respiratory syndrome coronavirus (MERS-CoV) infection in the United States, updated information on the epidemiology of MERS-CoV infection, and guidance for the public, clinicians, and public health authorities–May 2014. MMWR Morb Mortal Wkly Rep 2014;63(19):431–6.

38. Zaki AM, van Boheemen S, Bestebroer TM, et al. Isolation of a novel coronavirus from a man with pneumonia in Saudi Arabia. N Engl J Med 2012;367(19):1814–20.

39. Azhar EI, El-Kafrawy SA, Farraj SA, et al. Evidence for camel-to-human transmission of MERS coronavirus. N Engl J Med 2014;370(26):2499–505.

40. Muller MA, Meyer B, Corman VM, et al. Presence of Middle East respiratory syndrome coronavirus antibodies in Saudi Arabia: a nationwide, cross-sectional, serological study. Lancet Infect Dis 2015;15(6):629.

41. Assiri A, McGeer A, Perl TM, et al. Hospital outbreak of Middle East respiratory syndrome coronavirus. N Engl J Med 2013;369(5):407–16.

42. Drosten C, Meyer B, Muller MA, et al. Transmission of MERS-coronavirus in household contacts. N Engl J Med 2014;371(9):828–35.

43. Oboho IK, Tomczyk SM, Al-Asmari AM, et al. 2014 MERS-CoV outbreak in Jeddah–a link to health care facilities. N Engl J Med 2015;372(9):846–54.

44. Centers for Disease Control and Prevention. Update: severe respiratory illness associated with Middle East Respiratory Syndrome Coronavirus (MERS-CoV)–worldwide, 2012-2013. MMWR Morb Mortal Wkly Rep 2013;62(23):480–3.

45. Memish ZA, Al-Tawfiq JA, Assiri A, et al. Middle East respiratory syndrome coronavirus disease in children. Pediatr Infect Dis J 2014;33(9):904–6.

46. Corman VM, Muller MA, Costabel U, et al. Assays for laboratory confirmation of novel human coronavirus (hCoV-EMC) infections. Euro Surveill 2012;17(49) [pii: 20334].

47. Centers for Disease Control and Prevention. Interim laboratory biosafety guidelines for handling and processing specimens associated with Middle East respiratory syndrome coronavirus (MERS-CoV) – Version 2. 2015. Available at: https://www.cdc.gov/coronavirus/mers/guidelines-lab-biosafety.html. Accessed June 11, 2017.

48. Omrani AS, Saad MM, Baig K, et al. Ribavirin and interferon alfa-2a for severe Middle East respiratory syndrome coronavirus infection: a retrospective cohort study. Lancet Infect Dis 2014;14(11):1090–5.

49. Modjarrad K. MERS-CoV vaccine candidates in development: the current landscape. Vaccine 2016;34(26):2982–7.

50. Centers for Disease Control and Prevention. Interim infection prevention and control recommendations for hospitalized patients with Middle East Respiratory syndrome coronavirus (MERS-CoV). 2015. Available at: https://www.cdc.gov/coronavirus/mers/infection-prevention-control.html. Accessed August 9, 2017.

51. Lamson D, Renwick N, Kapoor V, et al. MassTag polymerase-chain-reaction detection of respiratory pathogens, including a new rhinovirus genotype, that caused influenza-like illness in New York State during 2004-2005. J Infect Dis 2006;194(10):1398–402.

52. Arden KE, McErlean P, Nissen MD, et al. Frequent detection of human rhinoviruses, paramyxoviruses, coronaviruses, and bocavirus during acute respiratory tract infections. J Med Virol 2006;78(9):1232–40.

53. Lau SK, Yip CC, Tsoi HW, et al. Clinical features and complete genome characterization of a distinct human rhinovirus (HRV) genetic cluster, probably representing a previously undetected HRV species, HRV-C, associated with acute respiratory illness in children. J Clin Microbiol 2007;45(11):3655–64.

54. Lauinger IL, Bible JM, Halligan EP, et al. Patient characteristics and severity of human rhinovirus infections in children. J Clin Virol 2013;58(1):216–20.

55. Mackay IM, Lambert SB, Faux CE, et al. Community-wide, contemporaneous circulation of a broad spectrum of human rhinoviruses in healthy Australian preschool-aged children during a 12-month period. J Infect Dis 2013;207(9): 1433–41.

56. Iwane MK, Prill MM, Lu X, et al. Human rhinovirus species associated with hospitalizations for acute respiratory illness in young US children. J Infect Dis 2011; 204(11):1702–10.

57. Mak RK, Tse LY, Lam WY, et al. Clinical spectrum of human rhinovirus infections in hospitalized Hong Kong children. Pediatr Infect Dis J 2011;30(9):749–53.

58. Calvo C, Casas I, Garcia-Garcia ML, et al. Role of rhinovirus C respiratory infections in sick and healthy children in Spain. Pediatr Infect Dis J 2010;29(8):717–20.

59. Khetsuriani N, Lu X, Teague WG, et al. Novel human rhinoviruses and exacerbation of asthma in children. Emerg Infect Dis 2008;14(11):1793–6.

60. Miller EK, Khuri-Bulos N, Williams JV, et al. Human rhinovirus C associated with wheezing in hospitalised children in the Middle East. J Clin Virol 2009;46(1):85–9.

61. Linder JE, Kraft DC, Mohamed Y, et al. Human rhinovirus C: age, season, and lower respiratory illness over the past 3 decades. J Allergy Clin Immunol 2013; 131(1):69–77.e1-6.

62. Martin EK, Kuypers J, Chu HY, et al. Molecular epidemiology of human rhinovirus infections in the pediatric emergency department. J Clin Virol 2015;62:25–31.

63. Cox DW, Bizzintino J, Ferrari G, et al. Human rhinovirus species C infection in young children with acute wheeze is associated with increased acute respiratory hospital admissions. Am J Respir Crit Care Med 2013;188(11):1358–64.

64. Harvala H, McIntyre CL, McLeish NJ, et al. High detection frequency and viral loads of human rhinovirus species A to C in fecal samples; diagnostic and clinical implications. J Med Virol 2012;84(3):536–42.

65. Fuji N, Suzuki A, Lupisan S, et al. Detection of human rhinovirus C viral genome in blood among children with severe respiratory infections in the Philippines. PLoS One 2011;6(11):e27247.

66. Bochkov YA, Palmenberg AC, Lee WM, et al. Molecular modeling, organ culture and reverse genetics for a newly identified human rhinovirus C. Nat Med 2011; 17(5):627–32.

67. Mello C, Aguayo E, Rodriguez M, et al. Multiple classes of antiviral agents exhibit in vitro activity against human rhinovirus type C. Antimicrob Agents Chemother 2014;58(3):1546–55.

68. McLean GR. Developing a vaccine for human rhinoviruses. J Vaccines Immun 2014;2(3):16–20.

69. Siegel JD, Rhinehart E, Jackson M, et al, Health Care Infection Control Practices Advisory Committee. 2007 guideline for isolation precautions: preventing transmission of infectious agents in health care settings. Am J Infect Control 2007; 35(10 Suppl 2):S65–164.

Updates on Influenza Vaccination in Children

Angela J.P. Campbell, MD, MPH*, Lisa A. Grohskopf, MD, MPH

KEYWORDS

- Influenza vaccination • Vaccine effectiveness • Immunogenicity • Safety • Antiviral

KEY POINTS

- Routine annual influenza vaccination is recommended for all persons without contraindications 6 months of age and older.
- Influenza is a source of substantial illness burden among children, especially younger children and those with certain chronic medical conditions.
- Vaccines licensed for children in the United States include various intramuscular inactivated influenza vaccines. Live attenuated influenza vaccine (LAIV) is licensed for children 2 years of age and older but as of "the 2017-18 influenza season", it is not recommended for use.
- Effectiveness of influenza vaccines varies from season to season.
- Influenza antiviral medications are an important adjunct to vaccination, particularly for children at high risk of severe illness.

Influenza viruses cause illness in millions of children annually. Although most infected children will recover without complications, influenza can cause serious illness, particularly among young children and those with chronic medical conditions. Since 2008, influenza vaccination has been recommended by the US Centers for Disease Control and Prevention (CDC) Advisory Committee on Immunization Practices (ACIP) for all children 6 months of age and older who do not have contraindications.[1]

EPIDEMIOLOGY

Seasonal influenza is an important cause of morbidity and mortality in children, with an estimated 600,000 to 2,500,000 influenza-associated outpatient medical visits and

Disclosure Statement: The authors have no conflicts of interest.

Disclaimers: The findings and conclusions in this report are those of the authors and do not necessarily represent the official position of the US Centers for Disease Control and Prevention. Use of trade names and commercial sources is for identification only and does not imply endorsement by the CDC, the Public Health Service, or the US Department of Health and Human Services.

Influenza Division, National Center for Immunization and Respiratory Diseases, Centers for Disease Control and Prevention, 1600 Clifton Road NE, Mailstop A32, Atlanta, GA 30329, USA

* Corresponding author.

E-mail address: app4@cdc.gov

Infect Dis Clin N Am 32 (2018) 75–89
https://doi.org/10.1016/j.idc.2017.11.005
0891-5520/18/Published by Elsevier Inc.

6000 to 26,000 hospitalizations per year among children younger than 5 years old during recent US seasons.[2] Since 2004, 37 to 171 influenza-associated deaths among children younger than 18 years have been reported during nonpandemic seasons, with 358 deaths reported during the 2009 pandemic.[3]

Children less than 5 years, and particularly those less than 2 years, are at higher risk for severe outcomes due to influenza, including influenza-associated hospitalizations and death.[4–7] Several studies have estimated that younger children, particularly infants and those younger than 5 years of age, are more likely to be hospitalized than older children.[4,7–9] Complications of influenza in children include pneumonia, asthma exacerbations, dehydration, and, less commonly, lung abscess/empyema, bacteremia/sepsis, acute renal failure, myocarditis, and neurologic complications such as encephalopathy and encephalitis.[10–12] Bacterial coinfection may occur, most commonly with *Staphylococcus aureus*, *Streptococcus pneumoniae*, and *Streptococcus pyogenes*.[10,11,13] Children with underlying medical conditions, such as immunosuppression; prematurity; and pulmonary, cardiac, hematologic, or neurologic/neuromuscular disorders are at higher risk for influenza complications.[14–16] However, many influenza-associated hospitalizations and deaths occur in healthy children without known high-risk conditions.[5,6,17]

HISTORY OF INFLUENZA VACCINES AND VACCINE RECOMMENDATIONS IN CHILDREN

In the United States, routine vaccination of healthy children has been recommended only relatively recently (**Table 1**). Vaccination of persons of any age with certain chronic medical conditions has been recommended as early as publication of US guidance for the use of influenza vaccines in the civilian population in 1960.[18] The description of conditions considered to confer risk of severe illness due to influenza has evolved over time (**Box 1**).

The recommendation to vaccinate healthy individuals in the United States (those without recognized risk factors for severe illness) was largely focused on persons aged 65 years of age and older from the early 1960s through the late 1990s (adults aged 50 through 64 years were added in 2000).[19] Routine vaccination was encouraged when feasible for all children 6 through 23 months of age starting with the 2002-03 season.[20] A full recommendation for vaccination of healthy children in this age group (as well as contacts and caregivers of children 0 through 23 months of age) was made for the 2004-05 season by ACIP[21] and the American Academy of Pediatrics.[22] This recommendation followed the 2003-04 influenza season, during which

Table 1
History of childhood influenza vaccination recommendations in the United States

Year	Child Group of Interest	Comment
1960	Those with chronic conditions considered as risk factors for severe influenza	US guidance for the use of influenza vaccines in the civilian population was published[18]
2002	6–23 months of age	Routine vaccination encouraged when feasible for this age group[20]
2004	6–23 months of age	Full vaccination recommended for healthy children in this age group, and household contacts and caregivers[21]
2006	6–59 months of age	[23]
2008	6–18 months of age	[1]

Box 1
Groups at increased risk for severe illness because of influenza

- Children aged 6 to 59 months;

- Adults aged 50 years or older;

- Persons with chronic pulmonary (including asthma), cardiovascular (except isolated hypertension), renal, hepatic, neurologic, hematologic, or metabolic disorders (including diabetes mellitus)

- Persons who are immunocompromised due to any cause (including medications or HIV infection)

- Women who are or will be pregnant during the influenza season

- Children and adolescents (aged 6 months through 18 years) receiving aspirin- or salicylate-containing medications and who might be at risk for experiencing Reye syndrome after influenza virus infection

- Residents of nursing homes and other long-term care facilities

- American Indians/Alaska Natives

- Persons who are extremely obese (body mass index ≥40)

From Grohskopf LA, Sokolow LZ, Broder KR, et al. Prevention and control of seasonal influenza with vaccines: recommendations of the Advisory Committee on Immunization Practices - United States, 2017-18 influenza season. MMWR Recomm Rep 2017;66(2):7.

---

153 deaths of children younger than 18 years of age were reported. Only 33% of these children had a recognized risk factor for severe influenza illness; 20% had other underlying medical conditions, and 47% had been previously healthy.[17] For subsequent influenza seasons, the recommendation for routine vaccination of healthy children was expanded first to all children 6 through 59 months of age in the 2006-07 season,[23] and to all children 6 months through 18 years of age in the 2008-09 season.[1]

INFLUENZA VACCINE IMMUNOGENICITY, EFFICACY, AND EFFECTIVENESS IN CHILDREN

Many studies have evaluated immune responses to influenza vaccines in adults and children. Serum antibody responses are traditionally regarded as correlates of vaccine-induced protection for inactivated influenza vaccines (IIVs).[24,25] However, an antibody titer considered to correlate with immunity on a population level may not predict protection from illness for an individual. Mucosal antibody response and cellular immunity have been associated with protection induced by live-attenuated influenza vaccine (LAIV); however, this varies by study, and clear correlates of immunity are currently lacking.[24,26,27]

Immunogenicity studies and controlled clinical trials of IIV have generally shown that children 6 months of age and older develop protective levels of specific antibody after receiving the recommended number of vaccine doses.[28–30] Studies involving seasonal IIV among young children indicate that 2 doses are needed for optimal benefit among younger children who are influenza vaccine-naive,[31–33] which is the basis for the recommendation that children 6 months through 8 years of age receiving vaccine for the first time should receive 2 doses separated by at least 4 weeks[34] (**Fig. 1**).

Vaccine efficacy studies evaluate how well vaccination prevents illness in persons enrolled in clinical trials. Among children, randomized controlled trials using laboratory-confirmed influenza as the outcome reported vaccine efficacy ranging

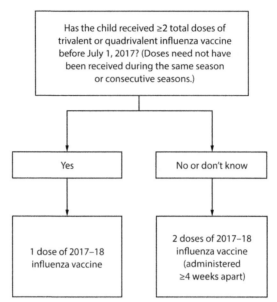

Fig. 1. Influenza vaccine dosing algorithm for children aged 6 months through 8 years, 2017-18 influenza season. (*From* Grohskopf LA, Sokolow LZ, Broder KR, et al. Prevention and control of seasonal influenza with vaccines: recommendations of the Advisory Committee on Immunization Practices - United States, 2017-18 influenza season. MMWR Recomm Rep 2017;66(2):9.)

from 43% to 91% for IIVs. For LAIV, estimates of vaccine efficacy against laboratory-confirmed influenza as the outcome ranged from 64% to 93%.[35]

Vaccine effectiveness reflects how well the vaccine works in the real-world setting (ie, not in randomized trials). Such estimates are obtained from observational studies, which are more subject to potential biases than randomized controlled trials. Many recent observational studies have used a test-negative study design (in which case/control status among participants who present with acute respiratory illness is assigned on the basis of influenza testing results) in order to control for biases that may occur when comparing outcomes among vaccinated and unvaccinated populations.

In a recent systematic review and meta-analysis of published test-negative design studies, analyses of the pediatric age groups (<20 years old) showed a pooled VE of 69% (95% confidence intervals [CI], 49% to 81%) against seasonal influenza A(H1N1)pdm09 virus and 56% (95% CI, 38% to 69%) against influenza B virus, similar estimates to the adult age groups. The pooled VE against influenza A(H3N2) virus was 43% (95% CI, 28% to 55%), highest in children and lowest in older adults.[36]

Recent studies have also evaluated VE in preventing severe outcomes in children. In a study examining effectiveness of seasonal vaccination against pediatric intensive care unit (PICU) admission in the 2010-11 and 2011-12 seasons, fully vaccinated children 6 months through 17 years old were 74% (95% CI, 19% to 91%) less likely to be admitted to the PICU for influenza than unvaccinated children.[37] Another study found that influenza vaccination reduced the likelihood of influenza-associated death among children by 65% (95% CI, 54% to 74%).[38] Neither of these studies assessed IIV and LAIV separately.

UPDATES IN PEDIATRIC INFLUENZA VACCINES AND INFLUENZA VACCINATION
Influenza Vaccines Licensed for Children

In recent years, many new influenza vaccines have been licensed in the United States; currently available vaccines are summarized in **Table 2**. Of 13 influenza vaccines licensed in the United States for the 2017-18 season, 8 vaccines are licensed for children.[34] Licensed products and approved ages for individual vaccines vary by country.

Quadrivalent versus Trivalent Influenza Vaccines

For the last several decades through the 2012-13 influenza season, US-licensed seasonal influenza vaccines were trivalent, containing hemagglutinin (HA) derived from 3 influenza viruses: an A(H1N1) virus, an A(H3N2) virus, and a B virus. Influenza B viruses consist of 2 lineages (Victoria and Yamagata), which have cocirculated during most seasons since the 1980s, generally with 1 lineage predominating.[39–41] Antibody cross-protection against influenza B viruses from 1 lineage to viruses from the opposite lineage is inconsistent.[41] Quadrivalent influenza vaccines, first available in the United States during the 2013-14 season, contain an influenza B virus from each lineage, and are thus intended to provide broader protection against circulating

Table 2
Types of influenza vaccines licensed in the United States, 2017-18 influenza season

Vaccine Type	Available Formulations	Licensed Age	Notes
Inactivated influenza vaccines	Quadrivalent • Standard-dose, intramuscular, unadjuvanted • Standard-dose, intradermal, unadjuvanted Trivalent • Standard-dose, intramuscular, unadjuvanted • Standard-dose, intramuscular, adjuvanted • High-dose, intramuscular unadjuvanted	Many brands available Quadrivalent and trivalent intramuscular vaccines are available for children as young as 6 months of age However, age indications vary. An age-appropriate vaccine should be used in all cases	As of October 2017, high-dose, adjuvanted and intradermal vaccines are not licensed for children <18 years of age
Recombinant influenza vaccines	• Quadrivalent, intramuscular • Trivalent, intramuscular	≥18 years	As of October 2017, not licensed for children <18 years of age
Live attenuated influenza vaccine	• Quadrivalent, intranasal	2 through 49 years	Not recommended for use in the United States during the 2016–2017 and 2017–2018 seasons due to concerns about effectiveness against H1N1pdm09-like viruses; consult current CDC/ACIP recommendations for future seasons

B viruses. As of the 2017-18 season, both trivalent and quadrivalent influenza vaccines are still available. No preferential recommendations are made for any specific product.

Dose Volume for Children 6 Through 35 Months of Age

Prior to the 2016-17 season, children 6 through 35 months of age in the United States were recommended to receive a smaller dose of IIV of 0.25 mL, half the 0.5 mL dose recommended for older children and adults. The basis of this recommendation was the observation during the 1970s of increased reactogenicity, particularly fever, among younger children.[42–44] These reactions were primarily noted with whole-virus IIVs, which are no longer used in the United States. Studies comparing 0.5 mL and 0.25 mL of currently licensed split-virus vaccines among children in this age group have reported a reassuring safety profile at the higher volume.[45,46]

Prior to 2016, the only US-licensed formulation of influenza vaccine for 6 through 35 month olds was a product approved to be given as a 0.25 mL dose. In 2016, an additional product was approved by US Food and Drug Administration (FDA), to be given at a 0.5 mL dose. Because there are 2 influenza vaccines licensed for this age group, with different approved doses, care should be taken to administer the appropriate product at the recommended dose.

Live Attenuated Influenza Vaccine

LAIV was initially licensed in the United States in 2003 for persons 5 through 49 years of age; subsequently the age indication was expanded to 2 through 49 years. LAIV was available as a trivalent vaccine through the 2012-13 season; a quadrivalent formulation was licensed in the United States in 2012 and was first available for the 2013-14 season.

Most clinical trials and observational studies comparing efficacy and effectiveness of trivalent IIV (IIV3) to trivalent LAIV (LAIV3) among adults have shown similar protection, or that IIV3 was more efficacious.[47] Prior to the 2009 pandemic, 3 randomized trials that directly compared LAIV3 and IIV3 suggested that LAIV3 provided increased protection in preventing laboratory-confirmed influenza among young children (under approximately 6 years of age).[48–50] Based upon review of this literature, in June 2014 CDC and ACIP made a preferential recommendation for LAIV over IIV for healthy children 2 through 8 years of age.[51]

However, analysis of observational studies of LAIV4 vaccine effectiveness from the US Influenza Vaccine Effectiveness Network showed low effectiveness of LAIV4 against influenza A(H1N1)pdm09 virus during the 2013-14 season (the first season that quadrivalent LAIV was available) among children 2 through 17 years old.[52–54] This was the first season since the start of the 2009 pandemic during which A(H1N1)pdm09 was the predominant circulating virus. Two other US case-control studies showed reduced effectiveness of LAIV4 among children 2 through 17 years old against H1N1pdm09 viruses. IIVs, however, demonstrated significant effectiveness against H1N1pdm09 virus among children in the 2013-14 season.[52–54] During the 2014-15 season, neither LAIV4 nor IIVs offered significant protection against antigenically drifted H3N2 viruses that predominated that season.[55–57] This contrasted with a large randomized trial during the 2004-05 season that demonstrated superior efficacy of LAIV3 compared with IIV3 against antigenically drifted H3N2 viruses.[49] During the 2015-16 season, LAIV4 effectiveness was lower than that for IIVs against influenza A(H1N1)pdm09 virus among children in the United States,[58] despite substitution of a different influenza A(H1N1)pdm09 vaccine virus component in LAIV4 to address concerns regarding stability and infectivity of the H1N1pdm09 virus in the vaccine for the 2013 to 2014 season. Based upon these data, ACIP recommended that LAIV not be used for any population for the 2016-17 season.[59] This recommendation has been extended into the 2017-18 US influenza season.[34]

Influenza Vaccination for Children with Egg Allergy

With the exception of the cell culture-based influenza vaccine (currently licensed for ages $\geq$4 years) and the recombinant influenza vaccines (currently licensed for adults $\geq$18 years), currently available influenza vaccines contain viruses that have been propagated in chicken eggs and may contain residual egg proteins. Only the recombinant influenza vaccines are considered egg-free. As of 2017-18, cell-based influenza vaccine contains some viruses for which the reference strain was initially derived in eggs. Residual egg protein is anticipated to be substantially less than for egg-based inactivated vaccines.[34]

Since the 2016-17 season, persons with egg allergy of any severity have been recommended for vaccination with any licensed, recommended, and age-appropriate influenza vaccine. For those who report reaction to egg consisting of only hives, no other measures are recommended. Those reporting reactions to egg including any other symptoms should be vaccinated in a medical setting, under the supervision of a health care provider who can recognize and manage severe allergic reactions. Personnel and equipment needed to treat severe allergic reactions should always be available in all vaccination settings.[34]

INFLUENZA VACCINE SAFETY IN CHILDREN

Currently licensed influenza vaccines for children are generally well-tolerated. Serious reactions are uncommon, and may not be observed during the course of prelicensure clinical studies. Therefore, ongoing safety monitoring for rare events is important for all vaccines. In the United States, monitoring of adverse events following vaccination occurs primarily via the Vaccine Adverse Event Reporting System (VAERS) and Vaccine Safety Datalink (VSD). Provider reporting to VAERS is encouraged for any adverse event regarded as clinically significant; reports are required by law for certain types of events. Detailed information and instructions for reporting may be found at https://vaers.hhs.gov/index.html.

Inactivated Influenza Vaccines

IIVs are generally well-tolerated by children. Among the more frequent adverse events reported in package inserts following administration of IIVs are local symptoms at the injection site, including injection site pain or tenderness, redness, and swelling or induration. Systemic symptoms, such as headache, myalgia, malaise, and fatigue may also occur, as well as irritability and drowsiness among younger children.[60–63]

Fever, which is generally more commonly among younger children, may occur following receipt of IIVs.[64] Fever was more commonly associated with older, whole-virus IIVs, and was more often observed in children than adults.[64,65] Whole virus IIVs are no longer used in the United States, having been replaced by split-virus and subunit vaccines.

Although febrile reactions remain of interest because of the potential for febrile seizures, febrile seizures may also occur in the context of viral illnesses, including influenza. However, IIVs have been associated with increased risk of febrile seizures during some seasons. In Australia, during the 2010 Southern Hemisphere influenza season, receipt of 1 particular vaccine (marketed as Afluria in the United States) was associated with an increased risk of febrile seizures.[66] Subsequent investigation into the causes of these reactions implicated residual lipid and viral RNA complexes following splitting of the influenza vaccine viruses. Testing of a modified formulation revealed no increased pyrogenicity in a clinical study among children 5 through 8 years of age.[67] Subsequently, an association of febrile seizures with receipt of IIV was observed through surveillance in VAERS and VSD in the United States during the 2010-11 season, with a lower risk than that observed in Australia. The risk was higher when IIV and 13-valent pneumococcal conjugate vaccine were administered concomitantly.[68,69] Investigations in the United States have found associations between receipt of IIVs and febrile seizures during later seasons, in general when coadministered with pneumococcal conjugate- or diphtheria/tetanus/acellular pertussis-containing vaccines.[70–73] No policy changes were made, and these vaccines may be given concomitantly.

Other serious reactions to influenza vaccines among children have been reported. Increased reports of narcolepsy among children and adults were noted during pandemic influenza vaccination campaigns in several European countries, mainly in association with ASO3-containing monovalent (H1N1)pdm09 vaccines.[64,74] No seasonal influenza vaccines that are licensed and commercially available in the United States contain ASO3.

Live-Attenuated Influenza Vaccines

As with IIVs, LAIV is generally well-tolerated among children; results of serious adverse events are uncommon.[75,76] Common reactions are generally self-limited and include runny nose, nasal congestion, sore throat, headache, vomiting, and myalgia; in general, symptoms are more severe with the first dose.[77–80]

Wheezing is a potential adverse event following LAIV, particularly among younger children. In a trial comparing LAIV3 with IIVs, wheezing was reported more frequently among LAIV3 recipients, and was mainly observed among those younger than 12 months of age.[49] LAIV is not currently licensed for children younger than 2 years of age in the United States.

LAIV contains live, attenuated, cold-adapted influenza viruses that replicate locally in the nasal mucosa. Shedding of vaccine viruses can occur following administration of LAIV. In a study of LAIV3 administered to persons 5 through 49 years of age, shedding was inversely correlated with age, and peak shedding occurred approximately 2 days after vaccination.[80] Shed virus can potentially be transmitted to unvaccinated persons, but has been rarely reported.[81]

ACIP has previously recommended that health care personnel who receive LAIV should avoid caring for severely immunocompromised patients (those requiring a protected environment).[82] Likewise, it has been recommended that LAIV not be administered to persons living with severely immunocompromised persons.[83]

FUTURE OF INFLUENZA VACCINES FOR CHILDREN

Improving influenza vaccine effectiveness is an important goal. Government agencies, academic institutions, and private companies are working toward development of improved vaccines. Potential novel approaches include strategies to improve immunogenicity, such as high-dose or adjuvanted vaccines, and nonegg-based production platforms including recombinant vaccines, cell culture-based or plant-based vaccines, and vaccines developed using virus-like particles, vectors, or DNA vaccines.[84–86]

Adjuvanted influenza vaccines, although shown to be immunogenic and efficacious in children in some studies,[87,88] are not currently licensed for children in the United States. A trivalent IIV containing MF59 (an oil-in-water emulsion adjuvant) and a high-dose trivalent IIV are licensed for adults 65 years of age and older.[89,90] Although all inactivated vaccines currently available for children are administered intramuscularly, 1 intradermal IIV4 is licensed in the United States for adults 18 through 64 years, which requires less HA antigen than standard-dose intramuscular IIVs.[91]

With respect to nonegg-based production platforms, trivalent and quadrivalent recombinant influenza vaccines are available in the United States for adults 18 years of age and older for the 2017-18 season. Recombinant vaccines are manufactured via production of HA in an insect cell culture, and are egg-free.[92,93] A quadrivalent inactivated vaccine produced via a cell culture-based platform was licensed for the 2016-17 season for persons 4 years of age and older. Although viruses for this product are not propagated in eggs, it is not considered egg-free because of the potential introduction of egg proteins via egg-derived reference viruses supplied to the manufacturer.[34]

Other strategies are underway to develop new influenza vaccines. Plant-based systems have been used to rapidly produce influenza virus-like particle vaccines, and a plant-derived quadrivalent virus-like particle influenza vaccine has been shown in a phase 1 to 2 clinical trial to produce a strong immune response with cross-reactive responses to antigenically different influenza viruses in adults.[94] Most other approaches to vaccines are in preclinical and phase I clinical trials, and include vector-based vaccines (eg, using adenovirus, poxvirus, and alphavirus systems), peptide-based vaccines, and DNA vaccines.[85,86] Even with newer vaccine approaches, most studies have been targeted to the influenza virus HA, similar to currently approved vaccines. The quest for a broadly protective, universal influenza vaccine has involved evaluation of conserved viral epitopes as targets, including more conserved portions of the HA stalk region, the extracellular portion of the M2 ion channel protein, and internal matrix and nucleoproteins.[84,85]

ANTIVIRALS AS AN IMPORTANT ADJUNCT TO INFLUENZA VACCINATION

Although influenza vaccination is the first line of defense against influenza, early antiviral treatment is important as a second line, and is recommended by CDC for children with suspected or confirmed influenza who are hospitalized for those who have severe or progressive illness, and for children at high risk for influenza complications (see **Box 1**). Timely antiviral treatment can shorten the duration of illness and may reduce the risk of complications.[95] Among critically ill children hospitalized in the intensive care unit, early treatment has been reported to reduce the length of hospitalization and to reduce the estimated risk of death.[96,97] A study of patients hospitalized with influenza over 5 seasons found that antiviral treatment in children was lower than in adults (72% vs 86%, respectively).[98]

Although room for improvement remains regarding antiviral treatment in hospitalized children, treatment among outpatient children for whom it is recommended is even more underprescribed. During the 2013-14 influenza season, only 28% of children 6 months to 2 years old who sought outpatient medical care for acute respiratory illness received antiviral treatment, despite presenting no more than 2 days from symptom onset and having a confirmed RT-PCR-positive influenza result (not necessarily known to the provider).[99] None of the 66 children younger than 2 years old with chronic medical conditions and acute respiratory illness were prescribed an influenza antiviral.[99] These data necessitate further efforts to understand factors that influence antiviral prescribing among providers caring for high-risk children in outpatient settings.

SUMMARY

Influenza continues to be a formidable seasonal foe for clinicians caring for children. Severe illness and death may occur, particularly among younger children and those with underlying medical conditions, but also in previously healthy children of any age. Moreover, seasonal influenza is associated with hundreds of thousands to millions more less severe illnesses and outpatient visits,[2] with missed school days among children and lost work among parents reported during influenza seasons.[100]

Although the effectiveness of vaccination varies annually, the best way to prevent seasonal influenza in children is to vaccinate before each season with recommended vaccines. Vaccination is also important for caregivers and other household members. This is particularly the case for children who are too young to be vaccinated or have conditions placing them at higher risk for influenza-related complications.

REFERENCES

1. Fiore AE, Shay DK, Broder K, et al. Prevention and control of influenza: recommendations of the Advisory Committee on Immunization Practices (ACIP), 2008. MMWR Recomm Rep 2008;57(RR-7):1–60.
2. Rolfes MA, Foppa IM, Garg S, et al. Annual estimates of the burden of seasonal influenza in the United States: a tool for strengthening influenza surveillance and preparedness. Influenza Other Respi Viruses 2017;00:1–6.
3. D'Mello T, Brammer L, Blanton L, et al. Update: influenza activity–United States, September 28, 2014-February 21, 2015. MMWR Morb Mortal Wkly Rep 2015; 64(8):206–12.
4. Poehling KA, Edwards KM, Weinberg GA, et al. The underrecognized burden of influenza in young children. N Engl J Med 2006;355(1):31–40.
5. O'Brien MA, Uyeki TM, Shay DK, et al. Incidence of outpatient visits and hospitalizations related to influenza in infants and young children. Pediatrics 2004; 113(3 Pt 1):585–93.
6. Wong KK, Jain S, Blanton L, et al. Influenza-associated pediatric deaths in the United States, 2004-2012. Pediatrics 2013;132(5):796–804.
7. Poehling KA, Edwards KM, Griffin MR, et al. The burden of influenza in young children, 2004-2009. Pediatrics 2013;131(2):207–16.
8. Coffin SE, Zaoutis TE, Rosenquist AB, et al. Incidence, complications, and risk factors for prolonged stay in children hospitalized with community-acquired influenza. Pediatrics 2007;119(4):740–8.
9. Ampofo K, Gesteland PH, Bender J, et al. Epidemiology, complications, and cost of hospitalization in children with laboratory-confirmed influenza infection. Pediatrics 2006;118(6):2409–17.
10. Dawood FS, Chaves SS, Perez A, et al. Complications and associated bacterial coinfections among children hospitalized with seasonal or pandemic influenza, United States, 2003-2010. J Infect Dis 2014;209(5):686–94.
11. Ampofo K, Herbener A, Blaschke AJ, et al. Association of 2009 pandemic influenza A (H1N1) infection and increased hospitalization with parapneumonic empyema in children in Utah. Pediatr Infect Dis J 2010;29(10):905–9.
12. Yildizdas D, Kendirli T, Arslankoylu AE, et al. Neurological complications of pandemic influenza (H1N1) in children. Eur J Pediatr 2011;170(6):779–88.
13. Centers for Disease Control and Prevention. Surveillance for pediatric deaths associated with 2009 pandemic influenza A (H1N1) virus infection - United States, April-August 2009. MMWR Morb Mortal Wkly Rep 2009;58(34):941–7.
14. Keren R, Zaoutis TE, Bridges CB, et al. Neurological and neuromuscular disease as a risk factor for respiratory failure in children hospitalized with influenza infection. JAMA 2005;294(17):2188–94.

15. Gill PJ, Ashdown HF, Wang K, et al. Identification of children at risk of influenza-related complications in primary and ambulatory care: a systematic review and meta-analysis. Lancet Respir Med 2015;3(2):139–49.
16. Dharan NJ, Sokolow LZ, Cheng PY, et al. Child, household, and caregiver characteristics associated with hospitalization for influenza among children 6-59 months of age: an emerging infections program study. Pediatr Infect Dis J 2014;33(6):e141–50.
17. Bhat N, Wright JG, Broder KR, et al. Influenza-associated deaths among children in the United States, 2003-2004. N Engl J Med 2005;353(24):2559–67.
18. Burney LE. Influenza immunization: statement. Public Health Rep 1960;75(10):944.
19. Bridges CB, Winquist AG, Fukuda K, et al. Prevention and control of influenza: recommendations of the Advisory Committee on Immunization Practices (ACIP). MMWR Recomm Rep 2000;49(RR-3):1–38 [quiz: CE31–37].
20. Bridges CB, Fukuda K, Uyeki TM, et al. Prevention and control of influenza. Recommendations of the Advisory Committee on Immunization Practices (ACIP). MMWR Recomm Rep 2002;51(RR-3):1–31.
21. Harper SA, Fukuda K, Uyeki TM, et al. Prevention and control of influenza: recommendations of the Advisory Committee on Immunization Practices (ACIP). MMWR Recomm Rep 2004;53(RR-6):1–40.
22. American Academy of Pediatrics Committee on Infectious Diseases. Recommendations for influenza immunization of children. Pediatrics 2004;113(5):1441–7.
23. Advisory Committee on Immunization Practices, Smith NM, Bresee JS, et al. Prevention and Control of Influenza: recommendations of the Advisory Committee on Immunization Practices (ACIP). MMWR Recomm Rep 2006;55(RR-10):1–42.
24. Ilyushina NA, Haynes BC, Hoen AG, et al. Live attenuated and inactivated influenza vaccines in children. J Infect Dis 2015;211(3):352–60.
25. Couch RB, Kasel JA. Immunity to influenza in man. Annu Rev Microbiol 1983;37:529–49.
26. Hoft DF, Babusis E, Worku S, et al. Live and inactivated influenza vaccines induce similar humoral responses, but only live vaccines induce diverse T-cell responses in young children. J Infect Dis 2011;204(6):845–53.
27. Wright PF, Hoen AG, Ilyushina NA, et al. Correlates of immunity to influenza as determined by challenge of children with live, attenuated influenza vaccine. Open Forum Infect Dis 2016;3(2):ofw108.
28. Wright PF, Cherry JD, Foy HM, et al. Antigenicity and reactogenicity of influenza A/USSR/77 virus vaccine in children–a multicentered evaluation of dosage and safety. Rev Infect Dis 1983;5(4):758–64.
29. Daubeney P, Taylor CJ, McGaw J, et al. Immunogenicity and tolerability of a trivalent influenza subunit vaccine (Influvac) in high-risk children aged 6 months to 4 years. Br J Clin Pract 1997;51(2):87–90.
30. Gonzalez M, Pirez MC, Ward E, et al. Safety and immunogenicity of a paediatric presentation of an influenza vaccine. Arch Dis Child 2000;83(6):488–91.
31. Neuzil KM, Jackson LA, Nelson J, et al. Immunogenicity and reactogenicity of 1 versus 2 doses of trivalent inactivated influenza vaccine in vaccine-naive 5-8-year-old children. J Infect Dis 2006;194(8):1032–9.
32. Ritzwoller DP, Bridges CB, Shetterly S, et al. Effectiveness of the 2003-2004 influenza vaccine among children 6 months to 8 years of age, with 1 vs 2 doses. Pediatrics 2005;116(1):153–9.
33. Eisenberg KW, Szilagyi PG, Fairbrother G, et al. Vaccine effectiveness against laboratory-confirmed influenza in children 6 to 59 months of age during the 2003-2004 and 2004-2005 influenza seasons. Pediatrics 2008;122(5):911–9.

34. Grohskopf LA, Sokolow LZ, Broder KR, et al. Prevention and control of seasonal influenza with vaccines: recommendations of the advisory committee on immunization practices - United States, 2017-18 influenza season. MMWR Recomm Rep 2017;66(2):1–20.

35. Lafond KE, Englund JA, Tam JS, et al. Overview of influenza vaccines in children. J Pediatr Infect Dis Soc 2013;2(4):368–78.

36. Belongia EA, Simpson MD, King JP, et al. Variable influenza vaccine effectiveness by subtype: a systematic review and meta-analysis of test-negative design studies. Lancet Infect Dis 2016;16(8):942–51.

37. Ferdinands JM, Olsho LE, Agan AA, et al. Effectiveness of influenza vaccine against life-threatening RT-PCR-confirmed influenza illness in US children, 2010-2012. J Infect Dis 2014;210(5):674–83.

38. Flannery B, Reynolds SB, Blanton L, et al. Influenza vaccine effectiveness against pediatric deaths: 2010-2014. Pediatrics 2017;139(5):e20164244.

39. Ambrose CS, Levin MJ. The rationale for quadrivalent influenza vaccines. Hum Vaccin Immunother 2012;8(1):81–8.

40. McCullers JA, Saito T, Iverson AR. Multiple genotypes of influenza B virus circulated between 1979 and 2003. J Virol 2004;78(23):12817–28.

41. Rota PA, Wallis TR, Harmon MW, et al. Cocirculation of two distinct evolutionary lineages of influenza type B virus since 1983. Virology 1990;175(1):59–68.

42. Wright PF, Thompson J, Vaughn WK, et al. Trials of influenza A/New Jersey/76 virus vaccine in normal children: an overview of age-related antigenicity and reactogenicity. J Infect Dis 1977;136(Suppl):S731–41.

43. Wright PF, Dolin R, La Montagne JR. From the National Institute of Allergy and Infectious Diseases of the National Institutes of Health, the Centers for Disease Control, and the Bureau of Biologics of the Food and Drug Administration. Summary of clinical trials of influenza vaccines–II. J Infect Dis 1976;134(6):633–8.

44. Wright PF, Sell SH, Thompson J, et al. Clinical reactions and serologic response following inactivated monovalent influenza type B vaccine in young children and infants. J Pediatr 1976;88(1):31–5.

45. Halasa NB, Gerber MA, Berry AA, et al. Safety and immunogenicity of full-dose trivalent inactivated influenza vaccine (TIV) compared with half-dose TIV administered to children 6 through 35 months of age. J Pediatr Infect Dis Soc 2015; 4(3):214–24.

46. Jain VK, Domachowske JB, Wang L, et al. Time to change dosing of inactivated quadrivalent influenza vaccine in young children: evidence from a phase III, randomized, controlled trial. J Pediatr Infect Dis Soc 2017;6(1):9–19.

47. Ambrose CS, Levin MJ, Belshe RB. The relative efficacy of trivalent live attenuated and inactivated influenza vaccines in children and adults. Influenza Other Respir Viruses 2011;5(2):67–75.

48. Ashkenazi S, Vertruyen A, Aristegui J, et al. Superior relative efficacy of live attenuated influenza vaccine compared with inactivated influenza vaccine in young children with recurrent respiratory tract infections. Pediatr Infect Dis J 2006;25(10):870–9.

49. Belshe RB, Edwards KM, Vesikari T, et al. Live attenuated versus inactivated influenza vaccine in infants and young children. N Engl J Med 2007;356(7): 685–96.

50. Fleming DM, Crovari P, Wahn U, et al. Comparison of the efficacy and safety of live attenuated cold-adapted influenza vaccine, trivalent, with trivalent inactivated influenza virus vaccine in children and adolescents with asthma. Pediatr Infect Dis J 2006;25(10):860–9.

51. Grohskopf LA, Olsen SJ, Sokolow LZ, et al. Prevention and control of seasonal influenza with vaccines: recommendations of the Advisory Committee on Immunization Practices (ACIP) – United States, 2014-15 influenza season. MMWR Morb Mortal Wkly Rep 2014;63(32):691–7.
52. CDC. Advisory committee on immunization practices (ACIP). Summary report: October 29–30, 2014 (meeting minutes). Atlanta (GA): U.S. Department of Health and Human Services, Centers for Disease Control and Prevention; 2014.
53. Gaglani M, Pruszynski J, Murthy K, et al. Influenza vaccine effectiveness against 2009 pandemic influenza A(H1N1) virus differed by vaccine type during 2013-2014 in the United States. J Infect Dis 2016;213(10):1546–56.
54. Chung JR, Flannery B, Thompson MG, et al. Seasonal effectiveness of live attenuated and inactivated influenza vaccine. Pediatrics 2016;137(2):e20153279.
55. CDC. Advisory committee on immunization practices (ACIP). Summary report: February 26, 2015 (meeting minutes). Atlanta (GA): US Department of Health and Human Services, CDC; 2015.
56. McLean HQ, Caspard H, Griffin MR, et al. Effectiveness of live attenuated influenza vaccine and inactivated influenza vaccine in children during the 2014-2015 season. Vaccine 2017;35(20):2685–93.
57. Zimmerman RK, Nowalk MP, Chung J, et al. 2014-2015 influenza vaccine effectiveness in the United States by vaccine type. Clin Infect Dis 2016;63(12):1564–73.
58. Jackson ML, Chung JR, Jackson LA, et al. Influenza vaccine effectiveness in the United States during the 2015-2016 season. N Engl J Med 2017;377(6):534–43.
59. Advisory Committee on Immunization Practices (ACIP). Summary report: June 22–23, 2016 (meeting minutes). Atlanta (GA): U.S. Department of Helath and Human Services, Centers for Disease Control and Prevention; 2016.
60. Afluria [package insert]. Parkville, Victoria, Australia: Seqirus; 2017.
61. Fluarix Quadrivalent [package insert]. Research Triangle Park, NC: GlaxoSmithKline; 2017.
62. Flulaval Quadrivalent [package insert]. Quebec City, QC, Canada: IB Biomedical Corporation of Quebec; 2017.
63. Fluzone Quadrivalent [package insert]. Swiftwater, PA: Sanofi Pasteur; 2017.
64. Halsey NA, Talaat KR, Greenbaum A, et al. The safety of influenza vaccines in children: an Institute for Vaccine Safety white paper. Vaccine 2015;33(Suppl 5): F1–67.
65. Barry DW, Mayner RE, Hochstein HD, et al. Comparative trial of influenza vaccines. II. Adverse reactions in children and adults. Am J Epidemiol 1976; 104(1):47–59.
66. Australian Government Department of Health, Therapeutic Goods Administration. Investigation into febrile reactions in young children following 2010 seasonal trivalent influenza vaccination. Woden, Australia: Australian Government Department of Health, Therapeutic Goods Administration; 2010. Available at: https://www.tga.gov.au/alert/seasonal-flu-vaccine-investigation-febrile-reactions-young-children-following-2010-seasonal-trivalent-influenza-vaccination.
67. Airey J, Albano FR, Sawlwin DC, et al. Immunogenicity and safety of a quadrivalent inactivated influenza virus vaccine compared with a comparator quadrivalent inactivated influenza vaccine in a pediatric population: a phase 3, randomized noninferiority study. Vaccine 2017;35(20):2745–52.
68. Leroy Z, Broder K, Menschik D, et al. Febrile seizures after 2010-2011 influenza vaccine in young children, United States: a vaccine safety signal from the vaccine adverse event reporting system. Vaccine 2012;30(11):2020–3.

69. Tse A, Tseng HF, Greene SK, et al. Signal identification and evaluation for risk of febrile seizures in children following trivalent inactivated influenza vaccine in the Vaccine Safety Datalink Project, 2010-2011. Vaccine 2012;30(11):2024–31.
70. Duffy J, Weintraub E, Hambidge SJ, et al. Febrile seizure risk after vaccination in children 6 to 23 months. Pediatrics 2016;138(1) [pii:e20160320].
71. Kawai AT, Martin D, Kulldorff M, et al. Febrile seizures after 2010-2011 trivalent inactivated influenza vaccine. Pediatrics 2015;136(4):e848–55.
72. Li R, Stewart B, McNeil MM, et al. Post licensure surveillance of influenza vaccines in the vaccine safety datalink in the 2013-2014 and 2014-2015 seasons. Pharmacoepidemiol Drug Saf 2016;25(8):928–34.
73. Yih WK, Kulldorff M, Sandhu SK, et al. Prospective influenza vaccine safety surveillance using fresh data in the Sentinel system. Pharmacoepidemiol Drug Saf 2016;25(5):481–92.
74. Wijnans L, Lecomte C, de Vries C, et al. The incidence of narcolepsy in Europe: before, during, and after the influenza A(H1N1)pdm09 pandemic and vaccination campaigns. Vaccine 2013;31(8):1246–54.
75. Izurieta HS, Haber P, Wise RP, et al. Adverse events reported following live, cold-adapted, intranasal influenza vaccine. JAMA 2005;294(21):2720–5.
76. Haber P, Moro PL, Cano M, et al. Post-licensure surveillance of quadrivalent live attenuated influenza vaccine United States, Vaccine Adverse Event Reporting System (VAERS), July 2013-June 2014. Vaccine 2015;33(16):1987–92.
77. Belshe RB, Ambrose CS, Yi T. Safety and efficacy of live attenuated influenza vaccine in children 2-7 years of age. Vaccine 2008;26(Suppl 4):D10–6.
78. Piedra PA, Yan L, Kotloff K, et al. Safety of the trivalent, cold-adapted influenza vaccine in preschool-aged children. Pediatrics 2002;110(4):662–72.
79. Redding G, Walker RE, Hessel C, et al. Safety and tolerability of cold-adapted influenza virus vaccine in children and adolescents with asthma. Pediatr Infect Dis J 2002;21(1):44–8.
80. Block SL, Yogev R, Hayden FG, et al. Shedding and immunogenicity of live attenuated influenza vaccine virus in subjects 5-49 years of age. Vaccine 2008;26(38):4940–6.
81. Vesikari T, Karvonen A, Korhonen T, et al. CAIV-T Transmission Study Group. A randomized, double-blind study of the safety, transmissibility and phenotypic and genotypic stability of cold-adapted influenza virus vaccine. Pediatr Infect Dis J 2006;25:590–5.
82. Pearson ML, Bridges CB, Harper SA, Healthcare Infection Control Practices Advisory Committee (HICPAC), Advisory Committee on Immunization Practices (ACIP). Influenza vaccination of health-care personnel: recommendations of the Healthcare Infection Control Practices Advisory Committee (HICPAC) and the Advisory Committee on Immunization Practices (ACIP). MMWR Recomm Rep 2006;55(RR-2):1–16.
83. Rubin LG, Levin MJ, Ljungman P, et al. 2013 IDSA clinical practice guideline for vaccination of the immunocompromised host. Clin Infect Dis 2014;58(3):e44–100.
84. Nachbagauer R, Krammer F. Universal influenza virus vaccines and therapeutic antibodies. Clin Microbiol Infect 2017;23(4):222–8.
85. Wong SS, Webby RJ. Traditional and new influenza vaccines. Clin Microbiol Rev 2013;26(3):476–92.
86. Nair H, Lau E, Brooks W, et al. An evaluation of the emerging vaccines against influenza in children. BMC Public Health 2013;13(Suppl 3):S14.
87. Vesikari T, Knuf M, Wutzler P, et al. Oil-in-water emulsion adjuvant with influenza vaccine in young children. N Engl J Med 2011;365(15):1406–16.

88. Vesikari T, Forsten A, Arora A, et al. Influenza vaccination in children primed with MF59-adjuvanted or non-adjuvanted seasonal influenza vaccine. Hum Vaccin Immunother 2015;11(8):2102–12.
89. Fluad [package insert]. Holly Springs, NC: Seqirus; 2017.
90. Fluzone High-Dose [package insert]. Swiftwater, PA: Sanofi Pasteur; 2017.
91. Fluzone Intradermal Quadrivalent [package insert]. Swiftwater, PA: Sanofi Pasteur; 2017.
92. Flublok [package insert]. Meriden, CT: Protein Sciences; 2017.
93. Flublok Quadrivalent [package insert]. Meriden, CT: Protein Sciences; 2017.
94. Pillet S, Aubin E, Trepanier S, et al. A plant-derived quadrivalent virus like particle influenza vaccine induces cross-reactive antibody and T cell response in healthy adults. Clin Immunol 2016;168:72–87.
95. Fiore AE, Fry A, Shay D, et al. Antiviral agents for the treatment and chemoprophylaxis of influenza -- recommendations of the Advisory Committee on Immunization Practices (ACIP). MMWR Recomm Rep 2011;60(1):1–24.
96. Coffin SE, Leckerman K, Keren R, et al. Oseltamivir shortens hospital stays of critically ill children hospitalized with seasonal influenza: a retrospective cohort study. Pediatr Infect Dis J 2011;30(11):962–6.
97. Louie JK, Yang S, Samuel MC, et al. Neuraminidase inhibitors for critically ill children with influenza. Pediatrics 2013;132(6):e1539–45.
98. Appiah GD, Chaves SS, Kirley PD, et al. Increased antiviral treatment among hospitalized children and adults with laboratory-confirmed influenza, 2010-2015. Clin Infect Dis 2017;64(3):364–7.
99. Havers F, Flannery B, Clippard JR, et al. Use of influenza antiviral medications among outpatients at high risk for influenza-associated complications during the 2013-2014 influenza season. Clin Infect Dis 2015;60(11):1677–80.
100. Neuzil KM, Hohlbein C, Zhu Y. Illness among schoolchildren during influenza season: effect on school absenteeism, parental absenteeism from work, and secondary illness in families. Arch Pediatr Adolesc Med 2002;156(10):986–91.

Pediatric Considerations for Postexposure Human Immunodeficiency Virus Prophylaxis

William J. Muller, MD, PhD*, Ellen G. Chadwick, MD

KEYWORDS

- Human immunodeficiency virus • Postexposure prophylaxis
- Blood-borne infections • Needlestick • Antivirals

KEY POINTS

- Recent Centers for Disease Control and Prevention guidelines for nonoccupational postexposure HIV prophylaxis (nPEP) include updated antiretroviral recommendations, recommendations for not initiating nPEP if the exposure was more than 72 hours earlier, and specific testing indicated for the exposed patient.
- Data supporting nPEP recommendations are expert opinion based on animal studies and case series in humans, because randomized trials are not feasible.
- Pediatric considerations include availability of antiretrovirals (ARV) in appropriate dose forms and drug formulations, which influence adherence to the nPEP regimen.

INTRODUCTION

Exposures to blood and body fluids confer a risk of transmission for blood-borne diseases, including human immunodeficiency virus (HIV), prompting a need for evidence-based recommendations to minimize the risk of acquisition of this infection in certain situations. Initial suggestions that antiretroviral (ARV) treatment could prevent transmission of HIV after sexual, intravenous (IV) drug use, or other nonoccupational exposure[1,2] were extrapolated from recommendations made for occupational exposure to HIV, which were themselves influenced by a retrospective case-control study demonstrating that health care workers with a documented percutaneous

Potential/Perceived Conflicts of Interest: None.
Statement of Financial Support: No financial assistance was received to support this study.
Division of Pediatric Infectious Diseases, Northwestern University Feinberg School of Medicine, Ann & Robert H. Lurie Children's Hospital of Chicago, 225 E. Chicago Avenue, Box 20, Chicago, IL 60611, USA
* Corresponding author. Department of Pediatrics, Northwestern University, 320 East Superior Street, Morton 4-685, Chicago, IL 60611.
E-mail address: wjmuller@northwestern.edu

Infect Dis Clin N Am 32 (2018) 91–101
https://doi.org/10.1016/j.idc.2017.10.006
0891-5520/18/© 2017 Elsevier Inc. All rights reserved.

id.theclinics.com

exposure to HIV-infected blood had a significantly reduced risk of HIV seroconversion associated with the exposure when they received zidovudine after the exposure.[3]

Although many practitioners offered nonoccupational postexposure prophylaxis (nPEP) to individuals with high-risk exposures, the number of unanswered questions regarding efficacy, toxicity, and other risks (eg, development of resistance, behavior changes, and cost)[4] delayed any official US recommendations for nPEP until 2005.[5] At that time the US Department of Health and Human Services Working Group on Nonoccupational Postexposure Prophylaxis recommended the following:

- A 28-day course of highly active ARV therapy for individuals with nonoccupational exposures to blood, genital secretions, or other potentially infected body fluids from an HIV-infected person, when the exposure occurred within 72 hours of starting ARVs;
- A case-by-case evaluation of the risks and benefits of highly active ARV therapy in individuals with similar nonoccupational exposures, when the HIV status of the source individual was unknown but the exposure represented a substantial potential risk for transmission;
- If the exposure did not represent a substantial potential risk for transmission or if the exposure was more than 72 hours before presentation, no ARVs were recommended;
- However, ARVs could be considered, weighing risks and benefits, if the exposure was more than 72 hours from the time of starting ARVs but represented a serious risk for transmission.

The preferred ARV nPEP regimen in the 2005 guidelines was either efavirenz plus (lamivudine or emtricitabine) plus (zidovudine or tenofovir), or lopinavir/ritonavir plus (lamivudine or emtricitabine) plus zidovudine.

The Department of Health and Human Services guidelines for nPEP were updated in 2016.[6] The changes in recommendations with this update included the following:

- Specifying that individuals being considered for nPEP be tested for HIV, preferably by a rapid test;
- nPEP in individuals with exposure more than 72 hours before presentation was specifically not recommended;
- Specific recommendations for additional testing and treatment that would be indicated based on the details of the exposure, and for counseling or intervention services in individuals at risk for frequently recurring HIV exposure, including consideration of pre-exposure prophylaxis (PrEP).

The 2016 guidelines also updated the preferred ARV regimen for healthy adults and adolescents to include tenofovir with emtricitabine plus raltegravir, or tenofovir with emtricitabine plus darunavir/ritonavir.

This article discusses some of the evidence informing the 2005 and 2016 guidelines for nPEP, with a specific focus on the pediatric population. In addition, possibilities for future interventions are presented.

EVIDENCE SUPPORTING THE RECOMMENDATIONS OF THE 2016 NONOCCUPATIONAL POSTEXPOSURE PROPHYLAXIS GUIDELINES
Data Supporting the Use of a 28-Day Course

The choice of 28-day nPEP treatment duration is largely based on studies in animal models and evidence of clinical efficacy from case series of patients. Macaque models using simian immunodeficiency virus (SIV) challenge have provided useful data demonstrating proof of principle for different PEP regimens.[7,8] For example, when a 28-day course of subcutaneous tenofovir was initiated either before, 4 hours after, or 24 hours after IV inoculation of macaques with SIV, no treated animals became infected, whereas 10 of 10 control animals who did not receive drug were infected.[7] Follow-up studies using a similar macaque model found that shorter treatment courses were less effective at preventing infection; when tenofovir was started 24 hours after IV inoculation of SIV, only half of animals treated for 10 days, and none of those treated for 3 days, were protected from infection.[8] Subcutaneous tenofovir started within 36 hours of inoculation and continued for 28 days has also been shown to protect macaques from SIV infection after intravaginal inoculation.[9] A systematic review and meta-analysis of 25 primate studies (macaques or cynomolgus monkeys) concluded that the risk of seroconversion of animals challenged with HIV or SIV was 89% lower in animals given PEP than control animals.[10]

Animal studies allow for control of conditions surrounding inoculation and antiviral dosing, and provide important insights into the potential benefits and limitations of nPEP. However, there are obvious limitations surrounding the extent to which animal models are directly applicable to humans. Importantly, observational studies and case reports in humans support the recommendation for continuing nPEP for a 28-day course. Among men who have sex with men, an estimated combined seroconversion rate of about 31 of 1000 persons who became infected with HIV despite nPEP has been reported; however, additional analysis suggested that many of these seroconversions may have been attributable to ongoing risk behavior after completion of nPEP.[6] In studies involving child and adolescent survivors of sexual assault, a pooled analysis of 10 studies identified no HIV infections in 472 individuals who initiated nPEP, although it was noted that return rates for these patients varied widely and that incident infections may have been underestimated.[6] A similar pooled analysis of studies involving patients who received nPEP for a variety of exposure indications identified only 1 of 2209 participants in whom seroconversion was attributed to failure of nPEP, with seroconversion in 18 other patients associated with additional high-risk exposures and/or poor adherence to nPEP.[6] Additionally, an analysis of combined reports involving 438 individuals, mostly children, who were exposed to sharps injuries, with unknown HIV status of the source individual in all but one report, found no HIV seroconversions among either the 149 individuals who accepted nPEP (not all of whom completed the regimen), or the six individuals who did not receive nPEP.[6] Taken together, the implications of these multiple analyses provide support for the rationale and efficacy of the recommended 28-day nPEP course.

Starting Nonoccupational Postexposure Prophylaxis Within 72 Hours of Exposure

In addition to providing evidence supporting the 28-day duration of nPEP treatment, animal models have also been informative for evaluating the time for initiating nPEP to optimize efficacy. Macaques treated daily with tenofovir for 28 days starting 24 hours after IV inoculation with SIV were protected from infection, whereas animals who started tenofovir 48 or 72 hours after similar SIV inoculation had evidence of infection.[8] In the intravaginal SIV inoculation model, macaques who received subcutaneous tenofovir starting by 36 hours of inoculation had no evidence of systemic infection, whereas some animals in the group starting tenofovir 72 hours after inoculation had systemic infection.[9] The previously cited meta-analysis of PEP studies in primate models also found a strong association between the timing of PEP initiation and seroconversion, supporting the importance of starting nPEP as early after exposure as possible.[10]

Data in humans also support that delaying the start of nPEP increases the risk of seroconversion. A case series of 776 patients receiving nPEP reported only one case of an individual seroconverting after completing a 28-day nPEP course; that course was started more than 72 hours after a high-risk exposure.[11]

Which Exposures Constitute a Substantial (or Serious) Risk for Transmission?

Although starting effective nPEP within the 72-hour window is clearly an important aspect of patient management, understanding which exposures constitute a signifi-cant enough risk of HIV acquisition to offer nPEP, and which do not, is critical to maxi-mizing the benefits of treatment while minimizing the risks of unnecessary exposure to ARVs. The initial information to establish is whether the exposed person is HIV-infected, and whether the source is known to be HIV-infected.[6] Testing of the exposed person is discussed in more detail in the next section, but an individual found to have HIV infection through baseline testing should be referred for HIV care rather than nPEP. Knowledge of the status of the source, along with the nature of the exposure, helps determine whether nPEP is or is not clearly recommended.

Per-act risk of acquisition of HIV from an infected source has been estimated for different exposure types (**Table 1**).[12,13] Among exposures for which nPEP is often rec-ommended in pediatric patients, needlestick injuries and condomless sexual expo-sure, specifically anal intercourse or penile-vaginal intercourse, confer the highest risks of transmission.[12] Importantly, biting or spitting are considered to have negligible risk of transmission.[14] However, a bite from an HIV-positive source that breaks the skin, is associated with a site of prior skin injury, or in which there is blood in the mouth of the source, has at least a theoretic but still low risk of transmission.[13,15–17] Recom-mendations for nPEP in such cases should be handled on a case-by-case basis.

Risks from needlestick or other sharps exposures where the status of the source is unknown represent another fairly common situation in which nPEP is considered in pediatrics, often involving injuries sustained in public places, such as parks. Small-bore needles have not been documented to result in HIV transmission,[6] and HIV is not thought to survive for long in discarded syringes.[18] However, as with human

Table 1 Risk of acquisition of HIV from an infected source, based on type of exposure	
Exposure	**Risk of Acquiring HIV, per 10,000 Exposures**
Blood transfusion	9250
Needle-sharing intravenous drug use	63
Percutaneous needlestick	23
Receptive anal intercourse	138
Insertive anal intercourse	11
Receptive penile-vaginal intercourse	8
Insertive penile-vaginal intercourse	4
Receptive oral sex	<2
Insertive oral sex	<2
Mother-to-child transmission without ARV use	2260
Human bite	Technically possible but unlikely

Data from Patel P, Borkowf CB, Brooks JT, et al. Estimating per-act HIV transmission risk: a system-atic review. AIDS 2014;28(10):1509–19; and Pretty IA, Anderson GS, Sweet DJ. Human bites and the risk of human immunodeficiency virus transmission. Am J Forensic Med Pathol 1999;20(3):232–9.

bite wounds, the risk of transmission cannot be considered to be absent, and recommendations for nPEP in these situations should be handled on a case-by-case basis.

Specific Recommendations for Human Immunodeficiency Virus Testing of Individuals Being Considered for Nonoccupational Postexposure Prophylaxis

Establishing the HIV status of the exposed individual is important, because the initial management of a newly HIV-positive person differs from management of patients offered nPEP. Because nPEP must be started on a timely basis, testing results must be available quickly. In the years following publication of the initial nPEP guidelines,[5] rapid testing has become more accurate and more widely available, allowing it to be incorporated into the more recent guidelines,[6] which recommend rapid combined antigen/antibody (Ag/Ab) testing or antibody blood tests for these patients. Results from these tests should be available within an hour; if results are not available during the initial evaluation and nPEP would be indicated if the patient were not previously infected, it should be started, and discontinued later if the patient is subsequently found to have been previously infected.[6]

There are several Food and Drug Administration–approved combined Ag/Ab tests with excellent sensitivity in early HIV infection. These immunoassays detect antibodies and the HIV p24 antigen to maximize sensitivity and specificity. HIV-specific IgM and IgG are detected using recombinant protein and peptide antigens, whereas p24 protein is detected using monoclonal anti-p24 antibodies[19]; the final detection step is the same for both reactions.[20] The advantage of this approach is that it can rapidly detect acute infection, even in the window before generation of a humoral response against HIV.[21] Positive tests are followed by immunoassays to determine HIV-1 versus HIV-2 serology, which may in turn be followed by nucleic acid testing.[21]

If combined Ag/Ab testing is not available, a rapid antibody test may be used in the initial evaluation of an exposed patient. These tests use similar methodology, but do not detect p24 antigen and are therefore less sensitive for early HIV infection as the combined assays, because they may be negative in the window before seroconversion.[19]

Recommendations for Additional Treatment, Testing, Counseling

Additional testing in patients at the time they are offered nPEP is also recommended, to screen for other infections associated with similar exposure risk and to obtain baseline creatinine and liver enzyme levels before ARV exposure.[6] Follow-up testing for HIV, hepatitis B virus, or hepatitis C virus seroconversion, sexually transmitted infections, and ARV toxicity at different time points is also recommended, depending on the exposure.

It is important to recognize that families and patients who need evaluation for possible acquisition of HIV or other infectious diseases through sexual assault or needlestick injury are experiencing a great deal of stress,[22] which may be magnified in the pediatric setting. In addition to proper testing, treatment, and medical referrals in these situations, referral for appropriate family and mental health counseling services is an important component of the acute care for these patients.

Recommendations for Pre-exposure Prophylaxis

Some adolescents who seek nPEP after high-risk sexual behavior or IV drug use could be candidates for PrEP. Initiation of PrEP requires documentation of a negative HIV status and completion of the nPEP course. Most patients for whom PrEP is indicated take a fixed-dose combination of tenofovir and emtricitabine once daily.[23] Referral to an experienced pediatric HIV provider is recommended for patients for whom PrEP is being considered.

Efficacy of Current First-Line Regimens

Recommendations for ARV regimens in nPEP are based largely on expert opinion; there are no randomized trials to inform treatment choices. Current recommendations in otherwise healthy adult and adolescent patients (**Table 2**) include the combination of tenofovir and emtricitabine, plus either an integrase strand transfer inhibitor (raltegravir or dolutegravir; preferred regimen) or the ritonavir-boosted protease

Table 2
Preferred regimens for nPEP

Drug	Dose	Most Common Side Effects
Preferred regimen for otherwise healthy adults, adolescents, and children weighing >35 kg		
Tenofovir disoproxil fumarate[a] AND	300 mg once daily	Weakness/lack of energy, headache, diarrhea, nausea, vomiting
Emtricitabine[a] AND	200 mg once daily	Hyperpigmented rash or skin discoloration
Raltegravir OR	400 mg twice daily	Insomnia, nausea, fatigue, headache
Dolutegravir	50 mg daily	Insomnia, headache
Preferred regimen for otherwise healthy children ages 2–12 y, weighing <35 kg		
Zidovudine AND	Syrup or capsules 4 to <9 kg: 12 mg/kg twice daily 9 to <30 kg: 9 mg/kg twice daily Tablet ≥30 kg: 300-mg tablet twice daily	Nausea, vomiting, headache, insomnia, and fatigue
Lamivudine AND	Oral solution 4 mg/kg (up to 150 mg) twice daily Scored 150-mg tablet 14 to <20 kg: one-half tablet twice daily 20 to <25 kg: one-half tablet in AM + 1 tablet in PM ≥25 kg: 1 tablet twice daily	Headache, nausea, malaise and fatigue, nasal signs and symptoms, diarrhea, and cough
Raltegravir[b]	Ages 6–12 y and weighing >25 kg 400-mg tablet twice daily OR Ages 2–12, chewable tablets dosed by weight 11 to <14 kg: 75 mg twice daily 14 to <20 kg: 100 mg twice daily 20 to <28 kg: 150 mg twice daily 28 to <40 kg: 200 mg twice daily ≥40 kg: 300 mg twice daily	Insomnia, nausea, fatigue, headache

Alternate regimens are also available, as are recommendations in cases where there is decreased renal function or in pregnancy.

[a] Usually given as a fixed-dose combination pill (Truvada).

[b] May be given as chewable tablet or suspension.

From Centers for Disease Control and Prevention. Updated guidelines for antiretroviral postexposure prophylaxis after sexual, injection drug use, or other nonoccupational exposure to HIV—United States, 2016. U.S. Department of Health and Human Services; 2016.

inhibitor darunavir (alternative regimen). Tenofovir-containing regimens are chosen in part because of an association with fewer side effects and higher nPEP completion rates,[24-27] discussed further in the next section. The addition of an integrase strand transfer inhibitor or boosted darunavir to the combination of tenofovir and emtricitabine mimics the preferred initial regimens in antiretroviral therapy–naive patients with newly diagnosed HIV infection.[28] The recommendations for initial ARV regimens are based on clinical trial data, which generally demonstrate no significant differences in HIV-related clinical end points or survival when comparing different initial treatment regimens.[28]

Recommendations for nPEP in younger children are similar to those in adult and adolescent patients and are based on expert opinion. Children who weigh more than 35 kg and are able to swallow tablets may be offered the combination pill containing tenofovir disoproxil fumarate and emtricitabine (Truvada) in combination with raltegravir. The availability of chewable tablet and oral suspension formulations of raltegravir allows this drug to also be used in younger patients less than 35 kg body weight, generally given in combination with liquid suspensions of zidovudine and lamivudine.[6]

SPECIAL SITUATIONS IN PEDIATRIC PATIENTS
Choice of Antiretroviral Regimens for Nonoccupational Postexposure Prophylaxis

In addition to efficacy of the ARV regimen against HIV, considerations for optimal adherence to nPEP are similar to those used in determining initial treatment regimens for newly infected patients. These include minimizing adverse effects of the drugs and decreasing the drug burden for the patient, in terms of the size of an individual dose (number of pills or volume of liquid) and the number of times per day drugs need to be taken. Studies comparing adherence to different nPEP regimens have noted that patients receiving regimens containing tenofovir, when compared with patients receiving regimens containing zidovudine, report fewer side effects and are more likely to complete the course.[24,25] As with zidovudine, protease inhibitor-containing regimens have also been associated with patient intolerance leading to discontinuation, when compared with regimens containing tenofovir in combination with lamivudine and stavudine.[29] Tenofovir in combination with raltegravir and lamivudine has similarly been associated with good adherence and fewer concerns for side effects, including drug interactions, than regimens containing a protease inhibitor.[30,31]

In pediatric patients, the availability of correct dosage forms, including liquid formulations in patients unable to swallow pills, and pills with an appropriate amount of drug based on a patient's size, are also important influences on the choice of an nPEP regimen. For liquid medications, the taste of the formulation impacts adherence[32]; palatability is a particular problem for liquid preparations of protease inhibitors.[33] In addition, liquid ARVs are not generally stocked in local pharmacies, so considering the importance of prompt initiation of nPEP, it is optimal to provide a 3-day supply of drugs at the time of the initial visit to allow time for the patient or caregiver to obtain a 1-month prescription.

Adherence to Nonoccupational Postexposure Prophylaxis and Follow-up in Children, Adolescents, and Young Adults

Adherence to nPEP ARV regimens and follow-up visits after starting nPEP have been repeatedly poor across numerous studies in different populations. Meta-analyses consistently find completion rates of less than 50% in nPEP studies involving victims of sexual assault,[34,35] compared with higher completion rates of about two-thirds of patients with other reasons for nPEP.[35] Completion rates seem to be higher in studies in resource-constrained countries compared with developed countries.[34] Most studies considered in these meta-analyses involved adults, although the results were similar in studies involving children and adolescent nPEP patients.[35–39]

LOOKING AHEAD: ARE THERE DEVELOPMENTS THAT MIGHT INFLUENCE NONOCCUPATIONAL POSTEXPOSURE PROPHYLAXIS RECOMMENDATIONS?

The challenges in adherence and follow-up of nPEP patients mirror similar issues with adherence in some HIV-positive patients and some patients on PrEP. Recent efforts to address these challenges have included development of longer acting ARVs, which are currently under study for treatment of HIV-positive patients and for PrEP.[40] If efficacy, safety, and tolerability are demonstrated for these indications, it is plausible that there may be a role for these interventions in nPEP.

The long-acting ARV that has advanced furthest in clinical trials is a nanoformulation of the integrase strand transfer inhibitor cabotegravir. An injectable depot form of this drug has an elimination half-life of more than 25 days, with plasma levels after a single 800-mg intramuscular (IM) injection achieving and maintaining therapeutic levels for many weeks.[41] A phase 2a study (HPTN 077) recently demonstrated safety and tolerability of a 600-mg IM dose in uninfected adults,[42] providing supporting data for trials of this formulation as PrEP (HPTN 083 and HPTN 084). A phase 2b open-label study of long-acting cabotegravir and rilpivirine used in combination in HIV-infected adults supported good tolerability and preliminary evidence of efficacy.[43]

If additional medications can be formulated as long-acting ARVs that may provide sufficient drug concentrations during a 28-day period, it is plausible that a future combination could provide effective nPEP as a single IM dose. In addition to cabotegravir and rilpivirine, drugs being tested in such formulations include the nucleoside reverse transcriptase inhibitor emtricitabine,[44] the novel nucleoside reverse transcriptase inhibitor 4'-ethynyl-2-fluoro-2'-deoxyadenosine (MK8591),[41,45] the protease inhibitor ritonavir-boosted atazanavir,[41] the strand transfer inhibitor raltegravir,[41] and the novel entry inhibitor combinectin.[41] Pharmacokinetic considerations suggest that at least some of these formulations can be appropriately dosed in children and adolescents.[46]

Similarly, broadly neutralizing antibodies are under study for treatment of HIV,[47] and early phase studies of their possible utility for preventing maternal-to-child transmission are underway.[48] The long half-life of antibodies might also suggest possible application for nPEP, although cost may be a barrier.

SUMMARY

Recently updated recommendations to Centers for Disease Control and Prevention guidelines for nPEP stress newer generation rapid testing for HIV; initiation of ARVs within 72 hours of exposure; and additional interventions, such as counseling, which are based on the details of the exposure.[6] These guidelines can be applied in the pediatric population, where considerations for the risks and benefits of ARV treatment may differ. Evidence is available to inform the recommendations for initiating treatment within 72 hours and continuing for 28 days, although adherence and follow-up remain problems in all populations studied. New developments in HIV treatment, which allow for significantly less frequent dosing, could eventually have an application for nPEP, although much additional research is needed.

REFERENCES

1. Carpenter CC, Fischl MA, Hammer SM, et al. Antiretroviral therapy for HIV infection in 1996. Recommendations of an international panel. International AIDS Society-USA. JAMA 1996;276(2):146–54.

2. Katz MH, Gerberding JL. Postexposure treatment of people exposed to the human immunodeficiency virus through sexual contact or injection-drug use. N Engl J Med 1997;336(15):1097–100.

3. Centers for Disease Control and Prevention. Case-control study of HIV seroconversion in health-care workers after percutaneous exposure to HIV-infected blood—France, United Kingdom, and United States, January 1988-August 1994. MMWR Morb Mortal Wkly Rep 1995;44(50):929–33.

4. Centers for Disease Control and Prevention. Management of possible sexual, injecting-drug-use, or other nonoccupational exposure to HIV, including considerations related to antiretroviral therapy. Public health service statement. MMWR Recomm Rep 1998;47(RR-17):1–14.

5. Smith DK, Grohskopf LA, Black RJ, et al. Antiretroviral postexposure prophylaxis after sexual, injection-drug use, or other nonoccupational exposure to HIV in the United States: recommendations from the U.S. Department of Health and Human Services. MMWR Recomm Rep 2005;54(RR-2):1–20.

6. Centers for Disease Control and Prevention. Updated guidelines for antiretroviral postexposure prophylaxis after sexual, injection drug use, or other nonoccupational exposure to HIV—United States, 2016. Atlanta (GA): U.S. Department of Health and Human Services; 2016.

7. Tsai CC, Follis KE, Sabo A, et al. Prevention of SIV infection in macaques by (R)-9-(2-phosphonylmethoxypropyl)adenine. Science 1995;270(5239):1197–9.

8. Tsai CC, Emau P, Follis KE, et al. Effectiveness of postinoculation (R)-9-(2-phosphonylmethoxypropyl) adenine treatment for prevention of persistent simian immunodeficiency virus SIVmne infection depends critically on timing of initiation and duration of treatment. J Virol 1998;72(5):4265–73.

9. Otten RA, Smith DK, Adams DR, et al. Efficacy of postexposure prophylaxis after intravaginal exposure of pig-tailed macaques to a human-derived retrovirus (human immunodeficiency virus type 2). J Virol 2000;74(20):9771–5.

10. Irvine C, Egan KJ, Shubber Z, et al. Efficacy of HIV postexposure prophylaxis: systematic review and meta-analysis of nonhuman primate studies. Clin Infect Dis 2015;60(Suppl 3):S165–9.

11. Rey D, Bendiane MK, Bouhnik AD, et al. Physicians' and patients' adherence to antiretroviral prophylaxis after sexual exposure to HIV: results from South-Eastern France. AIDS Care 2008;20(5):537–41.

12. Patel P, Borkowf CB, Brooks JT, et al. Estimating per-act HIV transmission risk: a systematic review. AIDS 2014;28(10):1509–19.

13. Pretty IA, Anderson GS, Sweet DJ. Human bites and the risk of human immunodeficiency virus transmission. Am J Forensic Med Pathol 1999;20(3):232–9.

14. Centers for Disease Control and Prevention. HIV/AIDS > HIV Risk and Prevention > HIV Risk and Prevention Estimates. Available at: https://www.cdc.gov/hiv/risk/estimates/riskbehaviors.html. Accessed June 29, 2017.

15. Richman KM, Rickman LS. The potential for transmission of human immunodeficiency virus through human bites. J Acquir Immune Defic Syndr 1993;6(4):402–6.

16. Deshpande AK, Jadhav SK, Bandivdekar AH. Possible transmission of HIV infection due to human bite. AIDS Res Ther 2011;8:16.

17. Vidmar L, Poljak M, Tomazic J, et al. Transmission of HIV-1 by human bite. Lancet 1996;347(9017):1762.
18. Rich JD, Dickinson BP, Carney JM, et al. Detection of HIV-1 nucleic acid and HIV-1 antibodies in needles and syringes used for non-intravenous injection. AIDS 1998;12(17):2345–50.
19. Centers for Disease Control and Prevention and Association of Public Health Laboratories. Laboratory testing for the diagnosis of HIV infection: updated recommendations. 2014; https://doi.org/10.15620/cdc.23447. Accessed July 5, 2017.
20. Weber B, Fall EH, Berger A, et al. Reduction of diagnostic window by new fourth-generation human immunodeficiency virus screening assays. J Clin Microbiol 1998;36(8):2235–9.
21. Alexander TS. Human immunodeficiency virus diagnostic testing: 30 years of evolution. Clin Vaccine Immunol 2016;23(4):249–53.
22. Gostin LO, Lazzarini Z, Alexander D, et al. HIV testing, counseling, and prophylaxis after sexual assault. JAMA 1994;271(18):1436–44.
23. US Public Health Service. Preexposure prophylaxis for the prevention of HIV infection in the United States–2014. A clinical practice guideline. Atlanta (GA): Department of Health and Human Services; 2014.
24. Mayer KH, Mimiaga MJ, Cohen D, et al. Tenofovir DF plus lamivudine or emtricitabine for nonoccupational postexposure prophylaxis (NPEP) in a Boston Community Health Center. J Acquir Immune Defic Syndr 2008;47(4):494–9.
25. Tosini W, Muller P, Prazuck T, et al. Tolerability of HIV postexposure prophylaxis with tenofovir/emtricitabine and lopinavir/ritonavir tablet formulation. AIDS 2010;24(15):2375–80.
26. Ford N, Shubber Z, Calmy A, et al. Choice of antiretroviral drugs for postexposure prophylaxis for adults and adolescents: a systematic review. Clin Infect Dis 2015;60(Suppl 3):S170–6.
27. Thomas R, Galanakis C, Vezina S, et al. Adherence to post-exposure prophylaxis (PEP) and incidence of HIV seroconversion in a major North American cohort. PLoS One 2015;10(11):e0142534.
28. Panel on Antiretroviral Guidelines for Adults and Adolescents. Guidelines for the use of antiretroviral agents in HIV-1-infected adults and adolescents. Available at: http://aidsinfo.nih.gov/contentfiles/lvguidelines/AdultandAdolescentGL.pdf. Accessed July 19, 2017.
29. Winston A, McAllister J, Amin J, et al. The use of a triple nucleoside-nucleotide regimen for nonoccupational HIV post-exposure prophylaxis. HIV Med 2005;6(3):191–7.
30. McAllister J, Read P, McNulty A, et al. Raltegravir-emtricitabine-tenofovir as HIV nonoccupational post-exposure prophylaxis in men who have sex with men: safety, tolerability and adherence. HIV Med 2014;15(1):13–22.
31. Mayer KH, Mimiaga MJ, Gelman M, et al. Raltegravir, tenofovir DF, and emtricitabine for postexposure prophylaxis to prevent the sexual transmission of HIV: safety, tolerability, and adherence. J Acquir Immune Defic Syndr 2012;59(4):354–9.
32. Lin D, Seabrook JA, Matsui DM, et al. Palatability, adherence and prescribing patterns of antiretroviral drugs for children with human immunodeficiency virus infection in Canada. Pharmacoepidemiol Drug Saf 2011;20(12):1246–52.
33. Chadwick EG, Rodman JH, Britto P, et al. Ritonavir-based highly active antiretroviral therapy in human immunodeficiency virus type 1-infected infants younger than 24 months of age. Pediatr Infect Dis J 2005;24(9):793–800.

34. Chacko L, Ford N, Sbaiti M, et al. Adherence to HIV post-exposure prophylaxis in victims of sexual assault: a systematic review and meta-analysis. Sex Transm Infect 2012;88(5):335–41.
35. Ford N, Irvine C, Shubber Z, et al. Adherence to HIV postexposure prophylaxis: a systematic review and meta-analysis. AIDS 2014;28(18):2721–7.
36. Olshen E, Hsu K, Woods ER, et al. Use of human immunodeficiency virus post-exposure prophylaxis in adolescent sexual assault victims. Arch Pediatr Adolesc Med 2006;160(7):674–80.
37. Du Mont J, Myhr TL, Husson H, et al. HIV postexposure prophylaxis use among Ontario female adolescent sexual assault victims: a prospective analysis. Sex Transm Dis 2008;35(12):973–8.
38. Neu N, Heffernan-Vacca S, Millery M, et al. Postexposure prophylaxis for HIV in children and adolescents after sexual assault: a prospective observational study in an urban medical center. Sex Transm Dis 2007;34(2):65–8.
39. Schremmer RD, Swanson D, Kraly K. Human immunodeficiency virus postexposure prophylaxis in child and adolescent victims of sexual assault. Pediatr Emerg Care 2005;21(8):502–6.
40. Lykins WR, Luecke E, Johengen D, et al. Long acting systemic HIV pre-exposure prophylaxis: an examination of the field. Drug Deliv Transl Res 2017;7(6):805–16.
41. Nyaku AN, Kelly SG, Taiwo BO. Long-acting antiretrovirals: where are we now? Curr HIV/AIDS Rep 2017;14(2):63–71.
42. HIV Prevention Trials Network. Long-acting injectable cabotegravir for PrEP well tolerated in HPTN 077. Available at: https://hptn.org/news-and-events/announcements/long-acting-injectable-cabotegravir-for-prep-well-tolerated-hptn-077. Accessed July 25, 2017.
43. Margolis DA, Gonzalez-Garcia J, Hans-Jurgen S, et al. Cabotegravir+Rilpivirine as long-acting maintenance therapy: LATTE-2 week 32 results. Conference on Retroviruses and Opportunistic Infections. Boston, MA, February 22-25, 2016.
44. Mandal S, Belshan M, Holec A, et al. An enhanced emtricitabine-loaded long-acting nanoformulation for prevention or treatment of HIV infection. Antimicrob Agents Chemother 2016;61(1):e01475–16.
45. Jacobson JM, Flexner CW. Universal antiretroviral regimens: thinking beyond one-pill-once-a-day. Curr Opin HIV AIDS 2017;12(4):343–50.
46. Rajoli RKR, Back DJ, Rannard S, et al. In silico dose prediction for long-acting rilpivirine and cabotegravir administration to children and adolescents. Clin Pharmacokinet 2017. [Epub ahead of print].
47. Margolis DM, Koup RA, Ferrari G. HIV antibodies for treatment of HIV infection. Immunol Rev 2017;275(1):313–23.
48. International Maternal Pediatric Adolescent AIDS Clinical Trials Network. P1112 (DAIDS ID 11903): Open-label, dose-escalating, phase I study to determine safety and pharmacokinetic parameters of subcutaneous (SC) VRC01 and VRC01LS, Potent anti-HIV neutralizing monoclonal antibodies, in HIV-1-exposed infants. Available at: http://impaactnetwork.org/studies/P1112.asp. Accessed July 25, 2017.

Norovirus Illnesses in Children and Adolescents

Minesh P. Shah, MD, MPH*, Aron J. Hall, DVM, MSPH

KEYWORDS

- Norovirus • Gastroenteritis • Diarrhea • Vomiting • Outbreaks

KEY POINTS

- Norovirus is a leading cause of both endemic and epidemic gastroenteritis in the United States and globally.
- Norovirus causes approximately 4.2 million illnesses; 815,000 outpatient visits; 130,000 emergency department visits; 24,600 hospitalizations; and 38 deaths annually in children in the United States.
- Most of the global childhood mortality from norovirus illness occurs in developing countries.
- Early assessment of dehydration status and treatment aimed at correcting fluid status are key to preventing severe outcomes from norovirus illness.
- Vaccines against norovirus illness and strategies for defining the target population, vaccination schedule, and delivery mechanism for vaccination are under development.

BACKGROUND

Norovirus is a leading cause of acute gastroenteritis in the United States[1] and globally[2]. Although norovirus infection causes illness in all age groups, incidence rates are highest among young children.[1,3] In several countries that have introduced national rotavirus vaccination programs, norovirus has replaced rotavirus as the leading cause of medically attended[4–8] and community[8,9] pediatric gastroenteritis. Approximately 99% of the 212,000 annual deaths caused by norovirus occur in developing countries.[10] Although deaths are rare in the United States, norovirus is responsible for approximately 24,000 hospitalizations; 132,000 emergency room visits; and 925,000 outpatient visits in children less than 18 years, at an estimated cost of more than $200 million.[11,12] With norovirus vaccines under development,[13] a review of the virology, epidemiology, clinical presentation, diagnosis, treatment, and prevention of pediatric norovirus is described herein.

Disclaimer: The findings and conclusions in this report are those of the authors and do not necessarily represent the official position of the Centers for Disease Control and Prevention.
Disclosure: The authors have no conflicts of interest to disclose.
Division of Viral Diseases, Centers for Disease Control and Prevention, 1600 Clifton Road Northeast, Atlanta, GA 30329, USA
* Corresponding author.
E-mail address: yxi8@cdc.gov

Infect Dis Clin N Am 32 (2018) 103–118
https://doi.org/10.1016/j.idc.2017.11.004   id.theclinics.com
0891-5520/18/Published by Elsevier Inc.

NOROVIRUS VIROLOGY

Noroviruses are a genetically diverse group of viruses in the *Caliciviridae* family that cause acute gastroenteritis.[14] The first norovirus was described when a viral particle was observed by electron microscopy in a stool sample derived from a 1968 outbreak in Norwalk, Ohio, leading to the initial name of Norwalk virus.[15] Norwalk virus was the first virus shown to cause gastroenteritis. Since then, other Norwalk-like viruses have been discovered; currently, noroviruses are classified into genogroups GI to GVII.[16] Genogroups GI, GII, and, to a lesser extent, GIV, are known to cause human disease. Globally, viruses of the GII.4 genotype are the leading cause of norovirus disease,[17] include new variants that emerge every 2 years to 4 years,[18,19] and are associated with greater symptom severity and health care burden.[20]

CLINICAL PRESENTATION AND DISEASE COURSE

Norovirus infections cause acute gastroenteritis, presenting as acute-onset vomiting and/or diarrhea. When present, diarrhea is typically watery and nonbloody and may be accompanied by abdominal cramps, nausea, and fever.[21] Constitutional symptoms, including low-grade fever, generalized myalgias, malaise, headache, and chills, frequently occur. The incubation period lasts 12 hours to 48 hours, and the duration of clinical symptoms is typically 12 hours to 72 hours. Asymptomatic norovirus infection, identified through stool shedding of norovirus in patients without gastroenteritis, has been found in 3% to 10% of children and adults.[22] Although most infections result in full recovery,[23] severe outcomes, such as hospitalization and death, occur, particularly among children ages less than 5 years, adults ages greater than 65 years, and immunocompromised hosts.[1,24–26]

Severity of Norovirus Illness in Children

A meta-analysis of norovirus-associated gastroenteritis in children aged less than 5 years worldwide found that approximately 70% of cases occur within the 6-month to 23-month age range, and fewer than 15% occur before 6 months.[27] In this analysis, the proportion of cases among children less than 12 months increased from community to outpatient to inpatient settings, suggesting that infants more often have severe disease or are more likely to seek medical care and be hospitalized. Gastroenteritis caused by norovirus is generally milder than illness caused by rotavirus.[28] Children less than 5 years diagnosed with norovirus gastroenteritis after presenting to 3 US children's hospitals participating in active surveillance had fewer days of diarrhea, fewer diarrhea episodes, less fever, fewer abnormal behavioral signs, and less hospitalization than those diagnosed with rotavirus.[29] In contrast, children with norovirus gastroenteritis had more days of vomiting and more vomiting episodes than those with an unknown etiology.

Norovirus in Immunocompromised Children

Typically, norovirus outbreaks in hospitalized children with immunocompromising conditions occur by community-acquired infection in an index patient followed by nosocomial transmission to other patients and hospital staff.[30–32] In both retrospective and prospective studies, children with norovirus infection after solid organ or stem cell transplantation are at risk for prolonged viral shedding,[33–37] diarrhea greater than 14 days,[33,34,36–40] and severe outcomes.[33,34,36,37,39,40] Hospitalizations from norovirus gastroenteritis in these studies did not follow the typical seasonal pattern of norovirus.

Children with primary immune deficiencies have also been found to have prolonged norovirus shedding after infection.[41,42]

NOROVIRUS TRANSMISSION

Norovirus is highly contagious, and the infectious dose can be as few as 20 viral particles.[43] The most common route for transmission is person to person, either directly through the fecal-oral route, by ingestion of aerosolized vomitus, or by indirect exposure via fomites or contaminated environmental surfaces.[44] Norovirus is also the leading known cause of both sporadic cases[2,45] and outbreaks of foodborne disease, with contamination occurring either from infected food handlers or directly from foods.[46] Foods often implicated in norovirus outbreaks include leafy greens, fresh fruits, and shellfish, but any food that is served raw or handled after being cooked can be contaminated. Waterborne transmission is less common but possible when drinking or recreational water is not chlorinated.[47]

Peak viral shedding occurs 2 days to 5 days after infection[44] and occurs primarily in stool but can also be present in vomitus. Although norovirus RNA has been detected in stool samples for up to 4 weeks to 8 weeks after symptom resolution in otherwise healthy individuals,[48] the infectivity of the virus beyond the symptomatic period is not well established.

IMMUNITY

Immunity to norovirus is an ongoing field of research relevant to prospects for vaccination. Acquired immunity after infection is likely of limited duration, with protection after volunteer challenge studies lasting for weeks up to 2 years,[49,50] whereas modeling studies suggest protection for up to 9 years.[51] Evidence to support a limited duration of immunity in children is the identification of multiple norovirus infections in children monitored in birth cohort studies, with 25% to 40% of children followed from birth to 3 years in various settings having at least 2 episodes of norovirus gastroenteritis.[52–55] When immunity is acquired, protection may be limited to the initial genotype, because repeat infections by other genotypes do occur.[54,56]

In addition to acquired immunity, innate immunity may be conferred by homozygous mutations in the alpha(1,2) fucosyltransferase (FUT2) gene, which control the expression of histo-blood group antigens on the gut surface epithelium that bind to norovirus.[52,57] These mutations vary by ethnicity and occur in approximately 5% to 50% of different populations worldwide.[58]

NOROVIRUS DIAGNOSIS

Although norovirus gastroenteritis can be suspected by clinical symptoms, confirmatory testing requires laboratory testing of stool specimens (**Table 1**). Molecular tests, including conventional reverse-transcriptase polymerase chain reaction (RT-PCR) and quantitative, real-time RT-PCR (RT-qPCR), are most sensitive and the gold standard for norovirus detection but are usually only available in public health laboratories and research facilities. RT-qPCR affords several advantages, because it is the most sensitive assay available, can detect GI and GII strains simultaneously, and can limit false-negative results. Interpretation of RT-qPCR results may be complicated by norovirus frequently detected in stool samples of healthy and asymptomatic individuals.[9,59,60] Detection of norovirus in asymptomatic individuals seems more common in developing countries.[22]

Table 1
Laboratory methods for detection of norovirus

Method	Characteristics	Availability	Use in Clinical Setting?	Use in Outbreak Setting?
Conventional RT-PCR, real-time RT-PCR	• Gold standard test • High sensitivity • Frequently detects viral RNA in asymptomatic and healthy patients	Public health and reference laboratories	Not widely[a]	Yes
Multiple enteric pathogen tests (PCR)	• Detects multiple viral, bacterial, and parasitic pathogens simultaneously • High sensitivity • Expensive	Public health and clinical laboratories	Yes	Yes
Enzyme immunoassay, Immunochromatographic	• Low sensitivity, high specificity	Public health and clinical laboratories	Not recommended for individual patients	Yes, for rapid screening of multiple samples
Electron microscopy	• Detect multiple viral pathogens • Low sensitivity • Expensive	Reference laboratories	No	No

Abbreviations: PCR, polymerase chain reaction; RNA, ribonucleic acid; RT-PCR, real-time polymerase chain reaction.

[a] Individual patient specimens can be tested, such as in an outbreak at a reference laboratory, and positive specimens genotyped, but due to lack of availability in the clinical setting is unlikely to provide results back to the patient in a timely fashion. Some commercial diagnostic laboratories, however, offer their own in-house RT-PCR as do some tertiary-care hospitals.

Laboratory diagnostics in the clinical setting have recently become more widely available. Molecular-based assays for multiple enteric pathogens, such as xTAG GPP (Luminex Corporation, Toronto, Canada),[61,62] FilmArray gastrointestinal panel (BioFire Diagnostics, Salt Lake City, Utah),[61,63] and Verigene Enteric Pathogens Test (Nanosphere, Northbrook, Illinois)[64] can detect multiple viral, bacterial, and parasitic pathogens simultaneously within a few hours. The equipment and testing can be expensive, however, and interpretation of positive results with mixed infections can pose challenges for appropriate treatment and management of patients. Norovirus-specific nucleic acid amplification tests are promising for having a short turn-around time for point-of-care testing and have recently received Food and Drug Administration clearance[65] but are not yet commonly used in practice. Other diagnostic tests include electron microscopy, enzyme immunoassay, and immunochromatographic lateral flow assays, although these tests are limited by moderate sensitivity or high cost.[16]

CLINICAL ASSESSMENT AND TREATMENT

The assessment and treatment of gastroenteritis caused by norovirus are similar to those of other causes of viral gastroenteritis. Treatment of diarrhea usually begins at home, with a focus on replacing fluid losses and maintaining adequate nutrition intake.[66] Medical evaluation of children is indicated with young age (eg, age <6 months or weight <8 kg), history of premature birth, chronic medical conditions or concurrent illness, fever, bloody stool, high volume and frequency of diarrhea, persistent vomiting, change in mental status, caregiver concern for dehydration, or poor response to home treatment.[66] At the time of medical evaluation, clinicians should conduct a thorough history and physical examination to assess the level of dehydration and loss of body weight.

Treatment should be based on the degree of dehydration and include 2 phases: rehydration and maintenance (**Box 1**).[66] The rehydration phase should occur in the first 3 hours to 4 hours of treatment with the goal of replacing the fluid deficit. The maintenance phase should focus on realimentation and returning the patient to an age-appropriate diet. Breastfed infants should continue to nurse throughout treatment. Oral-rehydration solutions (ORS), whose practical use was first studied during cholera outbreaks in Bangladesh and India,[67,68] should be the mainstay of rehydration treatment.[66] Although several ORS formulations are commercially

---

Box 1
Clinical assessment and treatment of acute diarrhea based on level of dehydration

Minimal or no dehydration (<3% loss of body weight)

- Examination findings: normal mental status, thirst, heart rate, respiratory rate, tears, moist mucosa, skin recoil, capillary refill, urine output, warm extremities

- Immediate rehydration: N/A

- Maintenance treatment: less than 10 kg body weight: 60 mL to 120 mL ORS for each diarrheal stool or vomiting episode; greater than 10 kg body weight: 120 mL to 240 mL ORS for each diarrheal stool or vomiting episode; continue breastfeeding or age-appropriate diet

Mild to moderate dehydration (3%–9% loss of body weight)

- Examination findings: irritable or fatigued mental status, increased thirst, normal to increased heart rate, respiratory rate, slightly sunken eyes, decreased tears, dry mucosa, skin recoil less than 2 seconds, prolonged capillary refill, decreased urine output, cool extremities

- Immediate rehydration: ORS, 50 mL/kg to 100 mL/kg body weight over 3 hours to 4 hours

- Maintenance treatment: same as for minimal or no dehydration

Severe dehydration (>9% loss of body weight)

- Examination findings: lethargic to unconscious mental status, poor thirst or unable to drink, tachycardia (bradycardia in very severe cases), deep breathing, deeply sunken eyes, absent tears, parched mucosa, skin recoil greater than 2 seconds, prolonged and minimal capillary refill, minimal urine output, cold to cyanotic extremities

- Immediate rehydration: iso-osmotic crystalloid intravenous fluids at 20 mL/kg body weight until perfusion and mental status improve; then ORS at 100 mL/kg body weight over 4 hours

- Maintenance treatment: same as for mild to moderate dehydration; if unable to drink, administer through nasogastric tube or intravenous

Adapted from King CK, Glass R, Bresee JS, et al, Centers for Disease Control and Prevention. Managing acute gastroenteritis among children: oral rehydration, maintenance, and nutritional therapy. MMWR Recomm Rep 2003;52(RR-16):6; with permission.

available, all are composed of a balance of carbohydrates, sodium, potassium, chloride, and bicarbonate to encourage rapid rehydration, electrolyte balance, and appropriate osmolarity, and glucose support.[69] Patients with minimal or no dehydration (<3% loss of body weight) may be managed conservatively with ORS provided at home. Patients with mild to moderate dehydration (3%–9%) should be initially medically supervised. Patients with severe dehydration (>9%) should be treated with ORS but may also require intravenous fluids to maintain fluid status. Intravenous fluids may also be required in cases of severe vomiting that precludes oral rehydration.

Aside from general supportive treatment of gastroenteritis, no specific antinorovirus therapy is recommended at this time. Research to identify antiviral treatment strategies is in progress[70,71] and should be bolstered by the recent discovery of human intestinal enteroid cultures to support norovirus replication in vitro.[72] Adjunctive treatments for diarrhea, including use of analgesic, antimotility, antiemetic, antisecretory, and probiotic agents, are commonly used but often without robust supportive evidence.[73]

NOROVIRUS EPIDEMIOLOGY: ENDEMIC DISEASE

The global prevalence of norovirus among cases of acute gastroenteritis is estimated at 17% in hospitalized patients and 24% in the community.[22] A World Health Organization–commissioned analysis estimated 685 million annual norovirus infections (95% uncertainty interval 491 million–1.1 billion) and 212,000 (95% uncertainty interval 161,00–278,000) annual norovirus deaths worldwide.[10] The wide uncertainty intervals reflect current gaps in country-level data, especially from low-income, high-mortality countries. More than half of global cases occur in winter months.[74] One factor in the seasonality of norovirus in high-income countries may be the start of the school year, with evidence to suggest that outbreaks in children begin with the school year and then spread to outbreaks in adults.[75] A systematic review found GII.4 the most common genotype in endemic norovirus gastroenteritis in children, identified in approximately two-thirds of cases.[76]

Estimated rates of norovirus disease in the community, outpatient, emergency, and inpatient settings and for deaths from norovirus in children in high-income countries are summarized in **Table 2**. Applying rates for studies conducted in the United States to 2016 population estimates from the US Census,[77] the authors estimate the burden from norovirus illness in children aged <18 years to be approximately 4.2 million total illnesses; 815,000 outpatient visits; 130,000 emergency department visits; 24,600 hospitalizations; and 38 deaths (**Fig. 1**).

EPIDEMIC NOROVIRUS GASTROENTERITIS

Norovirus is the leading etiology of gastroenteritis outbreaks reported to the National Outbreak Reporting System in the United States, accounting for 68% of outbreaks in which a single etiology is identified.[47] Norovirus is most commonly transmitted by person-to-person contact, reported in 66% to 77% of outbreaks, although can also be transmitted by food, water, and environmental routes.[47,78] Although long-term care facilities caring for adults are the most frequently reported setting, schools and day care centers have been reported in 2% to 5% of all norovirus outbreaks.[47,78] Periodic increases in norovirus outbreaks occur in association with the emergence of new GII.4 strains, observed every 2 to 4 years in the past 2 decades.[18]

Foodborne Disease Outbreaks

Norovirus is the leading cause of foodborne disease outbreaks in the United States.[46] Foodborne norovirus outbreaks occur year-round, and infectious food workers are implicated as the source of contamination in 70% of these outbreaks.[46] Globally, norovirus is the leading identified etiology of foodborne illnesses, causing almost 125 million illnesses annually, and the fifth leading identified etiology of foodborne deaths, with almost 35,000 deaths annually.[79] Among children aged less than 5 years, norovirus causes 35 million foodborne illnesses, the third highest after infections from *Campylobacter* and *Escherichia coli*, and 9000 foodborne deaths annually.[79]

Outbreak Prevention and Control

Principles of norovirus outbreak prevention and control include hand hygiene, exclusion of ill persons, and environmental disinfection.[44] For child care centers, the American Academy of Pediatrics offers additional guidelines for diapering and staff training.[80] Hand hygiene, beginning with proper hand washing with soap and running water for at least 20 seconds, is the most effective way to reduce norovirus contamination on the hands.[81] Alcohol-based sanitizers can be used when soap and water are unavailable but should not be a replacement for proper washing due to conflicting evidence.[81,82] Avoiding bare-hand contact with ready-to-eat foods (ie, food that is eaten raw or food eaten without further cooking) is recommended as an additional preventive strategy. Exclusion and isolation of infected persons are often the most practical means of disrupting norovirus transmission during an outbreak. Ill persons should be excluded during the symptomatic period of their illness as well as a period after recovery while the person is still shedding virus at high levels (typically 24–72 hours). Environmental disinfection is recommended using a chlorine bleach solution or other commercial product registered with the Environmental Protection Agency as effective against norovirus.[83] Particular attention should be given to areas of greatest potential contamination, such as bathrooms and high-touch surfaces. Specific regulations for outbreak prevention and control at child-care and school facilities are determined by state licensing agencies, and address practices, such as handwashing for staff and children, isolation and exclusion of ill children, exclusion of ill staff, diapering, and environmental cleaning.[84] Local school and public health authorities may also consider facility closure to control an outbreak, depending on factors, such as a rising case count, a high attack rate in a defined at-risk population, and input from local stakeholders.[85] Health care providers are encouraged to report suspected and confirmed outbreaks of norovirus to their local health department.

PROSPECTS FOR VACCINATION AGAINST NOROVIRUS

The ubiquity of norovirus in the environment and the high burden of norovirus infection make vaccination against norovirus an appealing prevention strategy. Norovirus vaccines in development have been based on virus-like particles (VLPs), which contain the major capsid antigen but lack genetic material for viral replication.[86] VLPs have been shown to induce humoral, mucosal, and cellular immune responses after oral and intranasal administration.[87] Several norovirus vaccines are currently under development in preclinical and clinical trials using VLPs and involving intranasal, oral, and intramuscular routes of administration.[13,88]

A norovirus vaccination strategy needs to address biological and programmatic challenges.[89] Biologically, norovirus vaccines need to protect against the diversity of norovirus strains that affect humans and the presence of emerging GII.4 strains.

Table 2
Studies estimating endemic norovirus incidence in children less than 18 years of age in developed countries, by outcome

	Country	Data Period Studied	Study Design	Population	Reported Incidence by Age Group
Deaths					Per 1,000,000 person-years
Hall et al,[92] 2012	US	1999–2007	Retrospective analysis using time-series regression models	Gastroenteritis-associated deaths from National Center for Health Statistics multiple cause-of-death mortality data	0–4 y: 1.3
Hospitalizations					Per 100,000 person-years
Lopman et al,[11] 2011	US	1996–2007	Retrospective analysis using time-series regression models	Gastroenteritis-associated hospital discharges from National Inpatient Sample	<5 y: 94 5–17 y: 11
Ruzante et al,[93] 2011	Canada	2001–2004	Retrospective database review	Norovirus hospital discharge codes and Canadian Institute for Health Information, Vital Statistics Registry, National Notifiable Diseases database	<1 y: 5.9 1–4 y: 2.0 5–9 y: 0.8 10–14 y: 0.3 15–19 y: 0.3
Emergency department visits					Per 10,000 person-years
Gastañaduy et al,[12] 2013	US	2001–2009	Retrospective analysis using time-series regression models	Gastroenteritis-associated health care encounters from MarketScan commercial claims and encounters database	0–4 y: 38 5–17 y: 10
Outpatient visits					Per 1000 person-years
Grytdal et al,[94] 2016	US	2012–2013	Retrospective laboratory-based cohort	AGE specimens submitted for routine clinical diagnostics from health maintenance organization in 2 US locations	<5 y: 26 5–15 y: 4
O'Brien et al,[24] 2016	UK	2008–2009	Prospective cohort (IID2 study)	AGE patients presenting for primary health care consultations nationwide	<5 y: 14 5–15 y: 1.5
Gastañaduy et al,[12] 2013	US	2001–2009	Retrospective analysis using time-series regression models	Gastroenteritis-associated health care encounters from MarketScan commercial claims and encounters database	0–4 y: 23 5–17 y: 8.5

Phillips et al,[3] 2010	UK	1993–1996	Prospective cohort (IID1 study)	AGE cases presenting to 70 general practitioner clinics nationwide	<2 y: 64 / 2–4 y: 15 / 5–14 y: 4
Bernard et al,[95] 2014	Germany	2001–2009	Retrospective analysis surveillance	National surveillance system for notifiable diseases, Federal Statistical Office, includes sporadic and outbreak cases	<5 y: 4–4.5[a] / 5–9 y: 1 / 10–14 y: 0.4 / 15–19 y: 0.4–0.6
Werber et al,[96] 2013	Germany	2004–2008	Retrospective analysis surveillance	National surveillance system for notifiable diseases, Federal Statistical Office	0–4 y: 5.4[a] / 5–9 y: 1.3 / 10–19 y: 0.5
Community					Per 1000 person-years
Grytdal et al,[94] 2016	US	2012–2013	Retrospective laboratory-based cohort	AGE specimens submitted for routine clinical diagnostics from health maintenance organization in 2 US locations	<5 y: 152 / 5–15 y: 22
O'Brien et al,[24] 2016	UK	2008–2009	Prospective cohort (IID2 study)	AGE cases in community nationwide	<1 y: 178 / 1–5 y: 137 / 5–15 y: 60
Phillips et al,[3] 2010	UK	1993–1996	Prospective cohort (IID study)	AGE cases in community nationwide	<2 y: 272 / 2–4 y: 167 / 5–14 y: 65
de Wit et al,[25] 2001	The Netherlands	1998–1999	Prospective cohort (Sensor)	AGE cases in sample of community practices	<1 y: 740 / 1–4 y: 900 / 5–11 y: 481 / 12–17 y: 157

Abbreviations: AGE, acute gastroenteritis; IID, infectious intestinal disease study; IID2, second infectious intestinal disease study.
[a] If point estimate was not reported in text or table, data points were extracted by digitizing plots.

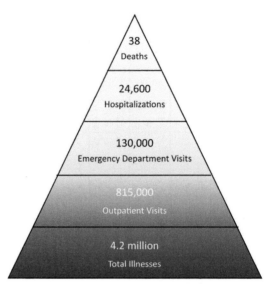

Fig. 1. Estimates of annual burden (annual number of illnesses and associated outcomes) for norovirus disease for children 0 to 17 years, United States. Data were derived from point estimates of rates of norovirus-associated deaths,[1] hospitalizations,[11] emergency department visits,[12] outpatient visits,[12,94] and illnesses.[94] Population size based on 2016 US Census estimates.

Immunity is currently thought to be of limited duration, estimated from 6 months to 9 years and to confer little protection across genogroups.[49,50] Programmatically, young children bear the highest overall incidence of disease and likely drive community transmission[90] and are thus an ideal target for vaccination. It is unknown, however, how norovirus vaccination might interact with other routine childhood vaccinations, and trials of norovirus vaccines have been mostly conducted in adults. Given prior exposure and underlying conditions, the immune response is likely to differ in young children, adolescents, adults, the elderly, and the immunocompromised.

Despite these challenges, norovirus vaccination has the potential to be highly beneficial to society. A simulation model estimated that vaccination could prevent 1 million to 2.2 million annual cases of norovirus gastroenteritis in the United States, resulting in savings of $2 billion over 4 years.[91] Given the high burden and higher mortality in low-income countries, norovirus vaccination would be of even greater benefit if adopted broadly by national immunization programs.

SUMMARY

Norovirus is the leading cause of acute gastroenteritis in the United States and globally, with higher incidence in children than in other age groups. In the United States, an estimated 4.2 million annual norovirus illnesses in children result in a high burden of medical care and hospitalization. Although deaths from norovirus in US children are rare, norovirus is a leading cause of death from childhood diarrhea in developing countries. Early assessment of dehydration status from diarrhea and appropriate treatment are advised to prevent complications, including death. Norovirus outbreaks should be managed with hand hygiene, exclusion of ill persons, and environmental control. Future prospects for prevention of norovirus include vaccination.

REFERENCES

1. Hall AJ, Lopman BA, Payne DC, et al. Norovirus disease in the United States. Emerg Infect Dis 2013;19(8):1198–205.
2. Kirk MD, Pires SM, Black RE, et al. World Health organization estimates of the global and regional disease burden of 22 foodborne bacterial, protozoal, and viral diseases, 2010: a data synthesis. PLoS Med 2015;12(12):e1001921.
3. Phillips G, Tam CC, Conti S, et al. Community incidence of norovirus-associated infectious intestinal disease in England: improved estimates using viral load for norovirus diagnosis. Am J Epidemiol 2010;171(9):1014–22.
4. Payne DC, Vinje J, Szilagyi PG, et al. Norovirus and medically attended gastro-enteritis in U.S. children. N Engl J Med 2013;368(12):1121–30.
5. Tam CC, O'Brien SJ, Tompkins DS, et al. Changes in causes of acute gastroenteritis in the United Kingdom Over 15 Years: microbiologic findings from 2 prospective, population-based studies of infectious intestinal disease. Clin Infect Dis 2012;54(9):1275–86.
6. McAtee CL, Webman R, Gilman RH, et al. Burden of norovirus and rotavirus in children after rotavirus vaccine introduction, Cochabamba, Bolivia. Am J Trop Med Hyg 2016;94(1):212–7.
7. Hemming M, Räsänen S, Huhti L, et al. Major reduction of rotavirus, but not norovirus, gastroenteritis in children seen in hospital after the introduction of RotaTeq vaccine into the National Immunization Programme in Finland. Eur J Pediatr 2013; 172(6):739–46.
8. Bucardo F, Reyes Y, Svensson L, et al. Predominance of norovirus and sapovirus in Nicaragua after implementation of universal rotavirus vaccination. PLoS One 2014;9(5):e98201.
9. Platts-Mills JA, Babji S, Bodhidatta L, et al. Pathogen-specific burdens of community diarrhoea in developing countries: a multisite birth cohort study (MAL-ED). Lancet Glob Health 2015;3(9):e564–75.
10. Pires SM, Fischer-Walker CL, Lanata CF, et al. Aetiology-specific estimates of the global and regional incidence and mortality of diarrhoeal diseases commonly transmitted through food. PLoS One 2015;10(12):e0142927.
11. Lopman BA, Hall AJ, Curns AT, et al. Increasing rates of gastroenteritis hospital discharges in US adults and the contribution of norovirus, 1996-2007. Clin Infect Dis 2011;52(4):466–74.
12. Gastañaduy PA, Hall AJ, Curns AT, et al. Burden of norovirus gastroenteritis in the ambulatory setting–United States, 2001-2009. J Infect Dis 2013;207(7):1058–65.
13. Aliabadi N, Lopman BA, Parashar UD, et al. Progress toward norovirus vaccines: considerations for further development and implementation in potential target populations. Expert Rev Vaccin 2015;14(9):1241–53.
14. Green KY. Caliciviridae: the noroviruses. In: Knipe DM, Howley PM, Cohen JI, et al, editors. Fields virology. 6th edition. Philadelphia: Lippincott Williams & Wilkins; 2013. p. 582–608.
15. Kapikian AZ, Wyatt RG, Dolin R, et al. Visualization by immune electron microscopy of a 27-nm particle associated with acute infectious nonbacterial gastroenteritis. J Virol 1972;10(5):1075–81.
16. Vinjé J. Advances in laboratory methods for detection and typing of norovirus. J Clin Microbiol 2015;53(2):373–81.
17. Siebenga JJ, Vennema H, Zheng DP, et al. Norovirus illness is a global problem: emergence and spread of norovirus GII.4 variants, 2001-2007. J Infect Dis 2009; 200(5):802–12.

18. Zheng D-P, Widdowson M-A, Glass RI, et al. Molecular epidemiology of genogroup II-genotype 4 noroviruses in the United States between 1994 and 2006. J Clin Microbiol 2010;48(1):168–77.

19. Vega E, Barclay L, Gregoricus N, et al. Genotypic and epidemiologic trends of norovirus outbreaks in the United States, 2009 to 2013. J Clin Microbiol 2014; 52(1):147–55.

20. Desai R, Hembree CD, Handel A, et al. Severe outcomes are associated with genogroup 2 genotype 4 norovirus outbreaks: a systematic literature review. Clin Infect Dis 2012;55(2):189–93.

21. Glass RI, Parashar UD, Estes MK. Norovirus gastroenteritis. N Engl J Med 2009; 361(18):1776–85.

22. Ahmed SM, Hall AJ, Robinson AE, et al. Global prevalence of norovirus in cases of gastroenteritis: a systematic review and meta-analysis. Lancet Infect Dis 2014; 14(8):725–30.

23. Rockx B, de Wit M, Vennema H, et al. Natural history of human calicivirus infection: a prospective cohort study. Clin Infect Dis 2002;35(3):246–53.

24. O'Brien SJ, Donaldson AL, Iturriza-Gomara M, et al. Age-specific incidence rates for norovirus in the community and presenting to primary healthcare facilities in the United Kingdom. J Infect Dis 2016;213(Suppl 1):S15–8.

25. de Wit MAS, Koopmans MPG, Kortbeek LM, et al. Sensor, a population-based cohort study on Gastroenteritis in the Netherlands: incidence and etiology. Am J Epidemiol 2001;154(7):666–74.

26. Bok K, Green KY. Norovirus gastroenteritis in immunocompromised patients. N Engl J Med 2012;367(22):2126–32.

27. Shioda K, Kambhampati A, Hall AJ, et al. Global age distribution of pediatric norovirus cases. Vaccine 2015;33(33):4065–8.

28. Riera-Montes M, O'Ryan M, Verstraeten T. Norovirus and Rotavirus disease severity in children: Systematic Review and Meta-Analysis. Pediatr Infect Dis J 2017. [Epub ahead of print].

29. Wikswo ME, Desai R, Edwards KM, et al. Clinical profile of children with norovirus disease in rotavirus vaccine era. Emerg Infect Dis 2013;19(10):1691–3.

30. Munir N, Liu P, Gastanaduy P, et al. Norovirus infection in immunocompromised children and children with hospital-acquired acute gastroenteritis. J Med Virol 2014;86(7):1203–9.

31. Schwartz S, Vergoulidou M, Schreier E, et al. Norovirus gastroenteritis causes severe and lethal complications after chemotherapy and hematopoietic stem cell transplantation. Blood 2011;117(22):5850–6.

32. Simon A, Schildgen O, Maria Eis-Hubinger A, et al. Norovirus outbreak in a pediatric oncology unit. Scand J Gastroenterol 2006;41(6):693–9.

33. Roos-Weil D, Ambert-Balay K, Lanternier F, et al. Impact of norovirus/sapovirus-related diarrhea in renal transplant recipients hospitalized for diarrhea. Transplantation 2011;92(1):61–9.

34. Ye X, Van JN, Munoz FM, et al. Noroviruses as a cause of diarrhea in immunocompromised pediatric hematopoietic stem cell and solid organ transplant recipients. Am J Transplant 2015;15(7):1874–81.

35. Osborne CM, Montano AC, Robinson CC, et al. Viral gastroenteritis in children in Colorado 2006-2009. J Med Virol 2015;87(6):931–9.

36. Patte M, Canioni D, Fenoel VA, et al. Severity and outcome of the norovirus infection in children after intestinal transplantation. Pediatr Transplant 2017;21(5): e12930.

37. Roddie C, Paul JP, Benjamin R, et al. Allogeneic hematopoietic stem cell transplantation and norovirus gastroenteritis: a previously unrecognized cause of morbidity. Clin Infect Dis 2009;49(7):1061–8.
38. Ghosh N, Malik FA, Daver RG, et al. Viral associated diarrhea in immunocompromised and cancer patients at a large comprehensive cancer center: a 10-year retrospective study. Infect Dis (Lond) 2017;49(2):113–9.
39. Brown JR, Shah D, Breuer J. Viral gastrointestinal infections and norovirus genotypes in a paediatric UK hospital, 2014-2015. J Clin Virol 2016;84:1–6.
40. Ueda R, Fuji S, Mori S, et al. Characteristics and outcomes of patients diagnosed with norovirus gastroenteritis after allogeneic hematopoietic stem cell transplantation based on immunochromatography. Int J Hematol 2015;102(1):121–8.
41. Frange P, Touzot F, Debre M, et al. Prevalence and clinical impact of norovirus fecal shedding in children with inherited immune deficiencies. J Infect Dis 2012;206(8):1269–74.
42. Woodward JM, Gkrania-Klotsas E, Cordero-Ng AY, et al. The role of chronic norovirus infection in the enteropathy associated with common variable immunodeficiency. Am J Gastroenterol 2015;110(2):320–7.
43. Teunis PF, Moe CL, Liu P, et al. Norwalk virus: how infectious is it? J Med Virol 2008;80(8):1468–76.
44. Division of Viral Diseases, National Center for Immunization and Respiratory Diseases, Centers for Disease Control and Prevention. Updated norovirus outbreak management and disease prevention guidelines. MMWR Recomm Rep 2011; 60(RR-3):1–18.
45. Scallan E, Hoekstra RM, Angulo FJ, et al. Foodborne illness acquired in the United States—Major pathogens. Emerg Infect Dis 2011;17(1):7–15.
46. Hall AJ, Wikswo ME, Pringle K, et al. Vital signs: foodborne norovirus outbreaks - United States, 2009-2012. MMWR Morb Mortal Wkly Rep 2014; 63(22):491–5.
47. Hall AJ, Wikswo ME, Manikonda K, et al. Acute gastroenteritis surveillance through the national outbreak reporting system, United States. Emerg Infect Dis 2013;19(8):1305–9.
48. Atmar RL, Bernstein DI, Harro CD, et al. Norovirus vaccine against experimental human Norwalk virus illness. N Engl J Med 2011;365(23):2178–87.
49. Parrino TA, Schreiber DS, Trier JS, et al. Clinical immunity in acute gastroenteritis caused by Norwalk agent. N Engl J Med 1977;297(2):86–9.
50. Johnson PC, Mathewson JJ, DuPont HL, et al. Multiple-challenge study of host susceptibility to Norwalk gastroenteritis in US adults. J Infect Dis 1990;161(1): 18–21.
51. Simmons K, Gambhir M, Leon J, et al. Duration of immunity to norovirus gastroenteritis. Emerg Infect Dis 2013;19(8):1260–7.
52. Lopman BA, Trivedi T, Vicuna Y, et al. Norovirus infection and disease in an Ecuadorian Birth Cohort: association of certain norovirus genotypes with host FUT2 secretor status. J Infect Dis 2015;211(11):1813–21.
53. Menon VK, George S, Sarkar R, et al. Norovirus Gastroenteritis in a Birth Cohort in Southern India. PLoS One 2016;11(6):e0157007.
54. Saito M, Goel-Apaza S, Espetia S, et al. Multiple norovirus infections in a birth cohort in a Peruvian Periurban community. Clin Infect Dis 2014;58(4):483–91.
55. O'Ryan ML, Lucero Y, Prado V, et al. Symptomatic and asymptomatic rotavirus and norovirus infections during infancy in a Chilean birth cohort. Pediatr Infect Dis J 2009;28(10):879–84.

56. Malm M, Uusi-Kerttula H, Vesikari T, et al. High serum levels of norovirus genotype-specific blocking antibodies correlate with protection from infection in children. J Infect Dis 2014;210(11):1755–62.

57. Kambhampati A, Payne DC, Costantini V, et al. Host genetic susceptibility to enteric viruses: a systematic review and metaanalysis. Clin Infect Dis 2016; 62(1):11–8.

58. Nordgren J, Sharma S, Kambhampati A, et al. Innate resistance and susceptibility to norovirus infection. PLoS Pathog 2016;12(4):e1005385.

59. Kotloff KL, Nataro JP, Blackwelder WC, et al. Burden and aetiology of diarrhoeal disease in infants and young children in developing countries (the Global Enteric Multicenter Study, GEMS): a prospective, case-control study. Lancet 2013; 382(9888):209–22.

60. Teunis PF, Sukhrie FH, Vennema H, et al. Shedding of norovirus in symptomatic and asymptomatic infections. Epidemiol Infect 2015;143(8):1710–7.

61. Khare R, Espy MJ, Cebelinski E, et al. Comparative evaluation of two commercial multiplex panels for detection of gastrointestinal pathogens by use of clinical stool specimens. J Clin Microbiol 2014;52(10):3667–73.

62. Wessels E, Rusman LG, van Bussel MJ, et al. Added value of multiplex Luminex Gastrointestinal Pathogen Panel (xTAG(R) GPP) testing in the diagnosis of infectious gastroenteritis. Clin Microbiol Infect 2014;20(3):O182–7.

63. Buss SN, Leber A, Chapin K, et al. Multicenter evaluation of the BioFire FilmArray gastrointestinal panel for etiologic diagnosis of infectious gastroenteritis. J Clin Microbiol 2015;53(3):915–25.

64. Huang RS, Johnson CL, Pritchard L, et al. Performance of the Verigene(R) enteric pathogens test, Biofire FilmArray gastrointestinal panel and Luminex xTAG(R) gastrointestinal pathogen panel for detection of common enteric pathogens. Diagn Microbiol Infect Dis 2016;86(4):336–9.

65. Gonzalez MD, Langley LC, Buchan BW, et al. Multicenter evaluation of the xpert norovirus assay for detection of norovirus genogroups I and II in fecal specimens. J Clin Microbiol 2016;54(1):142–7.

66. King CK, Glass R, Bresee JS, et al. Managing acute gastroenteritis among children: oral rehydration, maintenance, and nutritional therapy. MMWR Recomm Rep 2003;52(RR-16):1–16.

67. Pierce NF, Banwell JG, Rupak DM, et al. Effect of intragastric glucose-electrolyte infusion upon water and electrolyte balance in Asiatic cholera. Gastroenterology 1968;55(3):333–43.

68. Nalin DR, Cash RA, Islam R, et al. Oral maintenance therapy for cholera in adults. Lancet 1968;2(7564):370–3.

69. World Health Organization. Oral rehydration salts:production of the new ORS. 2006. Available at: http://www.who.int/maternal_child_adolescent/documents/fch_cah_06_1/en/. Accessed May 2017.

70. Prasad BV, Shanker S, Muhaxhiri Z, et al. Antiviral targets of human noroviruses. Curr Opin Virol 2016;18:117–25.

71. Thorne L, Arias A, Goodfellow I. Advances toward a norovirus antiviral: from classical inhibitors to lethal mutagenesis. J Infect Dis 2016;213(Suppl 1):S27–31.

72. Ettayebi K, Crawford SE, Murakami K, et al. Replication of human noroviruses in stem cell-derived human enteroids. Science 2016;353(6306):1387–93.

73. Churgay CA, Aftab Z. Gastroenteritis in children: part II. Prevention and management. Am Fam Physician 2012;85(11):1066–70.

74. Ahmed SM, Lopman BA, Levy K. A systematic review and meta-analysis of the global seasonality of norovirus. PLoS One 2013;8(10):e75922.

75. Kraut RY, Snedeker KG, Babenko O, et al. Influence of school year on seasonality of norovirus outbreaks in developed countries. Can J Infect Dis Med Microbiol 2017;2017:9258140.

76. Hoa Tran TN, Trainor E, Nakagomi T, et al. Molecular epidemiology of noroviruses associated with acute sporadic gastroenteritis in children: global distribution of genogroups, genotypes and GII.4 variants. J Clin Virol 2013;56(3):185–93.

77. US Census Bureau, Population Division. Annual estimates of the Resident Population for the United States, Regions, States and Puerto Rico: April 1, 2010 to July 1, 2016. Available at: https://www.census.gov/data/tables/2016/demo/popest/state-total.html. Accessed May 2017.

78. Shah MP, Wikswo ME, Barclay L, et al. Near real-time surveillance of U.S. Norovirus outbreaks by the norovirus sentinel testing and tracking network - United States, August 2009-July 2015. MMWR Morb Mortal Wkly Rep 2017;66(7):185–9.

79. Havelaar AH, Kirk MD, Torgerson PR, et al. World Health Organization global estimates and regional comparisons of the burden of Foodborne Disease in 2010. PLoS Med 2015;12(12):e1001923.

80. American Academy of Pediatrics APHA, National Resource Center for Health and Safety in Child Care and Early Education. Caring for our children: national health and safety performance standards; guidelines for early care and education programs. 3rd edition. Elk Grove Village (IL): American Academy of Pediatrics; 2011.

81. Sickbert-Bennett EE, Weber DJ, Gergen-Teague MF, et al. Comparative efficacy of hand hygiene agents in the reduction of bacteria and viruses. Am J Infect Control 2005;33(2):67–77.

82. Liu P, Yuen Y, Hsiao HM, et al. Effectiveness of liquid soap and hand sanitizer against Norwalk virus on contaminated hands. Appl Environ Microbiol 2010;76(2):394–9.

83. Environmental Protection Agency. EPA's Registered antimicrobial products effective against norovirus. Available at: https://www.epa.gov/pesticide-registration/list-g-epas-registered-antimicrobial-products-effective-against-norovirus. Accessed May 17, 2017.

84. Leone CM, Jaykus LA, Cates SM, et al. A review of state licensing regulations to determine alignment with best practices to prevent human norovirus infections in child-care centers. Public Health Rep 2016;131(3):449–60.

85. Centers for Disease Control and Prevention (CDC). Norovirus outbreaks on three college campuses - California, Michigan, and Wisconsin, 2008. MMWR Morb Mortal Wkly Rep 2009;58(39):1095–100.

86. Jiang X, Wang M, Graham DY, et al. Expression, self-assembly, and antigenicity of the Norwalk virus capsid protein. J Virol 1992;66(11):6527–32.

87. Tacket CO, Sztein MB, Losonsky GA, et al. Humoral, mucosal, and cellular immune responses to oral Norwalk virus-like particles in volunteers. Clin Immunol 2003;108(3):241–7.

88. Giersing BK, Vekemans J, Nava S, et al. Report from the World Health Organization's third Product Development for Vaccines Advisory Committee (PDVAC) meeting. Geneva, June 8–10, 2016. Vaccine.

89. Lopman BA, Steele D, Kirkwood CD, et al. The vast and varied global burden of norovirus: prospects for prevention and control. PLoS Med 2016;13(4):e1001999.

90. de Wit MA, Koopmans MP, van Duynhoven YT. Risk factors for norovirus, Sapporo-like virus, and group A rotavirus gastroenteritis. Emerg Infect Dis 2003;9(12):1563–70.

91. Bartsch SM, Lopman BA, Hall AJ, et al. The potential economic value of a human norovirus vaccine for the United States. Vaccine 2012;30(49):7097–104.

92. Hall AJ, Curns AT, McDonald LC, et al. The roles of Clostridium difficile and nor-ovirus among gastroenteritis-associated deaths in the United States, 1999–2007. Clin Infect Dis 2012;55(2):216–23.

93. Ruzante JM, Majowicz SE, Fazil A, et al. Hospitalization and deaths for select enteric illnesses and associated sequelae in Canada, 2001-2004. Epidemiol Infect 2011;139(6):937–45.

94. Grytdal SP, DeBess E, Lee LE, et al. Incidence of norovirus and other viral path-ogens that Cause Acute Gastroenteritis (AGE) among Kaiser Permanente Mem-ber Populations in the United States, 2012–2013. PLoS One 2016;11(4): e0148395.

95. Bernard H, Hohne M, Niendorf S, et al. Epidemiology of norovirus gastroenteritis in Germany 2001-2009: eight seasons of routine surveillance. Epidemiol Infect 2014;142(1):63–74.

96. Werber D, Hille K, Frank C, et al. Years of potential life lost for six major enteric pathogens, Germany, 2004-2008. Epidemiol Infect 2013;141(5):961–8.

Changing Epidemiology of *Haemophilus influenzae* in Children

David F. Butler, MD[a], Angela L. Myers, MD, MPH[b],*

KEYWORDS

• Children • *H influenzae* • Meningitis • Vaccination

KEY POINTS

- *Haemophilus influenzae* is a common cause of upper respiratory tract infections in children and a rare cause of meningitis, pneumonia, and bacteremia.
- Vaccination against *H influenzae* type b (Hib) should be provided for all children starting at 2 months of age.
- Hib meningitis should be considered in any unimmunized child presenting with signs of meningeal irritation.
- The first-line treatment of meningitis and/or invasive *H influenzae* infection is a third-generation cephalosporin.
- Postexposure chemoprophylaxis with rifampin is an important measure for the prevention of secondary illness, particularly in the childcare setting.

INTRODUCTION

Haemophilus influenzae is a gram-negative bacteria that commonly colonizes the nasopharynx of children. The bacteria exist in both encapsulated (typeable) and unencapsulated (nontypeable) forms. Before the development of vaccination, *H influenzae* type b (Hib) was the leading cause of bacterial meningitis in children. Since the introduction of the Hib vaccine, the epidemiology of invasive *H influenzae* infections has shifted and is now dominated by nontypeable *H influenzae* species. Additionally,

Disclosure Statement: The authors have nothing to disclose.
[a] Division of Pediatric Critical Care Medicine, Department of Pediatrics, Seattle Children's Hospital, University of Washington School of Medicine, FA.2.112, 4800 Sand Point Way NE, Seattle, WA 98105, USA; [b] Division of Pediatric Infectious Diseases, Children's Mercy, Kansas City, University of Missouri-Kansas City School of Medicine, 2401 Gillham Road, Kansas City, MO 64108, USA
* Corresponding author.
E-mail address: amyers@cmh.edu

Infect Dis Clin N Am 32 (2018) 119–128
https://doi.org/10.1016/j.idc.2017.10.005
id.theclinics.com

antibiotic resistance of *H influenzae* has steadily increased because of the emergence of β-lactamase–producing strains. *H influenzae* remains a common cause of morbidity and mortality for children, particularly in the developing world.

MICROBIOLOGY

H influenzae is a nonmotile gram-negative bacteria, most often appearing in the form of small coccobacilli. Isolates are further classified based on the presence of capsular polysaccharides (typeable) versus unencapsulated (nontypeable) strains. Typeable strains of *H influenzae* are subdivided by the expression of one of 6 antigenically distinct capsular polysaccharides (a through f). *H influenzae* is capable of both aerobic and anaerobic metabolism.[1,2]

H influenzae has several virulence factors important to the pathogenesis in human disease. The presence of a polysaccharide capsule is the most important virulence factor in typeable strains of *H influenzae*. The capsule confers resistance to phagocytosis and complement-mediated lysis. Other important virulence factors include noncapsular cell wall proteins, which aid in attachment and acquisition of iron; lipooligosaccharide, which is similar in property to lipopolysaccharide; and immunoglobulin A (IgA) proteases, which cleave and, thus, inactivate IgA1, increasing the ability of the bacteria to adhere to mucous membranes.[3]

Although nontypeable strains have often been thought of as less invasive, these strains are still capable of colonizing the nasopharynx and resisting the mucociliary clearance mechanism via adhesions, such as outer membrane protein P2 and P5, high-molecular-weight proteins 1 and 2, *H influenzae* adhesion protein, pili, and a nonpilus adhesion autotransporter protein (Hap). Hap has been shown to promote adhesion to the respiratory epithelium and increase bacterial aggregation.[3] Nontypeable *H influenzae* also possess IgA proteases.[4]

EPIDEMIOLOGY

H influenzae frequently colonizes the nasopharynx of humans, and the major reservoir is infants and toddlers. Transmission occurs through respiratory secretions via droplet inhalation and/or direct contact. Neonatal transmission can also occur through aspiration of amniotic fluid or contact with genital secretions.[1]

Before the Hib vaccine, most preschool-aged children developed intermittent colonization with Hib in the nasopharynx at some point in time.[2,5] Colonization declines after 18 months but occurs in up to 50% of children younger than 5 years of age.[6] During this time, Hib was the leading cause of bacterial meningitis in children younger than 5 years in the United States, with approximately 17,000 to 21,000 cases per year.[7] Hib was also a cause of bacterial pneumonia, epiglottitis, septic arthritis, and purulent pericarditis.[2]

Since the introduction of the Hib vaccine in 1985, the incidence of invasive Hib disease has dramatically decreased. The incidence among children younger than 5 years has decreased by approximately 99%, with 8 cases reported in the United States in 2015.[8] The rate of colonization with Hib has also decreased to less than 1%.[8] Disease due to Hib now primarily occurs in unimmunized children, including closed communities (eg, Amish).[9] Additional groups at risk for invasive Hib disease include those with human immunodeficiency virus (HIV), impaired splenic function, some immunodeficiencies, and impaired immune function secondary to malignancy and/or chemotherapy.[1] Hib remains a major cause of both meningitis and pneumonia in resource-poor and developing nations where vaccination is unavailable.

The epidemiology of invasive *H influenzae* has dramatically shifted after vaccine introduction. Nontypeable *H influenzae* is now the major cause of invasive disease across all age groups and causes 62.5% of invasive disease cases in children younger than 5 years (annual incidence of 1.73 per 100,000).[1,8] Although Hib had a predilection for causing meningitis, nontypeable *H influenzae* causes bacteremia alone in up to 75% of invasive infections.[10] Nontypeable *H influenzae* remains a common cause of localized upper respiratory infections, accounting for approximately 50% of acute sinusitis and otitis media in children.[1]

Non–type b (a–f) encapsulated strains have been shown to have an annual estimated incidence of 2.23 per 100,000 in children less than 1 year of age and 0.47 per 100,000 in children 1 to 4 years of age.[8] Recently, *H influenzae* type a has emerged as an important pathogen in certain North American populations, mainly Alaskan Natives and Native Americans. Epidemiologic data from 2002 to 2012 demonstrated a yearly incidence of *H influenzae* type a in Alaskan Native children of 18 per 100,000 versus 0.5 per 100,000 in the non-Native pediatric population. Although the specific reason for the increased risk in these populations is unknown, studies have suggested the influence of genetic alterations resulting in more virulent *H influenzae* type a strains and increased carrier rates within these communities.[8,11]

CLINICAL MANIFESTATIONS
Haemophilus influenzae Type B

Nearly all invasive Hib disease begins with bacteremia. The most common manifestation of invasive Hib disease is meningitis, occurring in approximately 40% to 75% of invasive disease cases.[12,13] Rarely, meningitis may occur from direct extension from otitis media or sinusitis. Patients typically present with symptoms, such as fever or hypothermia (especially in neonates), emesis, altered mental status, and/or irritability. Physical examination findings consistent with meningitis include the Kernig sign (pain elicited following flexion of the hip and extension of the knee), the Brudzinski sign (flexion of the hips caused by passive flexion of the neck), cranial nerve abnormalities, hyperreflexia, and inconsolability.[14] Suspected bacterial meningitis is a medical emergency, as mortality for untreated disease is nearly 100%. Bacterial complications of Hib meningitis include intracranial abscess, hydrocephalus, subdural effusion or empyema, and ventriculitis. Neurologic complications are listed in **Box 1**. The Centers for Disease Control and Prevention (CDC) report a mortality rate of Hib meningitis of 3% to 6%. An additional 15% to 30% of survivors will demonstrate neurologic sequelae, most commonly sensorineural hearing loss.[2]

Box 1
Neurologic sequelae

- Seizures
- Sensorineural hearing loss
- Language delay
- Developmental delay
- Gross motor abnormalities
- Vision impairment
- Behavioral abnormalities
- Syndrome of inappropriate antidiuretic hormone

In contrast to the young age in which Hib meningitis is seen, epiglottitis is classically seen in older children between 2 and 7 years of age. Epiglottitis, a potentially life-threatening condition, involves epiglottis and aryepiglottic folds; symptoms typically include high fever, sore throat, drooling, dysphagia, stridor, and acute airway obstruction. Patients often present in acute distress and appear anxious and/or agitated. Children may place themselves in a sitting position with extension of the neck to reduce airway obstruction. In cases of suspected epiglottitis, direct laryngoscopy with placement of an endotracheal tube in a controlled environment is indicated, as sudden deterioration can occur. Bacteremia is found in up to 90% of children, and mortality ranges from 5% to 10% and is caused by airway compromise.

Pneumonia related to Hib typically presents as a consolidative pulmonary process with empyema in up to 50% of cases. Complications include necrotizing pneumonia and invasion of the pericardium resulting in purulent pericarditis. It is important to note that up to 25% of Hib pneumonia cases are associated with comorbid meningitis or epiglottitis. Although Hib pneumonia typically resolves without any sequelae in developed nations, significant morbidity and mortality remain in developing nations.

Nontypeable Haemophilus influenzae

Nontypeable H influenzae most commonly causes upper respiratory tract infections, such as acute otitis media (AOM) and acute sinusitis. According to several studies since 2000, 44% to 59% of AOM in children is caused by nontypeable H influenzae.[15–17] Furthermore, nontypeable H influenzae has emerged as the main cause of persistent AOM and of clinical failures of AOM treatment. Since the development of the pneumococcal conjugate vaccine, the percent of persistent AOM caused by nontypeable H influenzae has increased from 38% to 57%. This increase coincided with a significant increase in β-lactamase-producing nontypeable H influenzae species isolated from children between 1998 and 2003.[18] Despite this increase, current data suggest that approximately 58% to 82% of H influenzae isolates are susceptible to regular and high-dose amoxicillin.[17]

Based on the current epidemiology, the American Academy of Pediatrics (AAP) recommends high-dose amoxicillin (90 mg/kg/d) as the recommended first-line treatment of most patients with AOM.[17] AOM secondary to nontypeable H influenzae can also occur in association with infection of the conjunctiva, termed the conjunctivitis-otitis syndrome. Accordingly, the AAP's 2013 guidelines for AOM recommend extended coverage for β-lactamase–producing nontypeable H influenzae in the setting of concurrent AOM and conjunctivitis.[17] Alternative treatment regimens for patients with penicillin allergy are included in Table 1.

Table 1
Recommended therapies for treatment of AOM

Recommended Antibiotic	Alternative Therapy (Penicillin Allergy)
AOM • Amoxicillin (80–90 mg/kg/d in 2 divided doses) or AOM with conjunctivitis • Amoxicillin-clavulanate (80–90 mg/kg/d of amoxicillin component and 6.4 mg/kg/d of clavulanate component in 2 divided doses)	• Cefdinir (14 mg/kg/d in 1 or 2 divided doses) • Cefuroxime (30 mg/kg/d in 2 divided doses) • Cefpodoxime (10 mg/kg/d in 2 divided doses) • Ceftriaxone (50 mg/kg/d IM or IV for 1–3 days)

Abbreviations: AOM, acute otitis media; IM, intramuscularly.

H influenzae is the causal organism in approximately 30% of acute bacterial sinusitis cases in children. Similar to AOM, the introduction of the Hib and pneumococcal conjugate vaccine (PCV-13) have resulted in a steady increase in the incidence of infections due to nontypeable *H influenzae*. The recommended first-line treatment of uncomplicated acute bacterial sinusitis is amoxicillin or amoxicillin-clavulanate, although the latter may be optimized in cases where antimicrobial resistance is suspected.[19,20]

In addition to upper respiratory tract infections, nontypeable *H influenzae* is an important neonatal pathogen, causing 2% to 8% of early onset sepsis. Neonatal infection occurs most frequently in premature infants and often presents within the first several hours of life. Acquisition of infection is primarily the maternal genital tract, and strain concordance has been found. However, disease has occurred in infants born via cesarean delivery as well. Mortality is nearly 50%.[21]

Non–Type B Haemophilus influenzae

Non–type b *H influenzae* causes disease and sequelae similar to Hib and has been identified as a major cause of invasive *H influenzae* infection in certain populations. *H influenzae* type a (Hia) invasive disease emerged in Native Alaskans, indigenous Canadians, and children in Navajo reservations in the previous decade.[22] Similar to Hib disease, Hia was most commonly seen in children less than 5 years of age.[22] Overall, the rate of invasive disease due to the combined non–type b *H influenzae* strains (a–f) is lower than that of nontypeable *H influenzae*. However, the rate of non–type b *H influenzae* infections exceeds the rate of invasive Hib infections for all ages in the United States. In 2015, the rate of invasive Hib infections was 0.02 per 100,000 persons and serotype non–type b was 0.42 per 100,000 persons. (CDC)[8] Unlike Hib, there is no recommendation for prophylaxis of close contacts following invasive infection with non–type b *H influenzae*, as secondary disease is rare, although non-b strains should be reported to the CDC through the state health department for epidemiologic purposes.

DIAGNOSIS

Diagnosis of invasive *H influenzae* disease is achieved by growth within infected body fluid, including cerebrospinal fluid (CSF), blood, pleural fluid, middle ear effusion, or synovial fluid. Optimal growth occurs with the use of either chocolate agar or Fildes medium. Aerobic growth of *H influenzae* appears as gram-negative pleomorphic coccobacilli requiring supplementation of both heat-stable factor X (hemin) and heat-labile factor V (nicotinamide-adenine-dinucleotide [NAD]). Both are readily available in chocolate agar plates, which have undergone heat or enzymatic lysis of red blood cells, thus, causing release of both hemin and NAD. Growth from the blood culture is seen in most patients with invasive disease. Although isolation from the CSF is the gold standard for diagnosis of meningitis, studies in children have described cases of Hib meningitis with normal CSF studies.[23] For this reason, normal CSF results do not eliminate the possibility of bacterial meningitis in the setting of high clinical suspicion. Once identified, it is recommended that all invasive *H influenzae* isolates be serotyped in order to facilitate earlier recognition of potential outbreaks and improve understanding of the current epidemiology.[8,9]

Diagnostic tools, such as enzyme immunoassay, immunoelectrophoresis, and slide agglutination serotyping, can aid in diagnosis through antigen detection of type b capsular polysaccharide, although sensitivity and specificity may not be optimal. Antigen testing can be performed on CSF, urine, and serum samples and may be useful in the setting of antimicrobial pretreatment. Recently, advances in polymerase chain reaction (PCR) testing have provided further means of capsular typing, with a diagnostic sensitivity of 72% to 92% for Hib.[1,24]

Typeable *H influenzae* is identified as type a through f using type-specific antisera in a slide agglutination serotyping (SAST) method. Depending on the reagents used, the sensitivity and specificity may be low for SAST; thus, PCR may be performed.[25] Serotyping is routinely performed at state health department microbiology laboratories. Further strain typing of both nontypeable and typeable strains of *H influenzae* may be performed by multi-locus sequence testing (MLST), which has been described previously.[26] Each isolate is identified by the allelic profile. Each unique allelic profile is deemed a clone and assigned a sequence type (ST). Clusters of related STs are termed *clonal complexes* or *lineages* and come from a common ancestor. The MLST database contains the allelic profiles and other information about *H influenzae* strains (https://pubmlst.org/hinfluenzae/) and is accessible to clinicians and researchers alike.

TREATMENT

Recommendations for first-line antibiotic treatment of invasive *H influenzae* have changed over the past 20 years because of the increasing rates of antibiotic resistance secondary to β-lactamase production. Although *H influenzae* was classically treated with aminopenicillins, such as ampicillin and/or amoxicillin, resistance to these agents has been reported as high as 40% to 50%. Resistance is known to be mediated by both plasmid-mediated β-lactamases and a decreased affinity of penicillin-binding protein.[1,27]

Current guidelines recommend empirical treatment of suspected *H influenzae* meningitis or invasive disease with a third-generation cephalosporin, such as ceftriaxone or cefotaxime. Intravenous therapy is typically continued for 7 to 10 days or longer depending on the nature of the infection (**Table 2**).[1] In the case of Hib meningitis, adjunctive treatment with dexamethasone is recommended because of the evidence of decreased rates of sensorineural hearing loss and other neurologic sequelae, such as ataxia and hemiparesis.[28] A dosage of 0.15 mg/kg every 6 hours for 2 to 4 days is currently recommended by the AAP Committee on Infectious Diseases. Treatment with dexamethasone should be initiated within 1 hour of the first dose of antibiotics.[1,24]

Despite increasing rates of antibiotic resistance in *H influenzae*, the recommended first-line treatment of AOM in children is amoxicillin, as the most common pathogen continues to be *Streptococcus pneumoniae*. If no improvement with amoxicillin is seen, use of a beta-lactam antibiotic with beta-lactamase, such as amoxicillin-clavulanate, or an oral second- or third-generation cephalosporin should be considered.[17] In the setting of sinusitis, amoxicillin or amoxicillin-clavulanate are both considered to be first-line agents.[19,20] Isolation of middle ear fluid for culture and susceptibility testing may be helpful for guiding therapy in refractory cases.[1]

Table 2	
Disease specific treatment length recommendations	
Disease Process	**Treatment Length**
• Meningitis	• 10 d (uncomplicated)
• Septic arthritis	• 10–14 d
• Pericarditis	• 3–6 wk
• Empyema	• 3–6 wk
• Osteomyelitis	• 3–6 wk

PREVENTION
Vaccination

The first Hib vaccine was introduced in the United States in 1985. It was a monovalent vaccine made from purified polyribosylribitol phosphate (PRP) capsular material from type b strains. Unfortunately, the vaccine did not produce an adequate antibody response in children less than 24 months of age. Despite promising initial clinical trials performed in Finland, reporting protection rates of 90% for children greater than 18 months of age, subsequent studies in the United States demonstrated poor protection rates.[2,29]

Based on the poor efficacy of the first-generation polysaccharide PRP vaccine, the AAP Committee on Infectious Diseases recommended a change to a Hib polysaccharide vaccine in 1987. Over the following 2 years, 3 monovalent conjugate Hib vaccines were developed and licensed by the Food and Drug Administration (FDA) for use in children 15 months of age and older. The FDA later approved the use of the conjugate Hib vaccines in infants. Currently there are 2 monovalent PRP conjugate vaccine options and 4 Hib containing combination vaccines that are licensed for use in the primary series (**Table 3**).[2]

The Advisory Committee on Immunization Practices recommends the administration of Hib vaccination starting at 2 months of age. The first dose of the vaccine series can be given as early as 6 weeks of age if needed. Following completion of the primary series (see **Table 3**), a booster dose is recommended at 12 to 15 months of age. It is recommended that vaccine doses be administered 8 weeks apart; however, a minimal interval of 4 weeks is acceptable. The recommended vaccination catch-up schedule is available through the CDC's Web site (available at http://www.cdc.gov/vaccines/schedules/hcp/imz/catchup.html).[2]

High-Risk Groups

In addition to unimmunized and underimmunized young children, certain children are at an increased risk to develop invasive *H influenzae* infection compared with the population at large. These high-risk groups include patients with impaired splenic function; such as sickle cell disease, asplenia, HIV, immunoglobulin deficiencies (including IgG

Table 3
Routine *Haemophilus influenzae* type b vaccine recommendations

Vaccine Product	Primary Series	Booster Dose	Caveats
Monovalent			
PRP-OMP (Pedvaxhib)	2, 4 mo	12–15 mo	Third dose needed to complete primary series if <2 doses of PRP-OMP
PRP-T (ActHib)	2, 4, 6 mo	12–15 mo	—
PRP-T (Hiberix)	2, 4, 6 mo±	12–15 mo	Newly licensed for primary series±[30] Does not protect against N meningitidis types A and W.
Combination			
PRP-OMP-HepB (Comvax)	2, 4 mo	12–15 mo	Third dose needed to complete primary series if <2 doses of PRP-OMP
DTaP/IPV-PRP-T (Pentacel)	2, 4, 6 mo	15–18 mo	May be given as early as 12 months
MenCY/PRP-T (MenHibRix)	2, 4, 6 mo	12–15 mo	

Abbreviations: DTaP, diphtheria, tetanus, and pertussis vaccine; HepB, hepatitis B; IPV, inactivated polio vaccine; MenCY, meningococcal vaccine types C and Y; OMP, outer membrane protein complex from Neisseria meningitidis; PRP-T, polyribosylribotol phosphate-tetanus toxoid.

subclass 2), and early complement component deficiencies. Additionally, patients with an oncologic diagnosis who have undergone hematopoietic stem cell transplant, chemotherapy, or radiation are at an increased risk of invasive infection with *H influenzae* infection. Finally, Native Americans and Alaskans and indigenous Canadians are known to be at a higher risk for invasive *Haemophilus* infection. In some situations, Hib vaccination is recommended beyond 59 months of age. For patients who are unimmunized (not completed primary series), a dose of Hib vaccine is recommended 2 weeks before splenectomy. Additionally, patients undergoing hematopoietic stem cell transplant should be revaccinated with a 3-dose series at least 4 weeks apart 6 or more months following transplant.

Postexposure Prophylaxis

Postexposure chemoprophylaxis is an important aspect of secondary case prevention. Populations at high risk for secondary infection include household contacts of the index case aged less than 48 months of age, especially those 12 months of age and younger. Prophylaxis with rifampin (20 mg/kg once daily for 4 days; maximum dose 600 mg) has been shown to eradicate nasopharyngeal carriage of Hib in approximately 95% of carriers.[1,2] The CDC recommends rifampin chemoprophylaxis for the index case, all household contacts in households with children less than 48 months of age who are unimmunized or underimmunized, and households with members less than 18 years of age who are immunocompromised.[2] Additionally, rifampin chemoprophylaxis is recommended for childcare attendees when 2 or more cases of invasive Hib disease occur in the same facility within a 60-day period. In this setting, prophylaxis should be given to all attendees and childcare providers.[2] Finally, immunization campaigns have been conducted to decrease the risk of secondary cases in the setting of Hib disease in closed, unimmunized populations.[9]

SUMMARY

Before the 1990s, *H influenzae* type b disease was a major cause of bacterial meningitis and other invasive infections, among children less than 5 years of age in the United States. Hib disease is now rare because of the introduction of Hib vaccine into the routine immunization schedule and maintenance of high vaccine coverage. However, cases of invasive Hib disease continue to be seen in children who are unimmunized or underimmunized, highlighting the need for continued immunization of all children to prevent Hib disease. Although Hib disease is now rare, invasive infections with nontypeable and with non–type b *H influenzae* still occur and should be considered in patients with growth of pleomorphic gram-negative coccobacilli on chocolate but not routine blood agar plates. Additionally, noninvasive infection with nontypeable *H influenzae* is a common cause of AOM and sinusitis in children. The length of treatment depends on the site of infection, and all invasive disease caused by non–type b *H influenzae* should be reported to the state health department for epidemiologic tracking.

REFERENCES

1. American Academy of Pediatrics. *Haemophilus influenzae* infections. In: Kimberlin D, Brady M, Jackson M, et al, editors. Red book 2015: report of the committee on infectious diseases. Elk Grove Village (IL): American Academy of Pediatrics; 2015. p. 368–76.
2. Briere EC, Rubin L, Moro PL, et al. Prevention and control of *Haemophilus influenzae* type b disease: recommendations of the Advisory Committee on Immunization Practices (ACIP). MMWR 2014;63(1):1–14.

3. Fink DL, Bescher AZ, Green B, et al. The *Haemophilus influenzae* Hap autotrans- porter mediates microcolony formation and adherence to epithelial cells and extracellular matrix via binding regions in the C-terminal end of the passenger domain. Cell Microbiol 2003;5(3):175–86.

4. Clementi CF, Murphy TF. Non-typeable *Haemophilus influenzae* invasion and persistence in the human respiratory tract. Front Cell Infect Microbiol 2011;1(1): 1–9.

5. Mohle-Boetani J, Ajello G, Breneman E, et al. Carriage of *Haemophilus influenzae* type b in children after widespread vaccination with conjugate *Haemophilus influenzae* type b vaccines. Pediatr Infect Dis J 1993;12:589–93.

6. Murphy TF, Granoff D, Chrane DF, et al. Pharyngeal colonization with *Haemophilus influenzae* type b in children in a day care center without invasive disease. J Pediatr 1985;106:712–6.

7. Cochi SL, Broome CV. Vaccine prevention of *Haemophilus influenzae* type b disease: past, present and future. Pediatr Infect Dis 1986;5(1):12–9.

8. Centers for Disease Control and Prevention. 2015. Active bacterial core surveillance report, Emerging Infections Program Network, Haemophilus influenza 2015. Available at: https://www.cdc.gov/abcs/reports-findings/survreports/hib15. html. Accessed July 21, 2017.

9. Myers AL, Jackson MA, Zhang L, et al. Haemophilus influenza type b invasive disease in Amish children, Missouri, USA, 2014. Emerg Infect Dis 2017;23(1): 112–4.

10. O'Neill JM, St. Geme JW, Cutter D, et al. Invasive disease due to nontypeable *Haemophilus influenzae* among children in Arkansas. J Clin Microbiol 2003; 41(7):3064–9.

11. Hammitt LL, Block S, Hennessy TW, et al. Outbreak of invasive *Haemophilus influenzae* serotype a disease. Pediatr Infect Dis J 2005;24:453–6.

12. Takala AK, Ekola J, Peltola H, et al. Epidemiology of invasive *Haemophilus influenzae* type b disease among children in Finland before vaccination with *Haemophilus influenzae* type b conjugate vaccine. Pediatr Infect Dis J 1989;8(5): 297–302.

13. Tozzi AE, Salmaso S, Ciofi degli Atti ML, et al. Incidence of *Haemophilus influenzae* type b disease in Italian children. Eur J Epidemiol 1997;13(1):73–7.

14. Kim KS. Acute bacterial meningitis in infants and children. Lancet Infect Dis 2010; 10(1):32–42.

15. Hendley JO. Otitis media. N Engl J Med 2002;347:1169–74.

16. Grubb MS, Spaugh DC. Microbiology of acute otitis media, Puget Sound region, 2005-2009. Clin Pediatr (Phila) 2010;49(8):727–30.

17. Lieberthal AS, Carroll AE, Chonmaitree T, et al. Clinical practice guideline: the diagnosis and management of acute otitis media. Pediatrics 2013;131:e964–99.

18. Casey JR, Pichichero ME. Changes in frequency and pathogens causing acute otitis media in 1995-2003. Pediatr Infect Dis J 2004;23:824–8.

19. Wald ER, Applegate KE, Bordley C, et al. Clinical practice guideline: clinical practice guideline for the diagnosis and management of acute bacterial sinusitis in children aged 1 to 18 years. Pediatrics 2013;132:e262–80.

20. Chow AW, Benninger MS, Brook I, et al. Infectious Diseases Society of America: IDSA clinical practice guideline for acute bacterial rhinosinusitis in children and adults. Clin Infect Dis 2012;54(8):e72–112.

21. Friesen CA, Cho CT. Characteristic features of neonatal sepsis due to *Haemophilus influenza*. Rev Infect Dis 1986;8(5):777–80.

22. Bruce MG, Zulz T, Debyle C, et al. Haemophilus influenzae serotype a invasive disease, Alaska, USA, 1983-2011. Emerg Infect Dis 2013;19:932–7.
23. Hegenbarth MA, Green M, Rowley AH, et al. Absent or minimal cerebrospinal fluid abnormalities in *Haemophilus influenza* meningitis. Pediatr Emerg Care 1990;6(3):191–4.
24. Swanson D. Meningitis. Pediatr Rev 2015;36(12):514–26.
25. LaClaire LL, Tondella ML, Beall DS, et al. Identification of Haemophilus influenzae serotypes by standard slide agglutination serotyping and PCR-based capsule typing. J Clin Microbiol 2003;41:393–6.
26. Meats E, Feil EJ, Stringer S, et al. Characterization of encapsulated and nonencapsulated haemophilus influenzae and determination of phylogenetic relationships by multilocus sequence typing. J Clin Microbiol 2003;41:1623–36.
27. Kishii K, Chiba N, Morozumi M, et al. Diverse mutations in the ftsI gene in ampicillin-resistant *Haemophilus influenzae* isolates from pediatric patients with acute otitis media. J Infect Chemother 2010;16(2):87–93.
28. Odio CM, Faingezicht I, Paris M, et al. The beneficial effects of early dexamethasone administration in infants and children with bacterial meningitis. N Engl J Med 1991;324:1525–31.
29. Ward JI, Broome CV, Harrison LH, et al. *Haemophilus influenzae* type b vaccines: lessons for the future. Pediatrics 1988;81(6):886–93.
30. Briere EC. Food and drug administration approval for use of hiberix as a 3-dose primary *Haemophilus influenzae* type b (Hib) vaccination series. MMWR Morb Mortal Wkly Rep 2016;65:418–9.

Syphilis in Children

Sarah Heston, MD, Sandra Arnold, MD, MSc*

KEYWORDS

- Syphilis • Congenital infection • Antibodies • Penicillin G

KEY POINTS

- Congenital and acquired syphilis are common infections around the world and cases are increasing in the United States after declining for many years.
- Syphilis is diagnosed using serology. Nontreponemal antibodies against cardiolipin are measured to screen for syphilis and the diagnosis is confirmed with treponemal specific antibodies.
- The drug of choice for treating syphilis is parenteral penicillin G; route and duration of therapy are determined by the stage of infection and neurologic involvement.
- All pregnant women should be screened for syphilis and treated as soon as possible after the diagnosis is confirmed.
- All neonates born to mothers who tested positive for syphilis should have maternal titers and treatment reviewed as well as a nontreponemal antibody titer and complete clinical evaluation.

INTRODUCTION

Syphilis is caused by *Treponema pallidum*, a spirochete that is transmitted sexually and transplacentally.[1] If untreated, syphilis is a progressive disease that may result in death or disability from cardiac or neurologic complications in adults.[2] Untreated congenital syphilis also results in death or significant neurologic and musculoskeletal disabilities.[3–5] The diagnosis of syphilis requires 2-stage serologic testing for nontreponemal and treponemal antibodies[1,6]; however, reverse testing algorithms allow the use of automated screening for treponemal antibodies.[7] A diagnosis of congenital syphilis requires careful review of maternal testing and treatment, comparison of maternal and neonatal nontreponemal antibody titers, and clinical evaluation of the neonate.[6,8,9] In this review, we present the current epidemiology of syphilis, and the clinical manifestations, diagnosis, and management of syphilis as they relate to

The authors have no conflicts of interest to disclose.
Department of Pediatrics, University of Tennessee Health Science Center, Le Bonheur Children's Hospital, Faculty Office Building, 49 North Dunlap Street, Room 293, Memphis, TN 38105, USA
* Corresponding author.
E-mail address: sarnold5@uthsc.edu

Infect Dis Clin N Am 32 (2018) 129–144
https://doi.org/10.1016/j.idc.2017.11.007
0891-5520/18/© 2017 Elsevier Inc. All rights reserved.

pediatric practice, specifically, congenital syphilis and acquired syphilis in adolescents and pregnant women.

ACQUIRED SYPHILIS
Epidemiology

The global burden of syphilis along with other sexually transmitted infections remains high with approximately 1 million new infections (syphilis, chlamydia, gonorrhea, and trichomoniasis) daily.[9,10] Worldwide, the rate of syphilis in 2015 was 25.7 cases per 100,000 adults. The burden of syphilis is highest among female sex workers and men who have sex with men (MSM), for whom the prevalence is 5%.[10]

After reaching an all-time low of 2.1 cases per 100,000 population in 2000, primary and secondary syphilis rates[11] have been increasing in the United States, reaching 7.5 cases per 100,000 in 2015, a 67% increase since 2011.[11] Cases in men account for 90% of this change across all ages (including adolescents), races, ethnicities, and regions; as in other countries, cases in MSM predominate.[11] In addition, a 27.3% increase in cases in women was seen in 2014 and 2015 to a rate of 1.4 cases per 100,000.[11] This increase has led to a call to action by the Centers for Disease Control and Prevention to federal and state agencies and health care providers to improve the identification of and access to treatment for at-risk individuals, and, to research and industry, to develop novel diagnostic tests and vaccines to combat syphilis.[12]

Clinical Disease

Acquired syphilis presents in a similar fashion regardless of age of acquisition, although signs of tertiary syphilis rarely present in childhood. Syphilis has 3 stages with varying clinical manifestations (**Table 1**). The hallmark of primary syphilis is 1 or more chancres (painless ulcers) at the site of primary inoculation. Secondary syphilis, resulting from dissemination of infection, typically presents as a polymorphous rash involving the palms and soles, fever, and lymphadenopathy along with other findings (see **Table 1**). Signs and symptoms of secondary syphilis overlap with other self-limited infectious conditions, often obscuring the diagnosis. Untreated syphilis enters a latent, asymptomatic, stage for a variable length of time, during which infected persons remain seropositive but not contagious. Signs of tertiary syphilis occur 10 to 30 years after initial infection. Manifestations include gummas (granulomatous skin and tissue growths), and cardiovascular and central nervous system involvement (see **Table 1**). Neurosyphilis may be diagnosed at any stage of symptomatic infection and is more common in individuals infected with the human immunodeficiency virus (HIV).[2,13]

Diagnosis

Although screening for syphilis is not routinely recommended for sexually active adolescents, it is recommended yearly in MSM and in all pregnant females at the first prenatal visit (including adolescents in both groups). A systematic review of screening for syphilis concluded that screening high risk-men (HIV positive or MSM) every 3 months improved early syphilis detection, but no data on the effect of screening on clinical outcomes was available.[14] Adolescents diagnosed with other sexually transmitted infections (chlamydia, gonorrhea, HIV) should be screened for syphilis.[6]

Darkfield microscopy of lesion scrapings to identify organisms is diagnostic, but is infrequently performed in practice.[1,6] Syphilis is diagnosed using serologic tests that are classified as nontreponemal and treponemal.[1,6] Nontreponemal tests detect

Table 1
Clinical features and diagnosis of acquired syphilis

Syphilis Stage	Clinical Manifestations	Diagnostic Tests
Primary	• One or more chancres (painless ulcers) at site of inoculation (genital, perianal, oral) • Occurs approximately 3 wk after exposure • Resolve spontaneously after weeks	• Nontreponemal test (RPR/VDRL) positive • Nontreponemal test may be negative in very early disease in ≤15% • Treponemal test positive • Organisms present on darkfield examination of chancre exudate

Secondary	• Dermatologic manifestations
	  ○ Polymorphous rash including palms and soles
	  ○ Condylomata lata (moist, flat, wartlike lesions)
	  ○ Mucous patches
	• Systemic manifestation
	  ○ Fever
	  ○ Nontender lymphadenopathy
	  ○ Headache, aseptic meningitis
	  ○ Arthralgia, myalgia
	  ○ Alopecia
	• Rarely nephropathy, hepatitis, gastritis, arthritis, periostitis, optic neuritis, uveitis neurosyphilis
	• Occurs 1–2 mo after primary syphilis and resolves in 1–3 mo
		• Nontreponemal test (RPR/VDRL) positive
		• Treponemal test positive
		• Organisms present on darkfield examination scrapings from mucocutaneous lesions or aspirates of lymph nodes
		• CSF VDRL may be positive in neurosyphilis (frequent false negative tests)
		• CSF cell count (>5 WBCs/mm^3 and protein elevated in neurosyphilis

Latent	• Asymptomatic • Classified as early latent (within 1 year of infections) and late latent (>1 year after infection) ○ Cases of unknown duration classified as late latent	• Nontreponemal test (RPR/VDRL) positive • Treponemal tests positive

Tertiary	• Occurs 15–30 y after primary infection
	• Neurologic
	  ○ Dementia
	  ○ Tables dorsalis
	  ○ Meningovascular (strokes)
	  ○ Visual impairment, hearing loss
	  ○ Gummas
	• Heart disease
	  ○ Ascending aortitis, aortic aneurysms
	• Gummas
	  ○ Granulomatous growths (cutaneous/subcutaneous) unique to tertiary syphilis involving skin, palate, nasal cartilage (saddle nose), liver, brain, heart, skin, bone, testis
		• Nontreponemal test (RPR/VDRL) positive in most but falsely negative in up to 25%
		• Treponemal test positive
		• Spirochetes not found in gummas

Abbreviations: CSF, cerebrospinal fluid; RPR, rapid plasma regain; VDRL, Venereal Disease Research Laboratory test; WBC, white blood cell.

antibody to cardiolipin and include the Venereal Disease Research Laboratory (VDRL) slide test and the rapid plasma reagin (RPR). Nontreponemal tests are used for screening because they have high sensitivity and the quantitative results can be used to assess response to therapy. Confirmatory testing is needed due to the low specificity of nontreponemal tests and is achieved by testing for antibodies directed against *T pallidum*, that is, treponemal tests (fluorescent treponemal antibody absorbed; *T pallidum* particle agglutination; and treponemal immunoassays, namely, enzyme immunoassays [EIA] and chemiluminescence assay [CIA]).[6] Two-stage testing has been used for decades and generally performs with high sensitivity and specificity[6]; however, it is labor intensive and not conducive to mass testing, RPR/VDRL are subject to the prozone phenomenon (false-negative result in the presence of high antibody titer), and RPR/VDRL may be falsely negative early in infection.[6]

Over the last 20 years, reverse sequence has evolved to evaluate nonpregnant individuals using EIA/CIA as the initial screen. This algorithm allows automated, high-throughput screening, which is more efficient and cost effective.[15] In reverse sequence testing, the initial test is a highly sensitive treponemal test (EIA or CIA) **(Fig. 1)**. If this test is negative, no further testing is required. If the test is positive, quantitative RPR is performed. If the RPR is positive, then the patient is determined to have syphilis, either past or present. If the RPR is negative (ie, discrepant result), a *T pallidum* particle agglutination is performed that, if negative, makes syphilis unlikely and, if positive, indicates past or present syphilis. Limitations of this algorithm include a high false-positive rate of the EIA/CIA tests and the confusion that results from discrepant results between EIA/CIA and RPR.[6,7,15–17]

The presence of neurologic symptoms such as cranial nerve dysfunction, ocular or auditory problems, meningitis, stroke, altered mental status, and loss of vibration sense should raise suspicion for neurosyphilis.[6,9,13] Individuals with these findings should be evaluated with a lumbar puncture for cell count, protein, and cerebrospinal fluid (CSF) VDRL, as well as ophthalmologic examination. Cell count and protein are very sensitive diagnostic tests for neurosyphilis, but lack specificity because they may be abnormal in early syphilis and spontaneously improve. CSF VDRL is a very specific but insensitive indicator of neurosyphilis; thus, neurosyphilis should still be strongly considered if there are clinical indicators of neurologic disease and reactive serology even if the CSF VDRL is negative. Some experts recommend evaluation for neurosyphilis in all patients with HIV and syphilis.[6,9,13]

Treatment

The drug of choice for the treatment of all stages of syphilis in all ages of patients is penicillin G, either benzathine, aqueous procaine, or aqueous crystalline.[6,18,19] The dose, route, and duration of treatment depend on the stage of disease with longer illness duration (latent disease of unknown duration, late latent, and tertiary) requiring more prolonged therapy **(Table 2)**. Alternative antibiotic therapies in nonpregnant children or adults who are allergic to penicillin include doxycycline 100 mg orally twice a day, tetracycline 500 mg 4 times a day for 14 days, and ceftriaxone (optimal dose and duration are not known).[6,20] Pregnant women with penicillin allergy must be desensitized and treated with penicillin.[6] Details of treatment dose, route, and duration are outlined in **Table 2**. All individuals diagnosed with syphilis should be screened for other sexually transmitted infections, including HIV.

Clinical and serologic follow-up is required to document treatment response because treatment failures can occur. Nontreponemal test titers should decrease 4-fold (eg, from 1:32 to 1:8) within 6 to 12 months of appropriate treatment. If this change fails to occur, patients should be followed for longer or retreated if follow-up

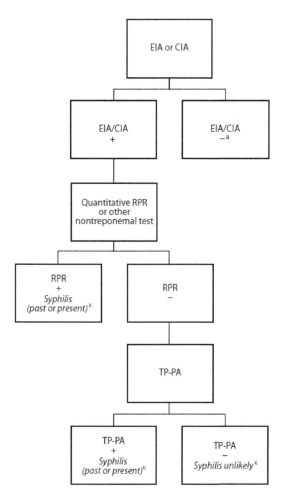

Fig. 1. Recommended algorithm for reverse sequence syphilis screening. EIA/CIA, enzyme immunoassay/chemiluminescence immunoassay; RPR, rapid plasma reagin; *T pallidum* particle agglutination, *Treponema pallidum* particle agglutination. Despite these recommendations for reverse sequence screening, the Centers for Disease Control and Prevention (CDC) continue to recommend the traditional algorithm with reactive nontreponemal tests confirmed by treponemal testing. [a] If incubating or primary syphilis is suspected, treat with benzathine penicillin G 2.4 million units intramuscularly in a single dose. [b] Evaluate clinically, determine whether treated for syphilis in the past, assess risk for infection, and administer therapy according to CDC's *2010 STD Treatment Guidelines* (available at: http://www.cdc. gov/std/treatment/2010). [c] If at risk for syphilis, repeat RPR in several weeks. (*From* Centers for Disease Control and Prevention. Discordant results from reverse sequence syphilis screening–five laboratories, United States, 2006–2010. MMWR Morb Mortal Wkly Rep 2011;60(5):133–7.)

is in doubt.[6] If a 4-fold increase in titer or new symptoms develop, treatment failure or reinfection has occurred and these patients need to be tested for HIV and neurosyphilis, then retreated with benzathine penicillin G 2.4 million units intramuscularly (IM) for weekly for 3 weeks or, if neurosyphilis is present, 10 to 14 days of intravenous penicillin G or daily IM procaine penicillin G with probenecid (see **Table 2**). Neurosyphilis

Table 2
Treatment of acquired and congenital syphilis

Acquired Syphilis	Treatment
Primary or secondary[a]	
Adult	Benzathine penicillin[b] G 2.4 million units IM in a single dose
Child	Benzathine penicillin G 50,000 U/kg IM to maximum of 2.4 million units in a single dose
Early latent[a]	
Adult	Benzathine penicillin[b] G 2.4 million units IM in a single dose
Child	Benzathine penicillin G 50,000 U/kg IM to maximum of 2.4 million units in a single dose
Late latent or unknown duration[a]	
Adult	Benzathine penicillin G 2.4 million units IM, weekly for 3 wk[c] (7.2 million units total)
Child	Benzathine penicillin G 50,000 U/kg IM to maximum of 2.4 million units weekly for 3 wk (150,000 U/kg up to 7.2 million units total)
Tertiary with normal CSF[a]	Benzathine penicillin G 2.4 million units IM, weekly for 3 wk (7.2 million units total)
Neurosyphilis or ocular syphilis[a]	Aqueous crystalline penicillin G 18–24 million U/d (3–4 million units IV every 4 h for 10–14 d) OR Procaine penicillin G 2.4 million units IM once daily with probenecid 500 mg by mouth QID both for 10–14 d
Congenital syphilis	
Proven or probable	Aqueous crystalline penicillin G 50,000 U/kg/dose given every 12 h for the first 7 d of life and every 8 h thereafter for 10 d[e] OR Procaine penicillin G 50,000 U/kg/d IM once daily for 10 d
Possible	Aqueous crystalline penicillin G 50,000 U/kg/dose given every 12 h the first 7 d of life and every 8 h thereafter for 10 d[e] OR Procaine penicillin G 50,000 U/kg/d IM once daily for 10 d OR Benzathine penicillin G 50,000 U/kg IM in a single dose[d]
Late	Aqueous crystalline penicillin G 50,000 U/kg/dose given every 4–6 h for 10 d with or without benzathine penicillin G 50,000 U/kg IM in a single dose at the end of therapy OR Procaine penicillin G 50,000 U/kg/d IM once daily for 10 d OR Benzathine penicillin G 50,000 U/kg IM once a week for 3 wk[e]

Abbreviations: CSF, cerebrospinal fluid; IM, intramuscularly.

[a] Persons with human immunodeficiency virus (HIV) infection should be treated in the same manner according to stage of disease. There should be a low threshold for evaluation and treatment of neurosyphilis in persons with HIV infection. Anyone diagnosed with syphilis should be screened for HIV infection.

[b] Alternatives to penicillin are found in the text. Pregnant women and those with neurosyphilis should only be treated with penicillin. Allergic subjects should be desensitized and treated with penicillin.

[c] If more than 10–14 d elapse between doses, the entire course must be restarted. In pregnant women, the dosing must occur at 7-d intervals or the course must be restarted.

[d] Should only be done if congenital syphilis is considered less likely or thorough evaluation is normal and mother has received adequate treatment. Usually given in the setting where follow-up is not well-assured to document appropriate fall in maternal and infant titers.

[e] This regimen should only be used if neurosyphilis has been excluded.

patients should have CSF examinations repeated every 6 months until the cell count is normal. If the cell count is not declining after 6 months, consideration should be given to retreatment.[6]

CONGENITAL SYPHILIS
Epidemiology

The World Health Organization closely monitors congenital syphilis and syphilis screening of pregnant women as part of their efforts toward global elimination of congenital syphilis. Between 2008 and 2012, a 30% worldwide reduction in cases of congenital syphilis occurred, coincident with increases in antenatal screening. Among screened women in regions monitored by the World Health Organization, the prevalence of syphilis remains high at 1%, indicating an ongoing, urgent need to increase antenatal screening.[10]

In the United States since 2012, a 46% increase in cases of congenital syphilis has occurred after a steady decrease for many years.[6,21] This increase parallels the increase in primary and secondary syphilis among women of reproductive age.[21] Congenital syphilis results from a lack of prenatal care and missed opportunities for screening.[22,23] A systematic review of interventions to improve screening for syphilis in pregnancy estimated that interventions to improve the coverage and effect of screening worldwide could reduce syphilis-associated stillbirth and perinatal death by 50%.[24]

Risk factors for congenital syphilis involve maternal and treatment-related factors, and include few prenatal visits, rural residence, previous pregnancy loss, indeterminate disease duration in the mother, treatment in the third trimester, high nontreponemal titer at the time of diagnosis, and younger gestational age of the infant at the time of the maternal diagnosis and treatment for syphilis.[25–28] These risk factors are confounded by maternal reinfection and inappropriate treatment regimens (eg, not receiving 3 doses for late latent infection).[25]

Syphilis can be transmitted to the fetus at any gestational age.[29] The stage of the mother's disease determines the likelihood of transmission; primary and secondary syphilis are associated with a 60% to 100% rate of transmission, early latent with a 40% rate, and late latent with an 8% rate.[28,30] A systematic review of adverse pregnancy outcomes associated with maternal seroreactivity to syphilis demonstrated that approximately 66% of pregnancies with syphilis were complicated by an adverse pregnancy outcome versus 14% without syphilis.[31] Overall, the prevalence of stillbirth and fetal loss, neonatal death, symptomatic congenital syphilis, and prematurity and low birthweight for syphilis-affected pregnancies were 25%, 12%, 15%, and 12%, respectively. In the United States, the case fatality rate of congenital syphilis (stillbirth and neonatal deaths) is 6.5%, with 85% of these stillbirths.[4,5] The majority of live born infants with congenital syphilis are asymptomatic at birth (80% by clinical examination and 54% if results of laboratory testing included),[5,21] but may develop symptoms within 3 to 8 weeks or later.[32,33] Live born infants with congenital syphilis are more likely to have low birth weight and be premature.[4]

Clinical Disease

The consequences of untreated congenital syphilis include chronic bone, joint, dental, and neurologic morbidities.[3,26,33,34] Early manifestations of congenital syphilis occur before the age of 2 years.[5,26,28,35–37] A complete list of clinical findings is presented in **Box 1**. Asymptomatically infected infants who are missed at birth present later but may not have typical signs and symptoms resulting in delayed diagnosis.[33] For the

Box 1
Clinical findings of congenital syphilis

Early Congenital Syphilis

General
- Prematurity
- Fetal demise
- Small for gestational age
- Nonimmune hydrops
- Fever

Hematologic
- Anemia
- Thrombocytopenia
- Hepatosplenomegaly

Mucocutaneous
- Snuffles/rhinitis
- Maculopapular rash that progresses to desquamation and is present on palms and soles

Skeletal
- Long-bone changes, commonly femur, tibia, and humerus
- Osteitis
- Localized demineralization of proximal tibia metaphysis (Wimberger sign)
- Diaphyseal periostitis

Neurologic/ophthalmologic
- Elevated protein, pleocytosis, positive VDRL of CSF
- Acute meningitis
- Hydrocephalus
- Chorioretinitis
- Cataract
- Glaucoma

Other systems
- Pneumonia
- Myocarditis
- Necrotizing enterocolitis
- Nephrotic syndrome

Late Congenital syphilis

Skeletal
- Frontal bossae of Parrot
- Short maxilla
- High palatal arch
- Saddle nose
- Saber shins
- Clutton's joints, symmetric arthritis of knees and elbows
- Higoumenaki's sign, thickening of clavicle at sternoclavicular joint

Oral
- Hutchison teeth, widely spaced, notched incisors[a]
- Mulberry molars, with multiple cusps
- Hard palate perforation

Neurologic/ophthalmologic
- Intellectual disability
- Sensorineural hearing loss[a]
- Hydrocephalus
- Cranial nerve palsy
- Interstitial keratitis[a]

Other systems
- Rhagades, perioral fissures
- Mucocutaneous gummas
- Paroxysmal cold hemoglobinuria

Abbreviations: CSF, cerebrospinal fluid; VDRL, Venereal Disease Research Laboratory test.
[a] These 3 features referred to as Hutchison's triad.

most part, the diagnosis of congenital syphilis requires a careful review of maternal serology and treatment because many infants with congenital syphilis will have only serologic evidence of disease (see sections on Maternal and Infant Testing).[1,8,9,28,32,38–41]

Late congenital syphilis occurs in individuals presenting with signs and symptoms after the age of 2 years. This late presentation is a result of missed diagnosis at birth in an asymptomatic newborn lacking appropriate review of maternal and infant serology, infants exposed to maternal infection a short time before delivery with negative nontreponemal testing at birth[41] (mother and infant), or failure to respond to neonatal treatment with inadequate follow-up. The findings of late congenital syphilis predominantly affect the central nervous system, bones and joints, teeth, eyes, and skin (see **Box 1**).[3,9,29,34]

Maternal Testing

All pregnant women should be screened for syphilis at the first prenatal visit, or, if follow-up is in doubt, at the time of confirmation of pregnancy.[6,42] Treatment should be initiated immediately to prevent transmission to the developing fetus.[31,38,43,44] Additional testing after 28 weeks and at delivery is indicated for women at higher risk and in specific geographic areas where syphilis is common.[6] Screening of pregnant women may be done using the traditional or reverse testing algorithms.[6,45] In geographic areas where syphilis is prevalent, the traditional screening algorithm should be used to limit unnecessary treponemal testing in women who have been previously diagnosed with and treated for syphilis.[6] Nontreponemal serologic titers should decrease 4-fold within 6 to 12 months after therapy[6,9]; however, depending on the timing of diagnosis and treatment in gestation, a reduction in titer may not be documented before delivery because insufficient time has elapsed. This circumstance complicates the determination of the infant's risk of congenital infection. This topic is discussed further in the section on Treatment Guidance. Women who deliver without prenatal care as well as women diagnosed with syphilis and treated in pregnancy should be tested at the time of delivery. Mothers and infants should not be discharged until results are reviewed.[6,9]

Prenatal ultrasound examination may reveal abnormalities suggestive of congenital syphilis.[38,43,46] Up to 31% of prenatal ultrasound examinations done before treatment demonstrated abnormalities including hepatomegaly, placentomegaly, polyhydramnios, ascites, and elevated middle cerebral artery velocimetry.[43] Women with abnormal ultrasound examinations were more likely to be diagnosed with syphilis later in pregnancy, to have fewer prenatal visits, and to be treated later in pregnancy.[43] After treatment, middle cerebral artery abnormalities, ascites, and polyhydramnios were of the first defects to resolve on ultrasound examination. Placentomegaly and hepatomegaly remained present the longest and, often, hepatomegaly was still present at the time of birth. There was no difference in the severity of ultrasound abnormalities and stage of maternal syphilis infection, and some congenitally infected infants had normal ultrasound findings.[43]

Infant Testing

Darkfield microscopy is the gold standard for identifying *T pallidum* in fluids or tissues; however, this test is rarely done in practice. Pathologic examination of the placenta might demonstrate compatible histology or spirochetes by Warthin Starry silver staining. Immunofluorescent staining of specimens may be done in place of darkfield microscopy. Failure to observe organism with any of these tests does not exclude a diagnosis of syphilis.[1,6,9,32] Diagnosis is usually made through review of neonatal nontreponemal antibody titers, although interpretation of results is complicated by maternal transfer of antibodies.[6,9,32,40] Additional tests that provide support for the diagnosis of congenital syphilis include polymerase chain reaction,[32] and a variety of IgM assays on maternal and infant serum, although none has been approved for the diagnosis of congenital syphilis in the United States.[30,32,40,46] The IgM immunoblot and the IgM enzyme-linked immunosorbent assay seem to be the most sensitive and specific tests, but a negative test does not exclude the diagnosis of congenital syphilis.[6] Umbilical cord blood should not be used for neonatal testing because there is a high risk of a false-negative test.[6,8] Results of maternal testing and treatment before and during pregnancy must be obtained and reviewed in conjunction with the newborn and current maternal nontreponemal titer to make treatment decisions for the baby.[6,9,40] Any concerning lesions or secretions should be evaluated with darkfield microscopy or immunofluorescent staining if available.[6] All infants should be evaluated for HIV infection.

The decision to treat a newborn and the type and duration of therapy is based upon the likelihood of congenital syphilis. The Centers for Disease Control and Prevention defines these risk groups as proven or highly probable congenital syphilis, possible congenital syphilis, congenital syphilis less likely, and congenital syphilis unlikely.[6] The diagnostic criteria for and evaluation and treatment of neonates in each category is outlined in detail in **Fig. 2**.[6]

Beyond review of nontreponemal titers and maternal therapy, the evaluation of an infant for congenital syphilis includes a thorough physical examination, complete blood count with differential, liver enzymes and bilirubin, ophthalmologic and audiologic evaluation, and diagnostic imaging, which may include long bone and chest radiographs, and neuroimaging.[6,9,47] Central nervous system imaging may reveal findings of meningovascular disease with or without infarction, leptomeningeal enhancement, and/or parenchymal masses.[48] Long bone films show metaphysitis (metaphyseal bands or bony destruction of the metaphyses) as well as periostitis (layered periosteal reaction)[49] and osteitis of the diaphysis, all of which result from changes in osseous development during the period of rapid growth during gestation.[47] Erosion of the inner aspects of the tibia is known as Wimberger's sign.[50] These bone findings are most commonly present in symptomatic infants and are rarely seen without other findings of congenital syphilis. Although of limited usefulness in the asymptomatic infection, these radiographs remain part of the recommended evaluation.[6] The chest radiograph in congenital syphilis may demonstrate coarse nodules throughout bilateral lungs, especially at the bases, with bands radiating from the hilar region, which is distinct from the radiographic findings in neonates with respiratory failure owing to hyaline membrane disease.[36] Lung diseases is a well-described but uncommon manifestation of early congenital syphilis.

CSF examination for cell count, protein, and VDRL is recommended for infants with probable or possible congenital syphilis[6,9,51]; however, the need for CSF examination has been questioned. In 2 studies, CSF VDRL was rarely positive and positive results did not influence treatment, because those with positive test results qualified for a full course of parenteral therapy based on infant and maternal RPR titers and maternal treatment history.[52,53] Many CSF specimens are of limited usefulness as a result of blood contamination or insufficient quantity. The CSF VDRL lacks sensitivity and is often negative in infants with neurosyphilis.[51] There are no universally agreed upon values for leukocyte count and protein for the diagnosis of neurosyphilis in the neonate. The recommended upper limits of normal for CSF leukocyte count is greater than 25 cells/mm^3 and for protein greater than 150 mg/dL; however, lower values (>5 leukocytes/mm^3 protein >40 mg/dL) could be abnormal, and values between these 2 levels overlap significantly in children with and without evidence of

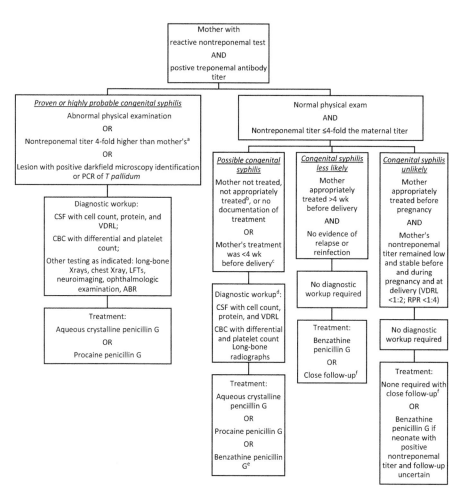

Fig. 2. Recommendations for evaluation and treatment of congenital syphilis. ABR, auditory brainstem response; CBC, complete blood count; CSF, cerebrospinal fluid; LFTs, liver function tests; PCR, polymerase chain reaction; RPR, rapid plasma reagin test; VDRL, Venereal Disease Research Laboratory test. Treatment regimen for aqueous crystalline penicillin G: 50,000 U/kg/dose IV every 12 hours in the first 7 days of life and every 8 hours thereafter for total of 10 days; procaine penicillin G: 50,000 U/kg/dose IM every 24 hours for total of 10 days; benzathine penicillin G: 50,000 U/kg/dose IM in single dose. [a] Lack of 4-fold or greater nontreponemal titer does not exclude congenital syphilis. [b] Not appropriately treated could mean inadequate dosing or duration of penicillin G therapy or non-penicillin G treatment. [c] If untreated, early syphilis at delivery, consider treating for 10 days with parenteral penicillin G, because these infants are at greatest risk of congenital syphilis. [d] Diagnostic workup not required if treated with 10 days of parenteral penicillin G therapy. [e] Diagnostic workup must be complete and normal, and follow-up must be ensured. [f] Close follow-up is defined as serologic titers every 2 to 3 months for 6 months and reevaluation and treatment if nontreponemal titers are positive. (Adapted from Workowski KA, Bolan GA, Centers for Disease Control and Prevention. Sexually transmitted diseases treatment guidelines, 2015. MMWR Recomm Rep 2015;64(RR-03):1–137.)

neurosyphilis.[6] The lumbar puncture is, thus, considered of limited value in the assessment of an infant at risk for congenital syphilis, despite recommendations from expert bodies.[6,9] Practically, most clinicians err on the side of treating with 10 days of penicillin G because the consequences of congenital syphilis are severe and appropriate follow-up is not easily ensured.

Treatment

Treatment recommendations and options are outlined in **Table 2**. Infants with proven or probable infection require 10 days of intravenous aqueous or intramuscular procaine penicillin G.[6] If treatment interruption occurs, treatment must be restarted for an additional 10 days. Treatment days on other antibiotics, even other penicillins such as ampicillin, cannot count toward therapy for congenital syphilis because there is insufficient data to support their use in congenital syphilis.[6] Ceftriaxone has been studied but is only recommended if a shortage of aqueous penicillin G exists.[6,20]

Neonates with possible congenital syphilis are usually treated with a full 10-day course of intravenous aqueous or IM procaine penicillin G. They may receive a single dose of IM benzathine penicillin G if the recommended evaluation for congenital infection (see **Fig. 2**) is complete and negative, and close follow-up is assured.[6] The guideline strongly recommends that if any results from the evaluation are missing or difficult to interpret, for example, CSF studies contaminated with blood, or if follow-up is in question, then a full 10-day course of penicillin G should be given.[6] If a 10-day course of therapy is planned, an infant need not necessarily be subjected to a complete evaluation (eg, CSF examination, long bone radiographs) because this treatment regimen provides appropriate therapy for neurosyphilis.

Neonates less likely to have congenital infection may receive IM benzathine penicillin G in a single dose or receive no treatment if follow-up for repeat nontreponemal serology every 2 to 3 months for 6 months is assured.[6] Newborns unlikely to have congenital syphilis require no treatment; however, close follow-up with repeat nontreponemal titers is required for those with a reactive nontreponemal antibody titer that is not more than 4-fold lower than the mother's titer. Benzathine penicillin G is an option for these infants as well.[6]

Follow-up

After nursery discharge, neonates born with reactive syphilis serology should undergo assessment with a physical examination and nontreponemal testing every 2 to 3 months until the titers are nonreactive.[6,9] For infants with maternal transfer of nontreponemal antibodies, titers will decrease by 3 months of age and usually be negative by 6 months of age.[6,9] Antibody titers in infected but treated infants should decrease by 4-fold within 6 to 12 months. Untreated infants with positive nontreponemal serology at 6 months after evaluation should undergo treatment. Those treated as a neonate who still have reactive serology at 6 to 12 months of age should be reevaluated (including CSF studies) and receive another course of penicillin.[6] If the nontreponemal titers were nonreactive at birth in an infant born to a mother with early syphilis infection, another nontreponemal assay should be performed at 3 months to ensure that infection of the infant did not occur near the time of delivery.[6]

In general, treponemal antibodies are of no diagnostic value in monitoring the response to treatment because they remain positive for life in infected infants. In infants who were evaluated and/or treated for congenital syphilis but were not actually infected, passively acquired maternal treponemal antibodies will revert to negative after approximately 15 months of age.[54] A positive treponemal test is only diagnostic of congenital syphilis if collected at or after 18 months of age,[9] which is too late to prevent possible further sequelae.

Neonates who underwent lumbar puncture in the nursery and had abnormal results should undergo repeat lumbar puncture every 6 months until results are normal. If the CSF VDRL remains positive or other parameters (white blood cell count or protein level) do not normalize, this is an indication for retreatment. Neuroimaging should be considered at this time as well.[6,9]

Congenital Syphilis in Older Infants and Children

Children with congenital syphilis missed at birth can present with symptomatic congenital syphilis at any time. If a reactive nontreponemal antibody is first discovered once the infant is older than 1 month of age, the infant or child should undergo complete workup for congenital syphilis, including lumbar puncture with VDRL on CSF, CBC with differential and platelet count, HIV testing, long bone radiographs, chest radiograph, liver function panel, abdominal ultrasound imaging, neuroimaging, ophthalmologic examination, and hearing evaluations.[6] Treatment consists of intravenous aqueous penicillin G, 200,000 to 300,000 U/kg/d divided every 4 to 6 hours for 10 days that may also be followed by 1 dose of IM benzathine penicillin 50,000 U/kg after the 10-day course.[6,9] However, if the examination and complete laboratory workup are negative for neurosyphilis, the infant or child may be treated with 3 weekly doses of IM benzathine 50,000 units per kilogram.[6,9]

SUMMARY

Acquired and congenital syphilis continue to cause disease in high-risk populations. Improved methods of screening these high-risk populations and preventive measures such as vaccines are needed if syphilis is to be eradicated. The World Health Organization has a goal to eradicate congenital syphilis. This goal will require high rates of compliance with current screening and treatment regimens and ongoing vigilance if achieved.

REFERENCES

1. Larsen SA, Steiner BM, Rudolph AH. Laboratory diagnosis and interpretation of tests for syphilis. Clin Microbiol Rev 1995;8(1):1–21.
2. Rockwell DH, Yobs A, Moore M Jr. The Tuskegee study of untreated syphilis: the 30th year of observation. Arch Intern Med 1964;114(6):792–8.
3. Fiumara NJ, Lessell S. Manifestations of late congenital syphilis. An analysis of 271 patients. Arch Dermatol 1970;102(1):78–83.
4. Gust DA, Levine WC, St Louis ME, et al. Mortality associated with congenital syphilis in the United States, 1992-1998. Pediatrics 2002;109(5):E79-9.
5. Su JR, Brooks LC, Davis DW, et al. Congenital syphilis: trends in mortality and morbidity in the United States, 1999 through 2013. Am J Obstet Gynecol 2016; 214(3):381.e1-9.
6. Workowski KA, Bolan GA, Centers for Disease Control and Prevention. Sexually transmitted diseases treatment guidelines, 2015. MMWR Recomm Rep 2015; 64(RR-03):1–137.
7. Centers for Disease Control and Prevention. Discordant results from reverse sequence syphilis screening–five laboratories, United States, 2006-2010. MMWR Morb Mortal Wkly Rep 2011;60(5):133–7.
8. Chhabra RS, Brion LP, Castro M, et al. Comparison of maternal sera, cord blood, and neonatal sera for detecting presumptive congenital syphilis: relationship with maternal treatment. Pediatrics 1993;91(1):88–91.

9. American Academy of Pediatrics. Syphilis. In: Kimberlin DW, Brady MT, Jackson MA, et al, editors. Red book: 2015 report of the committee on infectious diseases. Elk Grove Village (IL): American Academy of Pediatrics; 2015. p. 755–68.

10. World Health O. Report on global sexually transmitted infection surveillance. 2015. Available at: http://apps.who.int/iris/bitstream/10665/249553/1/9789241565301-eng.pdf?ua=1.

11. Centers for Disease Control and Prevention. Sexually transmitted disease surveillance 2016. Atlanta (GA): US Department of Health and Human Services; 2017.

12. Centers for Disease Control and Prevention. CDC call to action: let's work together to stem the tide of rising syphilis in the United States. 2017. Available at: https://www.cdc.gov/std/syphilis/SyphilisCalltoActionApril2017.pdf.

13. Radolf JD, Tramont EC, Salazar JC. Syphilis (*Treponema pallidum*). In: Bennett JE, Dolin R, Blaser MJ, editors. Mandell, Douglas, and Bennett's principles and practice of infectious diseases. 8th edition. New York: Elsevier; 2015. p. 2684–709.

14. Cantor AG, Pappas M, Daeges M, et al. Screening for syphilis: updated evidence report and systematic review for the us preventive services task force. Jama 2016;315(21):2328–37.

15. Tong ML, Lin LR, Liu LL, et al. Analysis of 3 algorithms for syphilis serodiagnosis and implications for clinical management. Clin Infect Dis 2014;58(8):1116–24.

16. Goswami ND, Stout JE, Miller WC, et al. The footprint of old syphilis: using a reverse screening algorithm for syphilis testing in a U.S. Geographic information systems-based community outreach program. Sex Transm Dis 2013;40(11): 839–41.

17. Rhoads DD, Genzen JR, Bashleben CP, et al. Prevalence of traditional and reverse-algorithm syphilis screening in laboratory practice: a survey of participants in the college of American pathologists syphilis serology proficiency testing program. Arch Pathol Lab Med 2017;141(1):93–7.

18. Walker GJ. Antibiotics for syphilis diagnosed during pregnancy. Cochrane Database Syst Rev 2001;(3):CD001143.

19. Clement ME, Okeke NL, Hicks CB. Treatment of syphilis: a systematic review. JAMA 2014;312(18):1905–17.

20. Zhou P, Gu Z, Xu J, et al. A study evaluating ceftriaxone as a treatment agent for primary and secondary syphilis in pregnancy. Sex Transm Dis 2005;32(8):495–8.

21. Bowen V, Su J, Torrone E, et al. Increase in incidence of congenital syphilis - United States, 2012-2014. MMWR Morb Mortal Wkly Rep 2015;64(44):1241–5.

22. Newman L, Kamb M, Hawkes S, et al. Global estimates of syphilis in pregnancy and associated adverse outcomes: analysis of multinational antenatal surveillance data. PLoS Med 2013;10(2):e1001396.

23. Patel SJ, Klinger EJ, O'Toole D, et al. Missed opportunities for preventing congenital syphilis infection in New York City. Obstetrics Gynecol 2012;120(4):882–8.

24. Hawkes S, Matin N, Broutet N, et al. Effectiveness of interventions to improve screening for syphilis in pregnancy: a systematic review and meta-analysis. Lancet Infect Dis 2011;11(9):684–91.

25. McFarlin BL, Bottoms SF, Dock BS, et al. Epidemic syphilis: maternal factors associated with congenital infection. Am J Obstet Gynecol 1994;170(2):535–40.

26. Lago EG, Vaccari A, Fiori RM. Clinical features and follow-up of congenital syphilis. Sex Transm Dis 2013;40(2):85–94.

27. Mobley JA, McKeown RE, Jackson KL, et al. Risk factors for congenital syphilis in infants of women with syphilis in South Carolina. Am J Public Health 1998;88(4): 597–602.

28. Wicher V, Wicher K. Pathogenesis of maternal-fetal syphilis revisited. Clin Infect Dis 2001;33(3):354–63.

29. Pessoa L, Galvao V. Clinical aspects of congenital syphilis with Hutchinson's triad. BMJ Case Rep 2011;2011 [pii:bcr1120115130].

30. Sanchez PJ, Wendel GD Jr, Grimprel E, et al. Evaluation of molecular methodologies and rabbit infectivity testing for the diagnosis of congenital syphilis and neonatal central nervous system invasion by Treponema pallidum. J Infect Dis 1993;167(1):148–57.

31. Gomez GB, Kamb ML, Newman LM, et al. Untreated maternal syphilis and adverse outcomes of pregnancy: a systematic review and meta-analysis. Bull World Health Organ 2013;91(3):217–26.

32. Herremans T, Kortbeek L, Notermans DW. A review of diagnostic tests for congenital syphilis in newborns. Eur J Clin Microbiol Infect Dis 2010;29(5): 495–501.

33. Dorfman DH, Glaser JH. Congenital syphilis presenting in infants after the newborn period. N Engl J Med 1990;323(19):1299–302.

34. Christian CW, Lavelle J, Bell LM. Preschoolers with syphilis. Pediatrics 1999; 103(1):E4.

35. Zhou Q, Wang L, Chen C, et al. A case series of 130 neonates with congenital syphilis: preterm neonates had more clinical evidences of infection than term neonates. Neonatology 2012;102(2):152–6.

36. Pieper CH, van Gelderen WF, Smith J, et al. Chest radiographs of neonates with respiratory failure caused by congenital syphilis. Pediatr Radiol 1995;25(3): 198–200.

37. Basu S, Kumar A. Varied presentations of early congenital syphilis. J Trop Pediatr 2013;59(3):250–4.

38. Hollier LM, Harstad TW, Sanchez PJ, et al. Fetal syphilis: clinical and laboratory characteristics. Obstetrics Gynecol 2001;97(6):947–53.

39. Risser WL, Hwang LY. Problems in the current case definitions of congenital syphilis. J Pediatr 1996;129(4):499–505.

40. Stoll BJ, Lee FK, Larsen S, et al. Clinical and serologic evaluation of neonates for congenital syphilis: a continuing diagnostic dilemma. J Infect Dis 1993;167(5): 1093–9.

41. Wozniak PS, Cantey JB, Zeray F, et al. Congenital syphilis in neonates with nonreactive nontreponemal test results. J Perinatol 2017;37(10):1112–6.

42. Wolff T, Shelton E, Sessions C, et al. Screening for syphilis infection in pregnant women: evidence for the U.S. Preventive Services Task Force reaffirmation recommendation statement. Ann Intern Med 2009;150(10):710–6.

43. Rac MW, Bryant SN, McIntire DD, et al. Progression of ultrasound findings of fetal syphilis after maternal treatment. Am J Obstet Gynecol 2014;211(4)(426):e421–6.

44. Shahrook S, Mori R, Ochirbat T, et al. Strategies of testing for syphilis during pregnancy. Cochrane Database Syst Rev 2014;(10):CD010385.

45. Mmeje O, Chow JM, Davidson L, et al. Discordant syphilis immunoassays in pregnancy: perinatal outcomes and implications for clinical management. Clin Infect Dis 2015;61(7):1049–53.

46. Nathan L, Twickler DM, Peters MT, et al. Fetal syphilis: correlation of sonographic findings and rabbit infectivity testing of amniotic fluid. J Ultrasound Med 1993; 12(2):97–101.

47. Moyer VA, Schneider V, Yetman R, et al. Contribution of long-bone radiographs to the management of congenital syphilis in the newborn infant. Arch Pediatr Adolesc Med 1998;152(4):353–7.
48. Parmar H, Ibrahim M. Pediatric intracranial infections. Neuroimaging Clin N Am 2012;22(4):707–25.
49. Coblentz DR, Cimini R, Mikity VG, et al. Roentgenographic diagnosis of congenital syphilis in the newborn. JAMA 1970;212(6):1061–4.
50. Stephens JR, Arenth J. Wimberger sign in congenital syphilis. J Pediatr 2015; 167(6):1451.
51. Michelow IC, Wendel GD Jr, Norgard MV, et al. Central nervous system infection in congenital syphilis. N Engl J Med 2002;346(23):1792–8.
52. Talati AJ, Koneru P. Neonates at risk for congenital syphilis: radiographic and cerebrospinal fluid evaluations. South Med J 2011;104(12):827–30.
53. Beeram MR, Chopde N, Dawood Y, et al. Lumbar puncture in the evaluation of possible asymptomatic congenital syphilis in neonates. J Pediatr 1996;128(1): 125–9.
54. Rawstron SA, Mehta S, Marcellino L, et al. Congenital syphilis and fluorescent treponemal antibody test reactivity after the age of 1 year. Sex Transm Dis 2001;28(7):412–6.

Encephalitis in US Children

Kevin Messacar, MD[a],*, Marc Fischer, MD, MPH[b],
Samuel R. Dominguez, MD, PhD[a], Kenneth L. Tyler, MD[c],
Mark J. Abzug, MD[a]

KEYWORDS

- Encephalitis • Meningoencephalitis • Myelitis • Herpes simplex virus • Enterovirus
- Anti-NMDA • Arbovirus

KEY POINTS

- Encephalitis is an uncommon and potentially devastating condition of neurologic dysfunction due to brain parenchymal inflammation.
- In the absence of brain biopsy, presence of encephalopathy with clinical findings suggestive of central nervous system inflammation infers a diagnosis of encephalitis.
- Viruses, including herpes simplex viruses and enteroviruses, are the most common causes in children in the United States, although immune-mediated etiologic factors are increasingly recognized and may respond to immune modulation.
- Given the broad differential diagnosis, a staged diagnostic approach can be initially targeted toward common, treatable, and at-risk etiologic factors, followed by broader, more invasive testing for unexplained persistent or severe disease.
- Supportive care with empiric therapy toward bacteria and herpes simplex viruses should be administered during diagnostic evaluation with definitive therapy ultimately tailored toward identified treatable etiologic factors.

INTRODUCTION

Encephalitis is a rare but serious condition of neurologic dysfunction due to inflammation of the brain parenchyma. A wide variety of infectious and noninfectious etiologies are associated with encephalitis, though the cause in more than half of cases remains unexplained despite extensive testing. Given the heterogeneous and wide differential

Disclosure Statement: None of the authors have any conflicts of interest to disclose. K. Messacar receives salary support from NIH 1K23AI128069-01. K.L. Tyler receives grant support from NIH 5R33AI101064, R56NS101208, R21NS103186, and VA MERIT 5I01BX000963. The views expressed in this document are those of the authors and do not necessarily reflect those of the Centers for Disease Control and Prevention.
[a] Department of Pediatrics, University of Colorado, Children's Hospital Colorado, B055, 13123 East 16th Avenue, Aurora, CO 80045, USA; [b] Surveillance and Epidemiology Activity, Arboviral Diseases Branch, Centers for Disease Control and Prevention, 3156 Rampart Road, Fort Collins, CO 80521, USA; [c] Department of Neurology, University of Colorado, 12700 East 19th Avenue, B182, Aurora, CO 80045, USA
* Corresponding author.
E-mail address: kevin.messacar@childrenscolorado.org

Infect Dis Clin N Am 32 (2018) 145–162
https://doi.org/10.1016/j.idc.2017.10.007
id.theclinics.com

diagnosis, epidemiologic, clinical, laboratory, and radiographic factors are necessary to guide the diagnostic evaluation and treatment. This article focuses on the most common causes of acute encephalitis in previously healthy children in the United States and introduces a practical approach to prioritizing diagnostic evaluation and treatment.

CASE DEFINITION

Brain parenchymal inflammation associated with neurologic dysfunction is the strict definition of confirmed encephalitis.[1] However, due to the rarity of premortem brain biopsy specimens available for histopathologic confirmation (particularly in children), clinical correlates are used to infer evidence of probable brain inflammation. Wide variability in criteria used and emphasized by pediatric neurologists and infectious diseases subspecialists was previously used to infer a clinical diagnosis of encephalitis.[2] In 2013, the International Encephalitis Consortium (IEC) created simplified consensus diagnostic criteria for a standardized case definition of encephalitis and encephalopathy of a presumed infectious or autoimmune etiology.[3] Altered mental status for more than 24 hours without an alternative cause is required as evidence of neurologic dysfunction. In addition, supplemental minor criteria must be present (2 for possible, ≥3 for probable or confirmed): fever greater than or equal to 38°C within 72 hours, seizures, new focal neurologic findings, cerebrospinal fluid (CSF) pleocytosis (≥5 white blood cells/μL), neuroimaging with brain parenchymal changes, or electroencephalogram (EEG) consistent with encephalitis (**Fig. 1**). Confirmed cases require pathologic confirmation on brain biopsy, evidence of infection with a microorganism associated with encephalitis, or laboratory evidence of an autoimmune condition associated with encephalitis.

The IEC case definition combines previously distinct categories of encephalopathy and encephalitis without differentiating infectious from postinfectious or noninfectious processes, which may have important therapeutic implications. In cases with altered mental status greater than or equal to 24 hours without signs of an inflammatory response (fever, CSF pleocytosis, parenchymal changes on neuroimaging), a clinical diagnosis of encephalopathy, rather than encephalitis, is appropriate. In cases meeting encephalitis criteria with CSF pleocytosis, meningeal signs, or leptomeningeal enhancement, a clinical diagnosis of meningoencephalitis may be more descriptive.[4]

Several factors should be considered when applying the IEC case definition to pediatric patients. Simple and complex febrile seizures are common occurrences in young children and, in isolation, do not necessitate pursuing a workup for encephalitis if the child has returned to baseline mental status. Normal CSF white blood cell (WBC) counts in infants are higher than those cited for adults and a 95th percentile cutoff of less than or equal to 19 WBCs/μL for infants less than or equal to 1 month and less than or equal to 9 WBCs/μL for infants 1 to 2 months are more commonly used to define pleocytosis in these age groups.[5] Young infants are more likely to have infectious encephalitis without pleocytosis, particularly with enterovirus (EV; ~50%) or human parechovirus (HPeV; pleocytosis uncommon).[6–8] Therefore, as the IEC criteria suggest, CSF pleocytosis is a supportive but not necessary criterion for encephalitis, particularly in young infants.

EPIDEMIOLOGY

Overall, there were 7.3 encephalitis cases per 100,000 person years in the United States during 2000 to 2010,[9] with peak incidence in infants less than 1 year (13.5 per 100,000) and lowest in children ages 10 to 14 years (4.1 per 100,000).[9] Hospital

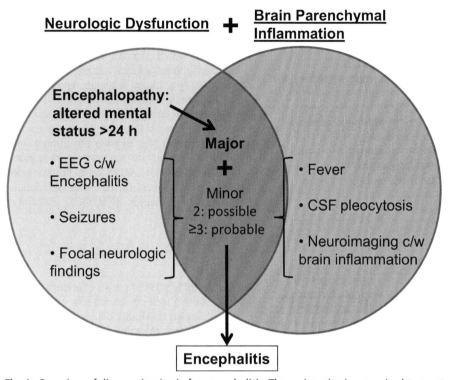

Fig. 1. Overview of diagnostic criteria for encephalitis. The major criterion required to meet the case definition for encephalitis is altered mental status greater than 24 hours without alternative cause identified. Two additional minor criteria are required for possible encephalitis, whereas 3 or more additional minor criteria are required for probable encephalitis. Confirmed encephalitis additionally requires brain tissue disease with inflammation, a diagnosis of a microorganism strongly associated with encephalitis, or laboratory evidence of an autoimmune condition strongly associated with encephalitis. c/w, consistent with.

admissions for encephalitis among the 44 free-standing children's hospitals in the Pediatric Health Information System network in the United States were 7298 from 2004 to 2013 (mean 18 per hospital annually).[10]

The reported incidence of encephalitis in children in the United States and England increased over the past 10 years,[9,10] which may be partially attributed to increasing use of immunosuppressive therapies and bone marrow and solid organ transplantation associated with an increased risk of encephalitis, as well as improved sensitivity of brain parenchymal imaging using MRI. Before this era, the number of encephalitis cases was decreasing following introduction of vaccines against poliovirus, measles virus, mumps virus, varicella virus, and pertussis.[11–13] Seasonal increases in the incidence of encephalitis in children occur over the summer to fall months, largely driven by epidemic and endemic circulation of arboviruses and EVs.[9]

PATHOGENESIS

Though poorly understood for some etiologies a variety of mechanisms contribute to encephalitis. The 2 main forms of encephalitis are primary infectious encephalitis, resulting from direct invasion of the central nervous system (CNS; most commonly gray matter) by the pathogen, and immune-mediated encephalitis, resulting from CNS damage from the immune system (most commonly white matter).[14] Viruses can invade the CNS via viremia, subsequently crossing the blood-brain barrier (eg, arboviruses) or retrograde axonal transport (eg, rabies virus) and infect neurons, leading to cytotoxicity (eg, herpes simplex virus [HSV]). Additionally, pathogens can cause inflammation leading to tissue damage (eg, West Nile virus [WNV]) or cause vasculitis, leading to tissue ischemia (eg, varicella zoster virus [VZV]), or a combination of these mechanisms.[15] Alternatively, primarily nonneuroinvasive pathogens infecting non-CNS sites (eg, *Mycoplasma pneumoniae*, influenza virus respiratory infections), neuroinvasive pathogens infecting the CNS (eg, HSV), tumors (eg, ovarian teratomas), and potentially some vaccinations may trigger CNS autoimmunity due to aberrant immune response against brain antigens. Direct CNS viral infection and triggering of immune-mediated disease may coexist, as illustrated with HSV encephalitis cases with subsequent or concurrent anti–N-methyl-D-aspartate receptor (NMDAR) antibodies identified.[16,17]

DIAGNOSIS
Overview of Etiologies

In the clinical setting, a cause is identified in roughly 50% of cases of encephalitis in children.[9,11] Of unexplained cases, more than 60% lack an identifiable cause even with comprehensive research testing using advanced molecular diagnostic technologies.[18] A broad array of infectious, immune-mediated, rheumatologic, endocrinological, neoplastic, and toxicologic causes all may cause or mimic encephalitis. Infectious causes, including viruses, atypical bacteria, fungi, and parasites are most common, with viruses accounting for most infectious encephalitis cases in children (**Box 1**). Immune-mediated causes of encephalitis include demyelinating conditions, such as acute disseminated encephalomyelitis (ADEM), and neuronal autoantibody–mediated conditions, such as anti-NMDAR encephalitis, and account for an increasing proportion of unexplained encephalitis cases (**Box 2**).[19]

Confirming the Syndromic Diagnosis

The first step in the diagnostic evaluation of a child with suspected encephalitis is to confirm the syndromic diagnosis by looking for evidence of neurologic dysfunction and brain parenchymal inflammation, while ruling out clinical mimickers (eg, toxic ingestion). A comprehensive, detailed history and physical examination is of utmost importance to characterize neurologic deficits, assess for meningeal signs and symptoms, and elicit risk factors. Typical alterations in speech, behavior, and cognition in older individuals with encephalopathy may be more challenging to detect in infants and young children, who present more commonly with irritability, lethargy, or loss of interest in feeding.

Diagnostic testing should include brain MRI, lumbar puncture, and EEG in all suspected cases of encephalitis (**Table 1**). MRI of the brain, with and without contrast using diffusion-weighted, T2-weighted, and fluid-attenuated inversion recovery (FLAIR) sequences, is the modality of choice to assess for changes consistent with brain parenchymal inflammation. After assessing for contraindications, a lumbar puncture with opening pressure measurement should be performed to obtain CSF for characterization of cell counts with differential, glucose, protein, and diagnostic testing. CSF in viral encephalitis typically has a mild to moderate mononuclear pleocytosis (predominantly lymphocytic, though can be neutrophilic early in course), increased protein, and normal glucose; though early in the course or with EV and HPeV infections

---

Box 1
Summary of common viral causes of encephalitis in children

Herpes simplex virus

HSV is the most common infectious cause of encephalitis in children, driven largely by cases of perinatally acquired HSV-2 encephalitis.[9] Neonatal HSV encephalitis is most common in the first month of life with fever, temperature instability, lethargy, seizures, vesicles, or sepsis-like illness. Pregnant women with active genital HSV lesions at delivery should receive acyclovir and deliver via Caesarean section, when possible, to decrease risk of perinatal transmission.[49] Infants born to mothers with active genital HSV lesions at delivery should receive acyclovir while undergoing HSV evaluation.[49,62] HSV evaluation in neonates includes CSF HSV polymerase chain reaction (PCR), as well as surface swab and blood HSV testing, and liver function testing (LFT).[49] Older children commonly present with lethargy, fever, confusion, and seizures. Most children with HSV encephalitis eventually have abnormal CSF with mild lymphocytic pleocytosis and elevated protein, though early samples can be normal.[63] MRI may demonstrate temporal and extratemporal lobe lesions and/or hemorrhage.[29] Diagnosis of HSV encephalitis is made by PCR of CSF (or brain tissue), which may be negative early in the course.[63] Treatment is 3 weeks of intravenous acyclovir, which in neonates should be followed by 6 months of oral acyclovir.[40] Though early antiviral treatment improves outcomes, HSV encephalitis carries a significant risk of mortality and many surviving neonates and children will have neurodevelopmental sequelae.

Enterovirus

EV is the second most common cause of encephalitis in children, most frequently occurring in the first year of life, and largely driven by the predominant circulating serotypes for the given year.[9,61] Neonatal EV encephalitis typically follows maternal EV illness preceding or immediately following delivery as part of a systemic neonatal EV sepsis syndrome. Children with humoral immunodeficiencies (eg, hypogammaglobulinemia) are at higher risk of EV encephalitis and may have chronic infections that are difficult to clear. Children with EV meningoencephalitis can present with fever, headaches, meningism, exanthema, and/or enanthem, with seizures, focal neurologic changes, or alterations in consciousness.[64] EV encephalitis is diagnosed by PCR of CSF, though with certain EVs (eg, poliovirus, EV-A71, EV-D68) CSF may be negative and detection may require testing of throat, rectal, blood, or respiratory specimens.[23] IVIG has not been studied specifically in children with encephalitis, though has shown efficacy in hypogammaglobulinemic children with chronic EV encephalitis. No effective antivirals are currently available.[64] Supportive care remains the mainstay of treatment. Unlike meningitis due to EVs, encephalitis carries increased risk of neurologic compromise.[65]

Human parechovirus

HPeV is recently recognized as an important and common cause of viral encephalitis in young infants. Infants may present with high fevers, sepsis-like illness, seizures, or lethargy. Peripheral leukopenia, elevated LFTs, and a palm-sole rash can be suggestive of HPeV infection.[66,67] CSF typically lacks pleocytosis. Periventricular white matter lesions on MRI are characteristic of HPeV encephalitis.[68] HPeV encephalitis is diagnosed by HPeV-specific CSF PCR and can also be detected from blood, throat, and rectal swabs. Supportive care is the mainstay of therapy because there are no known effective treatments. Though most infants will show short-term improvement, long-term neurodevelopmental sequelae have been described.[58]

Arboviruses[25]

Arboviruses, such as La Crosse virus (LACV), WNV, Eastern equine encephalitis virus (EEEV), Powassan virus (POWV), and St Louis encephalitis virus (SLEV), remain an important cause of seasonal encephalitis in children. LACV is the most common cause of arboviral encephalitis in US children, primarily affecting younger children (mean age 7 years) in Appalachian and Midwestern regions. WNV encephalitis is much less common in children than adults and has widespread distribution throughout the United States. EEEV is a rare cause of severe encephalitis in children (33% case-fatality rate), mostly along the Atlantic and Gulf coasts. POWV is an increasingly recognized tickborne arboviral cause of encephalitis, most common in the upper midwestern United States in the spring months. SLEV caused intermittent epidemics of encephalitis every 10 to 20 years in the United States but may be replaced by WNV due to cross-reactive immunity in birds, the zoonotic host. Arbovirus diagnosis is made by virus-specific IgM testing of serum (probable case) and CSF (confirmed case). Clinical management is supportive because there are no specific treatments.

in young infants abnormalities may be absent.[6-8] Repeat lumbar puncture should be considered if persistent or worsening symptoms for repeat diagnostic testing to assess for evolution of these findings. EEG should be used to look for evidence of encephalopathy, localizing signs, characteristic patterns (eg, periodic localizing epileptiform discharges), or subclinical seizure activity.

Box 2
Summary of selected immune-mediated causes of encephalitis in children

Acute disseminated encephalomyelitis

ADEM is an inflammatory demyelinating CNS condition; it is the most commonly identified immune-mediated encephalitis with highest incidence in early childhood (mean 5–8 years).[69,70] A temporal association with a prodromal illness (commonly upper respiratory tract infection), or rarely vaccination, in the preceding 3 weeks can often be identified.[71,72] Clinical symptoms include acute-onset encephalopathy with multifocal sensory and motor deficits, which depend on the location of the lesions in the brain and spinal cord.[71] MRI of the brain and spine demonstrate asymmetric, bilateral, poorly marginated, hyperintense lesions in the subcortical white and deep gray matter.[70] More than half have abnormal CSF, most commonly mild lymphocytic pleocytosis with elevated protein.[72] Oligoclonal bands are rarely found, unlike in multiple sclerosis.[70,73] Approximately 25% of children will have myelin oligodendrocyte glycoprotein antibodies, which are associated with relapse and optic neuritis.[70] First-line therapy is high-dose intravenous corticosteroids with second-line intravenous immune globulin (IVIG) or plasma exchange (PLEX).[70] Mortality is rare with approximately 80% of children fully recovering with treatment.[71]

Anti-N-methyl-D-aspartate receptor encephalitis

Anti-NMDAR encephalitis is the second leading cause of identified immune-mediated encephalitis in children.[74] In teenagers, a prodromal illness is followed days to weeks later by psychiatric and behavioral symptoms progressing to encephalopathy, seizures, and abnormal movements. Young children eventually develop a similar syndrome but may have more prominent initial behavioral changes (particularly agitation and aggression), speech changes, personality changes, sleep changes, seizures, and movement disorders (particularly gait disturbance).[60,69] Dysautonomia and hypoventilation are less common in children than in adults.[60] MRI is abnormal in less than half of cases but CSF is abnormal in most (lymphocytic pleocytosis and possibly elevated protein or oligoclonal bands) and EEG is abnormal in nearly all (diffuse background slowing, focal slowing, or seizures).[69] Diagnosis is confirmed by antibodies to the NR1 subunit of NMDAR found in serum or CSF, the latter being more specific, with level of titer correlating with prognosis. Though tumor is rare in children[60] (particularly males), if identified, removal improves outcome.[69] Immunotherapy includes first-line treatment with corticosteroids, IVIG, PLEX, or a combination, and secondary options include rituximab and cyclophosphamide.[46,69] Approximately 80% of patients have substantial recovery,[46] though relapse is seen in approximately 25% of children.[60]

Table 1
Diagnostic and therapeutic approach to encephalitis in United States children

	TIER 1		TIER 2
	a. Common and/or Treatable Causes	**b. Selected Testing for Etiologies More Likely Based on Risk Factors**	**Unexplained Persistent or Severe Disease**
Diagnostic Evaluation			
Procedures	• MRI brain ± spinal cord • Lumbar puncture • EEG	• Dilated ophthalmologic examination	• Consider repeat lumbar puncture • Consider brain biopsy: histopathology and immunohistochemical staining, flash-freeze for directed PCRs
CSF Testing	• Cell count and differential, glucose, protein • Culture • HSV PCR • EV PCR (or multiple PCR panels)	• Antineuronal Ab panel • HPeV PCR • VZV PCR • WNV, other arbovirus serology • Wet mount and ameba PCRs • Mycobacterial culture and PCR	• Metagenomic sequencing
Blood Testing	• CBC; CRP, ESR, or PCT; LFTs • Bacterial culture • HSV PCR (neonate) • EV PCR (neonate)	• Antineuronal Ab panel • WNV, other arbovirus serology • HIV serology or PCR • EBV, CMV serology	
Other Site Testing	• Surface swabs (neonate): HSV PCR or culture • Throat or rectal swab: EV PCR	• Respiratory specimen: PCR testing for influenza, mycoplasma, adenovirus (or multiplex panel) • Vesicle: EV, HSV, VZV PCR or culture • Urine toxicology panel • Nape of neck Skin biopsy: rabies PCR	• Brain tissue: Repeat HSV PCR, amebic PCRs • Brain tissue: metagenomic sequencing
Therapeutic Considerations			
Supportive Care	• Manage airway • Manage ICPs or cerebral edema • Control seizures • Rehabilitation therapies • Neuropsychiatric support		
Medications	• Acyclovir until HSV ruled out • Antibiotics until bacterial meningitis ruled out	• Targeted therapy based on identified etiologic causes • Corticosteroids or IVIG or PLEX if immune-mediated encephalitis suspected and potential for active infection sufficiently assessed	

Abbreviations: CMV, cytomegalovirus; DFA, direct fluorescent antibody; EBV, Epstein-Barr virus; HIV, human immunodeficiency virus; ICP, intracranial pressure; IVIG, intravenous immune globulin; LFT, liver function testing; PCR, polymerase chain reaction; PLEX, plasma exchange.

Diagnostic Approach to Identifying an Etiology

The identification of a specific cause may allow initiation of effective, targeted therapies for certain treatable causes, and limit unnecessary diagnostic testing or empiric therapies. Varying levels of evidence establishing a potential etiologic agent as a cause of encephalitis may be present.[20] For established causes of encephalitis, evidence of an etiologic agent in brain tissue specimens or CSF (eg, HSV DNA), or intrathecal antibody production for pathogens in which polymerase chain reaction (PCR) is not the study of choice (eg, WVN IgM antibodies), is considered a confirmed cause. Serologic evidence (eg, serum *Bartonella henselae* IgM antibodies) without PCR confirmation of an established cause that can sometimes be detected directly in CSF or detection of a not well-established cause in brain tissue or CSF by PCR (eg, human herpes virus-6 DNA) are examples of situations that meet the definition of probable cause. Finding suggestive serologic evidence (eg, WVN IgM antibodies in serum) or detection of a well-established pathogen at a site outside the CNS (eg, influenza RNA in respiratory specimens) is considered a possible cause. It is imperative that the clinical presentation and epidemiologic profile are consistent with the etiology detected for all levels of causality to avoid erroneous attribution of causality.

Given the broad array of causes of encephalitis, it is essential to prioritize the differential diagnosis for a targeted, staged diagnostic evaluation (**Table 2**). The authors advocate a 2-tiered approach: (1a) testing for common and/or treatable causes and (1b) selective testing for etiologic agents more likely based on risk factors, and (2) broader and/or more invasive testing for unexplained persistent or severe disease. Additionally, testing and reporting to state public health departments should be considered for certain etiologic agents that carry public health significance (eg, arboviruses, rabies virus, free-living ameba).

Tier 1a: Testing for Common and Treatable Etiologies

The most common infectious pathogens in children include HSV-1, HSV-2, and EVs, which can be identified in CSF, blood, and nonsterile sites (skin lesions and either pharynx or rectum for EVs, or eye, pharynx, or rectum for HSV in neonates). Given that HSV is treatable and carries high morbidity and mortality, all children with encephalitis should be tested for HSV by PCR testing of CSF, with consideration of repeat testing if clinical findings are suggestive and no alternative cause identified.[21] Testing of nonsterile sites increases sensitivity of detection, particularly for HSV in neonates and for EVs uncommonly found in CSF (eg, EV-A71, EV-D68, poliovirus), but must be interpreted with caution.[22,23] Multiplex PCR testing allows for rapid detection of multiple infectious agents, including HSV and EV, using a single test from a small amount of CSF.[24] Given the similar clinical presentations of infectious causes of encephalitis, rapid syndromic testing for a panel of common pathogens using a small volume of CSF may be advantageous. Bacterial meningitis mimicking meningoencephalitis should be considered in any child presenting with fever, headache, meningeal signs and/or encephalopathy, with blood and CSF sent for bacterial cultures.

Tier 1b: Selected Testing for Etiologies More Likely Based on Risk Factors

Targeted diagnostic testing can be directed by assessing host factors, epidemiologic factors, and clinical characteristics (see **Box 1**). The patient's age, immune status, and vaccinations; seasonality, travel, and exposures; as well as clinical signs and symptoms, and localizing findings on imaging and EEG, can all be used to prioritize testing for etiologic agents for which the patient is particularly at-risk.

Table 2
Directed differential diagnosis of encephalitis in United States children

Risk Category	Established Causes	Rare Cause or Mimic[a]
Age		
Neonates or infants	**HSV, CMV**, EV, HPeV	*Toxoplasma gondii, Treponema pallidum*, Zika virus
Teenagers	**HIV**, EBV, WNV	*Treponema pallidum*
Vaccination History		
Unvaccinated	Measles, mumps, rubella, **VZV**, poliovirus	
Recently vaccinated	**ADEM**	
Season		
Summer or fall	EV, WNV, LACV	*Rickettsia, Ehrlichia, Anaplasma, Borrelia burgdorferi*
Winter	**Influenza**, adenovirus	Respiratory viruses
International Travel		
Endemic regions	**Rabies**, JEV, TBEV, Measles	**TB**, dengue, chikungunya, Zika, *Plasmodium*
Animal Exposure		
Bat or Skunk bite	**Rabies**	
Raccoon feces	*Baylisascaris procyonis*	
Rodent	LCMV	
Cat	*Bartonella henselae*	
Mosquito	WNV, LACV, EEEV, SLEV	
Tick	Powassan	*Rickettsia, Ehrlichia, Anaplasma, Borrelia burgdorferi*
Activity		
Freshwater swimming	*N fowleri, Acanthamoeba*	
Eating unpasteurized dairy	*Listeria monocytogenes*	*Toxoplasma, Brucella, Coxiella*
Eating undercooked meat		*Toxoplasma*
Eating undercooked seafood, unwashed vegetables	*Angiostrongylus* **spp**	
Clinical Findings		
Vesicular Rash	**HSV, VZV, EV**	
Lymphadenopathy	**Generalized**: EBV, **CMV, HIV** **Localized**: Bartonella	
Psychiatric or behavioral changes	**Rabies, anti-NMDAR**	
Respiratory symptoms	*Mycoplasma*, **influenza**, adenovirus	Respiratory viruses
Retinitis or keratitis	WNV, **CMV, Bartonella**	*Toxoplasma gondii, Treponema pallidum, Toxocara canis,* or *Toxocara cati*
Parotitis	Mumps, **influenza**, respiratory viruses	

(continued on next page)

Table 2 (continued)		
Risk Category	**Established Causes**	**Rare Cause or Mimic[a]**
Eosinophilic CSF	*Angiostrongylus* spp	*Baylisascaris procyonis, N fowleri, Balamuthia mandrillaris, Acanthamoeba,* **TB, fungi,** *Toxocara canis* or *Toxocara cati*
Imaging or EEG Localization		
Frontal lobe	*N fowleri*	
Temporal lobe	**HSV**	
Thalamus or basal ganglia	WNV, **influenza**	**Respiratory viruses**
Cerebellum	**VZV**	
Brainstem or basilar	*Listeria monocytogenes,* **EV-A71, HSV**	**TB**
Myelitis	Poliovirus, nonpolio EVs, WNV, JEV	

Bold font indicates organisms that are potentially treatable pathogens.

Abbreviations: EEEV, eastern equine encephalitis virus; JEV, Japanese encephalitis virus; LACV, La Crosse virus; LCMV, lymphocytic choriomeningitis virus; SLEV, St Louis encephalitis virus; TB, tuberculosis; TBEV, tickborne encephalitis virus.

[a] Pathogens that are rare causes of encephalitis in immunocompetent US children or that cause a clinical syndrome that mimics encephalitis.

Host factors

In addition to HSV and EV, evaluating for HPeVs in young infants with encephalitis by PCR testing of CSF and potentially blood, throat, and/or rectal samples should be considered.[8,22] Consideration of congenital infections in neonates, such as cytomegalovirus (CMV), syphilis, Zika virus, and toxoplasma, based on clinical characteristics is also warranted. Human immunodeficiency virus (HIV) testing by serology should be considered in all patients at risk, with additional RNA PCR testing conducted in adolescents with concern for acute retroviral syndrome or infants in whom serologic testing may be confounded by maternal antibody. Syphilis also should be considered in adolescent patients with serologic screening followed by CSF VDRL (Venereal Disease Research Laboratory) testing to confirm neurosyphilis. Mumps, measles, varicella, influenza, and polio viruses, are more likely in children who lack immunization and have travel or exposure risk factors for these pathogens. The diagnostic evaluation of a child with a known or concerning history for immunodeficiency or who is receiving immunosuppressive medications warrants a broader diagnostic workup for opportunistic pathogens.

Epidemiologic factors

Seasonality in the spring to fall months, geographic location, and exposure to mosquitoes or ticks can be used to guide testing for arboviruses (eg, La Crosse virus, WVN, Eastern equine encephalitis virus, Powassan virus, and St Louis encephalitis virus),[25] *Rickettsia, Borrelia* (Lyme disease), *Ehrlichia,* or *Anaplasma.* In immunocompetent children, these insect-borne pathogens are best assessed by serologic testing of blood and CSF to detect intrathecal antibody production confirming neuroinvasive disease. A travel history to endemic areas warrants additional testing for exotic arboviruses (eg, chikungunya, dengue, Japanese encephalitis, tickborne encephalitis, or Zika viruses). During the winter months, influenza virus, adenovirus, and other seasonal respiratory viruses associated with encephalitis should be evaluated by PCR testing of respiratory specimens. When tuberculosis risk factors are present, tuberculin skin testing, or interferon-gamma release assay testing, a chest radiograph, and CSF mycobacterial culture and PCR should be obtained.

Exposures

History of animal contact can help guide testing for rabies virus following bites (eg, bats, skunks), *Baylisascaris procyonis* following exposure to raccoon feces or latrines, lymphocytic choriomeningitis virus following rodent exposure, and *Bartonella henselae* following feline exposure. Dietary history can help guide testing for pathogens transmitted via unpasteurized dairy, undercooked meat, seafood, or unwashed vegetables (see **Table 2**). Recreational activities in freshwater are a risk factor for leptospirosis, and *Naegleria fowleri* amebic encephalitis (also transmitted via nonsterile sinus rinses).[26] In contrast, freshwater exposure is typically absent in cases of *Balamuthia mandrillaris* amebic encephalitis, which can be transmitted by soil exposure.[27] A wet mount of CSF looking for free-living ameba can be conducted only on fresh CSF specimens. Specific PCR testing for ameba in CSF or brain tissue (more sensitive) can be conducted through the Centers for Disease Control and Prevention.[28]

Findings on physical examination

The presence of a vesicular rash should prompt HSV, EV, and VZV testing by PCR, or viral culture of an unroofed vesicle swab with CSF PCR testing to confirm a diagnosis. Regional lymphadenopathy can be suggestive of *Bartonella henselae*, whereas diffuse adenopathy may warrant serologic evaluation for systemic viral illnesses such as HIV, Epstein-Barr virus (EBV), or CMV. Ophthalmologic examination can detect characteristic retinitis or keratitis patterns, which may prompt testing for WNV, CMV, or *Bartonella henselae*. Respiratory symptoms should prompt testing for respiratory pathogens associated with encephalitis, including influenza virus, *M pneumoniae*, and adenovirus, many of which can be assessed through PCR testing of respiratory specimens. Parotitis is most commonly found with mumps virus but can be seen with HIV, CMV, EBV, influenza virus, and other respiratory viruses also associated with encephalitis. Hydrophobia and hypersalivation are suggestive, though not sensitive, signs of rabies encephalitis. Prominent behavior or psychiatric changes, abnormal limb movements, and dysautonomia should prompt testing for neuronal autoantibodies, including anti-NMDAR, in serum and CSF.

Findings on diagnostic studies

Certain laboratory, electrophysiological, and imaging patterns can be suggestive of particular etiologies. Eosinophilia in the CSF is always an abnormal finding and should prompt testing for parasites (eg, *Angiostrongylus cantonensis*, *Taenia solium*, *Baylisascaris procyonis*, *Toxocara canis* or *Toxocara cati*, *Toxoplasma gondii*, free-living ameba), tuberculosis, or fungal etiologies, if the patient has exposure risk factors. EEG with periodic localizing epileptiform discharges or temporal lobe-localizing EEG activity or neuroimaging are suggestive but not specific for HSV and can be seen with a spectrum of infectious pathogens, including tuberculosis and VZV.[29] Ring-enhancing lesions can be associated with *Toxoplasma gondii*, ameba, fungi, and tuberculosis. Respiratory viruses, especially influenza virus, have been associated with thalamic and basal ganglia lesions.[30] Rhombencephalitis, or brainstem involvement, has been described with *Listeria monocytogenes* and mycobacteria, as well as EVs, particularly EV-A71, and HSV. Cerebellitis can follow a variety of viral infections but is most commonly seen with VZV in areas without widespread VZV vaccination.

The presence of myelitis with encephalitis on imaging is suggestive of an EV (eg, EV-A71 or EV-D68) or flavivirus (eg, WNV, Japanese encephalitis virus).[31,32] A presumptive diagnosis of ADEM can be made based on neuroimaging findings of multifocal, diffuse, poorly demarcated, demyelinating lesions in the white matter or deep gray matter in the setting of encephalitis.[33]

Tier 2: Broader, More Invasive Testing

When no cause has been identified despite clinical testing for common, treatable, and at-risk etiologies, and the patient is not improving or has severe disease, consideration should be given to broader and more invasive diagnostic testing. This is particularly important in immunocompromised children because the identification of an etiology is challenging given the broad differential diagnosis. In addition to further pathogen-directed testing, metagenomic sequencing of CSF or brain tissue enables unbiased assessment for bacteria, viruses, fungi, and parasites not suspected or detected using traditional clinical testing, as well as novel pathogens. Potentially treatable pathogens, such as *Leptospira*, *Brucella*, and *Balamuthia mandrillaris,* as well as untreatable pathogens, such as astroviruses and novel viruses, that were not suspected clinically have been identified using this technology.[34–38] Testing of CSF can miss pathogens present in CNS tissue that may require a brain biopsy to identify. Neuroimaging should be used for stereotactic brain biopsy localization with consideration given to targeting affected areas with the least chance of affecting functional outcomes. Brain biopsy specimens should undergo histopathologic evaluation, staining for pathogens, cultures, and flash-freezing for targeted PCR testing or metagenomic sequencing.

THERAPEUTIC APPROACH

Supportive care is the mainstay of encephalitis therapy with careful management of the airway in cases of severely altered mental status or loss of bulbar function, management of intracranial pressure and cerebral edema, fluid and electrolyte management, and seizure control with antiepileptic medications. Although targeted therapies should be tailored toward the specific cause ultimately identified, a structured approach to administering empiric therapies for common treatable causes is warranted while diagnostic evaluation is in process. In patients in whom it is difficult to differentiate bacterial meningitis from viral meningoencephalitis, intravenous antibiotics (eg, vancomycin and a third-generation cephalosporin at meningeal dosing) should be promptly initiated. Antibiotics should be initiated after lumbar puncture and CSF cultures are obtained, if deemed safe and performed immediately. All children with suspected encephalitis should be started on empiric intravenous acyclovir (20 mg/kg per dose every 8 hours for age <3 months and 10 mg/kg per dose every 8 hours for age >3 months in the presence of normal renal function) while undergoing diagnostic evaluation for HSV.[1,39] Acyclovir should be continued until HSV testing is negative, and consideration should be given to continuing acyclovir while pursuing repeat CSF testing and/or brain biopsy in cases with high clinical suspicion with no alternative cause identified.[1,21]

Few viral causes of encephalitis have therapies proven to be effective for immunocompetent children. If HSV is detected (or highly suspected), intravenous acyclovir should be administered for 3 weeks with repeat lumbar puncture and HSV PCR testing near the end of therapy to ensure clearance before stopping therapy.[1,39] In neonates, this should be followed by 6 months of oral acyclovir suppressive therapy to reduce recurrences and improve neurodevelopmental outcomes.[40] In patients aged greater than 12 years, a 3-month course of oral valacyclovir did not provide added neuropsychological benefit following standard intravenous treatment with acyclovir.[41] Acyclovir is frequently administered for VZV-associated encephalitis; however, efficacy is unproven and it remains unclear if this is a direct viral infection or an immune-mediated postinfectious process. Oral influenza antivirals, such as oseltamivir, are recommended for hospitalized children with influenza identified in respiratory specimens, including those with encephalitis, though effectiveness for CNS disease is unknown. No effective therapies are currently available for the treatment of encephalitis due to EVs, most noninfluenza respiratory viruses, arboviruses, or rabies virus in immunocompetent children; experimental treatments are potential options for some agents (eg, adenovirus, rabies virus).

Identified bacterial, fungal, and parasitic CNS infections warrant treatment with targeted antimicrobial therapy, based on known antimicrobial susceptibilities when available. Treatment of non-CNS bacterial infections associated with encephalitis or encephalopathy, such as *M pneumoniae* and *Bordetella pertussis* respiratory infections, can be considered, though impact on the course of CNS disease has not been studied.

The use of corticosteroids, intravenous immune globulin (IVIG), and plasma exchange (PLEX) has not been systematically studied with controlled trials in encephalitis.[42] Due to differing pathophysiology among the various etiologies (ie, active CNS infection vs postinfectious or noninfectious immune-mediated), care should be taken when considering immunosuppressive therapies such as corticosteroids, and potentially PLEX, until the potential for active infections has been sufficiently assessed or is being treated with effective antimicrobial therapy. During the process of diagnostic evaluation for potential infectious encephalitis, IVIG carries the least potential immunosuppressive risk of these modalities. Additionally, IVIG may assist with pathogen clearance in children with humoral immunodeficiency, as well as immune modulation with certain pathogens, such as EV-A71.[43] When a diagnosis of ADEM is probable, first-line therapy is high-dose intravenous corticosteroids, with PLEX and IVIG considerations for refractory disease.[42,44,45] Immunotherapy, including corticosteroids, IVIG and PLEX alone or combined, and tumor removal (if present) are the mainstays of treatment of anti-NMDAR encephalitis, with second-line options, including rituximab and cyclophosphamide.[46]

PREVENTION

Vaccination against poliovirus, measles virus, mumps virus, seasonal influenza virus, and pertussis is recommended as part of the immunization series for children and likely provide protection against encephalitis associated with these pathogens. Travelers should be evaluated for eligibility to receive immunization against vaccine-preventable endemic diseases associated with encephalitis in the region to which they are traveling (ie, Japanese encephalitis virus, rabies virus, EV A71, and tickborne encephalitis virus). Protection against mosquito and tick bites, including staying in screened facilities; wearing long sleeves; use of repellants with proven efficacy; public health measures, such as standing-water pool mitigation; and pesticide application in outbreak situations, is recommended to decrease the risk of arboviral encephalitis.[47] Use of sterile water for sinus irrigation and avoiding recreational activities in warm freshwater are the only certain methods of prevention for *N fowleri* encephalitis.[48] Postexposure prophylaxis is recommended with rabies vaccine series and rabies immunoglobulin for rabies-prone animal bites, valacyclovir for Old World macaque monkey bites to decrease risk of herpes B encephalitis, albendazole for exposure to raccoon feces or latrines to decrease risk of baylisascariasis, and acyclovir for neonates born to mothers with active genital herpes lesions at the time of delivery.[49]

DISEASE COURSE, PROGNOSIS, AND OUTCOMES

Nearly all children with encephalitis in the United States are hospitalized with 40% requiring critical care in an intensive care unit. Prolonged length of stay, averaging 16 days and up to 25 days in those requiring intensive care, and the need for inpatient rehabilitation services (~20%–40%) are common.[10,50] The average cost of acute hospitalization of a child with encephalitis in the United States is estimated to be between $64,000 to $260,000, depending on the level of care and rehabilitation needs required.[10,51]

Most children with encephalitis have incomplete recovery at discharge and those who fully recover are most likely to do so within 6 to 12 months.[50,52] Though there are limited data on long-term neurologic outcomes in children, persistent long-term neurologic sequelae, including learning problems, developmental delays, and behavioral problems, are common.[50–53] The subsequent development of epilepsy is more common in those who presented initially with seizures and is correlated with long-term neurologic sequelae.[50,53,54] Children with abnormal neuroimaging are less likely to fully recover and report poorer quality of life at long-term follow-up.[50,51]

Outcomes differ greatly based on etiology. Many children with HSV encephalitis have long-term neurologic impairment, particularly those with delayed initiation of acyclovir.[52,55–57] Neonates with EV encephalitis have variable outcomes, ranging from full recovery to significant long-term deficits, whereas older infants and children with EV encephalitis tend to demonstrate significant recovery (with the exception of EV-A71).[52] Encephalitis due to HPeVs in young, particularly preterm, infants may have more long-term neurodevelopmental sequelae than encephalitis due to EVs.[58,59] Nearly 80% of children with anti-NMDAR encephalitis will have full or substantial response to immunotherapy, though 25% will have subsequent relapse.[60]

Recent population-based studies estimate a 3% mortality rate of encephalitis in children in the United States.[9,10] Complications requiring intensive care, including respiratory failure, intubation, sepsis, and pneumonia, are predictors of mortality.[9] HSV is the most common cause of pediatric death due to encephalitis, though some rare causes, such as amebic and rabies encephalitis, are nearly uniformly fatal.[9,26] Mortality is rare from most EVs (except EV-A71), HPeVs, arboviruses (except eastern equine encephalitis virus), and autoantibody-mediated encephalitides in children.[8,25,60,61]

REFERENCES

1. Tunkel AR, Glaser CA, Bloch KC, et al. The management of encephalitis: clinical practice guidelines by the Infectious Diseases Society of America. Clin Infect Dis 2008;47(3):303–27.
2. Flett KB, Rao S, Dominguez SR, et al. Variability in the diagnosis of encephalitis by pediatric subspecialists: the need for a uniform definition. J Pediatric Infect Dis Soc 2013;2(3):267–9.
3. Venkatesan A, Tunkel AR, Bloch KC, et al. Case definitions, diagnostic algorithms, and priorities in encephalitis: consensus statement of the International Encephalitis Consortium. Clin Infect Dis 2013;57(8):1114–28.
4. Sejvar JJ, Kohl KS, Bilynsky R, et al. Encephalitis, myelitis, and acute disseminated encephalomyelitis (ADEM): case definitions and guidelines for collection, analysis, and presentation of immunization safety data. Vaccine 2007;25(31): 5771–92.

5. Kestenbaum LA, Ebberson J, Zorc JJ, et al. Defining cerebrospinal fluid white blood cell count reference values in neonates and young infants. Pediatrics 2010;125(2):257–64.

6. Seiden JA, Zorc JJ, Hodinka RL, et al. Lack of cerebrospinal fluid pleocytosis in young infants with enterovirus infections of the central nervous system. Pediatr Emerg Care 2010;26(2):77–81.

7. Abzug MJ, Levin MJ, Rotbart HA. Profile of enterovirus disease in the first two weeks of life. Pediatr Infect Dis J 1993;12(10):820–4.

8. Renaud C, Harrison CJ. Human parechovirus 3: the most common viral cause of meningoencephalitis in young infants. Infect Dis Clin North Am 2015;29(3): 415–28.

9. George BP, Schneider EB, Venkatesan A. Encephalitis hospitalization rates and inpatient mortality in the United States, 2000-2010. PLoS One 2014;9(9):e104169.

10. Bagdure D, Custer JW, Rao S, et al. Hospitalized children with encephalitis in the United States: a pediatric health information system database study. Pediatr Neurol 2016;61:58–62.

11. Iro MA, Sadarangani M, Goldacre R, et al. 30-year trends in admission rates for encephalitis in children in England and effect of improved diagnostics and measles-mumps-rubella vaccination: a population-based observational study. Lancet Infect Dis 2017;17(4):422–30.

12. Wickstrom R, Fowler A, Bogdanovic G, et al. Review of the aetiology, diagnostics and outcomes of childhood encephalitis from 1970 to 2009. Acta Paediatr 2017; 106(3):463–9.

13. Pahud BA, Glaser CA, Dekker CL, et al. Varicella zoster disease of the central nervous system: epidemiological, clinical, and laboratory features 10 years after the introduction of the varicella vaccine. J Infect Dis 2011;203(3):316–23.

14. Lewis P, Glaser CA. Encephalitis. Pediatr Rev 2005;26(10):353–63.

15. Britton PN, Dale RC, Booy R, et al. Acute encephalitis in children: progress and priorities from an Australasian perspective. J Paediatr Child Health 2015;51(2): 147–58.

16. Pruss H, Finke C, Holtje M, et al. N-methyl-D-aspartate receptor antibodies in herpes simplex encephalitis. Ann Neurol 2012;72(6):902–11.

17. Armangue T, Moris G, Cantarin-Extremera V, et al. Autoimmune post-herpes simplex encephalitis of adults and teenagers. Neurology 2015;85(20):1736–43.

18. Glaser CA, Gilliam S, Schnurr D, et al. In search of encephalitis etiologies: diagnostic challenges in the California Encephalitis Project, 1998-2000. Clin Infect Dis 2003;36(6):731–42.

19. Gable MS, Sheriff H, Dalmau J, et al. The frequency of autoimmune N-methyl-D-aspartate receptor encephalitis surpasses that of individual viral etiologies in young individuals enrolled in the California Encephalitis Project. Clin Infect Dis 2012;54(7):899–904.

20. Glaser CA, Honarmand S, Anderson LJ, et al. Beyond viruses: clinical profiles and etiologies associated with encephalitis. Clin Infect Dis 2006;43(12): 1565–77.

21. Weil AA, Glaser CA, Amad Z, et al. Patients with suspected herpes simplex encephalitis: rethinking an initial negative polymerase chain reaction result. Clin Infect Dis 2002;34(8):1154–7.

22. de Crom SC, Obihara CC, de Moor RA, et al. Prospective comparison of the detection rates of human enterovirus and parechovirus RT-qPCR and viral culture in different pediatric specimens. J Clin Virol 2013;58(2):449–54.

23. Perez-Velez CM, Anderson MS, Robinson CC, et al. Outbreak of neurologic enterovirus type 71 disease: a diagnostic challenge. Clin Infect Dis 2007;45(8): 950–7.
24. Leber AL, Everhart K, Balada-Llasat JM, et al. Multicenter Evaluation of BioFire FilmArray Meningitis/Encephalitis Panel for Detection of Bacteria, Viruses, and Yeast in Cerebrospinal Fluid Specimens. J Clin Microbiol 2016;54(9):2251–61.
25. Gaensbauer JT, Lindsey NP, Messacar K, et al. Neuroinvasive arboviral disease in the United States: 2003 to 2012. Pediatrics 2014;134(3):e642–50.
26. Capewell LG, Harris AM, Yoder JS, et al. Diagnosis, clinical course, and treatment of primary amoebic meningoencephalitis in the United States, 1937-2013. J Pediatric Infect Dis Soc 2015;4(4):e68–75.
27. Schuster FL, Yagi S, Gavali S, et al. Under the radar: balamuthia amebic encephalitis. Clin Infect Dis 2009;48(7):879–87.
28. Cope JR, Ali IK. Primary amebic meningoencephalitis: what have we learned in the last 5 years? Curr Infect Dis Rep 2016;18(10):31.
29. Chow FC, Glaser CA, Sheriff H, et al. Use of clinical and neuroimaging characteristics to distinguish temporal lobe herpes simplex encephalitis from its mimics. Clin Infect Dis 2015;60(9):1377–83.
30. Beattie GC, Glaser CA, Sheriff H, et al. Encephalitis with thalamic and basal ganglia abnormalities: etiologies, neuroimaging, and potential role of respiratory viruses. Clin Infect Dis 2013;56(6):825–32.
31. Kincaid O, Lipton HL. Viral myelitis: an update. Curr Neurol Neurosci Rep 2006; 6(6):469–74.
32. Messacar K, Schreiner TL, Van Haren K, et al. Acute flaccid myelitis: a clinical review of US cases 2012-2015. Ann Neurol 2016;80(3):326–38.
33. Krupp LB, Banwell B, Tenembaum S, International Pediatric MS Study Group. Consensus definitions proposed for pediatric multiple sclerosis and related disorders. Neurology 2007;68(16 Suppl 2):S7–12.
34. Wilson MR, Naccache SN, Samayoa E, et al. Actionable diagnosis of neuroleptospirosis by next-generation sequencing. N Engl J Med 2014;370(25):2408–17.
35. Greninger AL, Messacar K, Dunnebacke T, et al. Clinical metagenomic identification of *Balamuthia mandrillaris* encephalitis and assembly of the draft genome: the continuing case for reference genome sequencing. Genome Med 2015;7:113.
36. Naccache SN, Peggs KS, Mattes FM, et al. Diagnosis of neuroinvasive astrovirus infection in an immunocompromised adult with encephalitis by unbiased next-generation sequencing. Clin Infect Dis 2015;60(6):919–23.
37. Phan TG, Messacar K, Dominguez SR, et al. A new densovirus in cerebrospinal fluid from a case of anti-NMDA-receptor encephalitis. Arch Virol 2016;161(11): 3231–5.
38. Mongkolrattanothai K, Naccache SN, Bender JM, et al. Neurobrucellosis: unexpected answer from metagenomic next-generation sequencing. J Pediatric Infect Dis Soc 2017. [Epub ahead of print].
39. Kimberlin DW, Lin CY, Jacobs RF, et al. Safety and efficacy of high-dose intravenous acyclovir in the management of neonatal herpes simplex virus infections. Pediatrics 2001;108(2):230–8.
40. Kimberlin DW, Whitley RJ, Wan W, et al. Oral acyclovir suppression and neurodevelopment after neonatal herpes. N Engl J Med 2011;365(14):1284–92.
41. Gnann JW Jr, Skoldenberg B, Hart J, et al. Herpes simplex encephalitis: lack of clinical benefit of long-term valacyclovir therapy. Clin Infect Dis 2015;61(5): 683–91.

42. Esposito S, Picciolli I, Semino M, et al. Steroids and childhood encephalitis. Pediatr Infect Dis J 2012;31(7):759–60.

43. Wang SM, Lei HY, Huang MC, et al. Modulation of cytokine production by intravenous immunoglobulin in patients with enterovirus 71-associated brainstem encephalitis. J Clin Virol 2006;37(1):47–52.

44. Schwartz J, Winters JL, Padmanabhan A, et al. Guidelines on the use of therapeutic apheresis in clinical practice-evidence-based approach from the Writing Committee of the American Society for Apheresis: the sixth special issue. J Clin Apher 2013;28(3):145–284.

45. Graus F, Titulaer MJ, Balu R, et al. A clinical approach to diagnosis of autoimmune encephalitis. Lancet Neurol 2016;15(4):391–404.

46. Titulaer MJ, McCracken L, Gabilondo I, et al. Treatment and prognostic factors for long-term outcome in patients with anti-NMDA receptor encephalitis: an observational cohort study. Lancet Neurol 2013;12(2):157–65.

47. Centers for Disease Control and Prevention. Mosquito prevention. 2017. Available at: https://www.cdc.gov/features/stopmosquitoes/. Accessed July 19, 2017.

48. Centers for Disease Control and Prevention. Prevention of *Naegleria fowlerii*. 2017. Available at: https://www.cdc.gov/parasites/naegleria/prevention.html. Accessed July 19, 2017.

49. Committee on Infectious Diseases. Red book. 30th edition. Elk Grove Village (IL): American Academy of Pediatrics; 2015.

50. Rao S, Elkon B, Flett KB, et al. Long-term outcomes and risk factors associated with acute encephalitis in children. J Pediatric Infect Dis Soc 2017;6(1):20–7.

51. DuBray K, Anglemyer A, LaBeaud AD, et al. Epidemiology, outcomes and predictors of recovery in childhood encephalitis: a hospital-based study. Pediatr Infect Dis J 2013;32(8):839–44.

52. Fowler A, Stodberg T, Eriksson M, et al. Long-term outcomes of acute encephalitis in childhood. Pediatrics 2010;126(4):e828–35.

53. Rismanchi N, Gold JJ, Sattar S, et al. Neurological outcomes after presumed childhood encephalitis. Pediatr Neurol 2015;53(3):200–6.

54. Rismanchi N, Gold JJ, Sattar S, et al. Epilepsy after resolution of presumed childhood encephalitis. Pediatr Neurol 2015;53(1):65–72.

55. Rautonen J, Koskiniemi M, Vaheri A. Prognostic factors in childhood acute encephalitis. Pediatr Infect Dis J 1991;10(6):441–6.

56. Ward KN, Ohrling A, Bryant NJ, et al. Herpes simplex serious neurological disease in young children: incidence and long-term outcome. Arch Dis Child 2012;97(2):162–5.

57. Lahat E, Barr J, Barkai G, et al. Long term neurological outcome of herpes encephalitis. Arch Dis Child 1999;80(1):69–71.

58. Britton PN, Dale RC, Nissen MD, et al. Parechovirus encephalitis and neurodevelopmental outcomes. Pediatrics 2016;137(2):e20152848.

59. Vergnano S, Kadambari S, Whalley K, et al. Characteristics and outcomes of human parechovirus infection in infants (2008-2012). Eur J Pediatr 2015;174(7):919–24.

60. Florance NR, Davis RL, Lam C, et al. Anti-N-methyl-D-aspartate receptor (NMDAR) encephalitis in children and adolescents. Ann Neurol 2009;66(1):11–8.

61. Fowlkes AL, Honarmand S, Glaser C, et al. Enterovirus-associated encephalitis in the California encephalitis project, 1998-2005. J Infect Dis 2008;198(11):1685–91.

62. Kimberlin DW, Baley J, Committee on Infectious Diseases, Committee on Fetus and Newborn. Guidance on management of asymptomatic neonates born to women with active genital herpes lesions. Pediatrics 2013;131(2):383–6.
63. To TM, Soldatos A, Sheriff H, et al. Insights into pediatric herpes simplex encephalitis from a cohort of 21 children from the California Encephalitis Project, 1998-2011. Pediatr Infect Dis J 2014;33(12):1287–8.
64. Abzug MJ. The enteroviruses: problems in need of treatments. J Infect 2014; 68(Suppl 1):S108–14.
65. Sells CJ, Carpenter RL, Ray CG. Sequelae of central-nervous-system enterovirus infections. N Engl J Med 1975;293(1):1–4.
66. Messacar K, Breazeale G, Wei Q, et al. Epidemiology and clinical characteristics of infants with human parechovirus or human herpes virus-6 detected in cerebrospinal fluid tested for enterovirus or herpes simplex virus. J Med Virol 2015;87(5): 829–35.
67. Karsch K, Obermeier P, Seeber L, et al. Human parechovirus infections associated with seizures and rash in infants and toddlers. Pediatr Infect Dis J 2015; 34(10):1049–55.
68. Verboon-Maciolek MA, Groenendaal F, Hahn CD, et al. Human parechovirus causes encephalitis with white matter injury in neonates. Ann Neurol 2008; 64(3):266–73.
69. Armangue T, Petit-Pedrol M, Dalmau J. Autoimmune encephalitis in children. J Child Neurol 2012;27(11):1460–9.
70. Pohl D, Alper G, Van Haren K, et al. Acute disseminated encephalomyelitis: updates on an inflammatory CNS syndrome. Neurology 2016;87(9 Suppl 2):S38–45.
71. Murthy SN, Faden HS, Cohen ME, et al. Acute disseminated encephalomyelitis in children. Pediatrics 2002;110(2 Pt 1):e21.
72. Davis LE, Booss J. Acute disseminated encephalomyelitis in children: a changing picture. Pediatr Infect Dis J 2003;22(9):829–31.
73. Sejvar JJ. Acute disseminated encephalomyelitis. Curr Infect Dis Rep 2008;10(4): 307–14.
74. Granerod J, Ambrose HE, Davies NW, et al. Causes of encephalitis and differences in their clinical presentations in England: a multicentre, population-based prospective study. Lancet Infect Dis 2010;10(12):835–44.

Fever in the Returning Traveler

Felicia A. Scaggs Huang, MD*, Elizabeth Schlaudecker, MD, MPH

KEYWORDS

• Fever • Child • International travel • Tropical infections • Returning traveler

KEY POINTS

- The initial workup of a febrile child without a clear source will be based on the history, physical examination, and potential risk factors but commonly includes laboratory testing.
- Malaria, enteric fever, and dengue fever are some of the most common and serious tropical infections in pediatric travelers.
- Clinicians need to remain up-to-date on potential etiologic factors for febrile illnesses to develop a focused plan best suited to the patient's clinical picture.

INTRODUCTION

Millions of children travel annually, whether they are refugees, international adoptees, visitors, or vacationers.[1–4] In 2015, the International Tourism Organization reported 1.2 billion overseas trips.[5,6] Although most young travelers do well, many develop febrile illnesses during or shortly after their journeys.[7] In a study of European children, 53% of all pediatric patients with travel-related infections were visiting friends and relatives (VFRs), 43.4% were tourists, and 2.4% were immigrants.[8] Most illnesses are self-limited childhood infections that do not require subspecialist consultation. However, 28% of 24,920 ill American travelers sought care at travel clinics after returning home.[9] Additionally, young children with fevers can present a diagnostic dilemma because they may not report symptoms and can be at risk for severe disease, such as malaria. As awareness of tropical illnesses rise in parents, such as the increase in multidrug-resistant bacteria worldwide or the emergence of epidemics with Zika virus in South America, families may be more anxious about serious infections as an etiologic factor of fevers.

Approaching fevers in the returning traveler requires an appropriate index of suspicion to diagnose and treat the child in a timely manner. This article offers a framework

Disclosure Statement: The authors do not have any commercial or financial conflicts of interest.
Division of Infectious Diseases, Cincinnati Children's Hospital Medical Center, Cincinnati, OH, USA
* Corresponding author. 240 Albert Sabin Way, MLC 7017, Cincinnati, OH 45229.
E-mail address: Felicia.ScaggsHuang@cchmc.org

on how to address these issues by discussing diseases based on geography, incubation period, and affected organ systems, as well as risk factors, diagnostic techniques, and resources.

GENERAL APPROACH

A thorough history is an important initial step when evaluating a pediatric traveler with a fever (**Table 1**). Discussing a detailed travel itinerary develops a timeline of exposures that can be unique to an urban or rural setting (**Table 2**).

Many children receive vaccinations and/or antimicrobial prophylaxis, but reported adherence does not preclude an illness with a particular pathogen. Up to 75% of travelers do not adhere to the recommended malaria prophylaxis.[10] Many travel vaccines, including typhoid vaccine, provide only partial protection despite proper administration of these immunizations.[11]

A medically complex individual may have sought care outside of the United States due to necessity or medical tourism, which can increase the risk of infection through body fluid exposures. Multidrug-resistant pathogens can also be associated with health care exposure. Up to half of hospitalized children in Zimbabwe are colonized with extended spectrum beta lactamase producing *Enterobacteriaceae* on admission to the hospital,[12] a problem that is increasingly seen worldwide. Underlying medical conditions, such as asplenia or immunosuppression from chemotherapy, may predispose children to overwhelming infections and sepsis. Refugee children from countries such as Syria are susceptible to vaccine-preventable diseases such as polio due to infrastructure breakdown.[13]

CLINICAL FINDINGS, DIAGNOSIS, AND MANAGEMENT

Fever is a common and anxiety-provoking sign for parents that can be exacerbated by overseas travel. Up to 34% of patients with recent travel history are diagnosed with routine infections.[3] Of the 82,825 cases of infection in travelers from 1996 to 2011 reported to GeoSentinel, a worldwide data collection network on travel-related diseases, 4% of cases were considered to be life-threatening.[14] A study in Swiss children showed that 0.45% of emergency room visits were due to travel-related morbidities with fever and gastrointestinal symptoms being the most common complaints in 63% and 50% of patients, respectively.[8] The temporality of travel to the onset of fever can offer important clues to the etiologic factors of fevers (**Table 3**). Because the causes and clinical outcomes associated with fevers in pediatric travelers vary from self-limited to deadly, a systems-based approach can lead to prompt diagnosis and treatment that evaluates for the most likely and serious diseases early in the illness course.

Fever

According to GeoSentinel, 91% of patients with an acute, life-threatening illness will present with fever.[14] There are a broad range of potential tropical infections, including malaria, dengue fever, and enteric fever. The incidence of emerging infections such as Zika virus and chikungunya are not yet known. In both adults and children, pneumonia, sepsis, meningococcemia, and urinary tract infections that were acquired at home or overseas should be on the differential diagnosis.

The initial workup of a febrile child without a clear source will be based on the history, physical examination, and risk factors but commonly includes a complete blood count, liver function tests, creatinine, urinalysis, and blood cultures.[1,3] Malaria smears are also frequently helpful. Other tests to consider include serologies for dengue fever

Table 1
Patient history for the returning traveler with fever

History	Implications
Travel itinerary	Offers information on potential diseases based on geography and other exposures
Diet history (improperly cooked meats, unpasteurized dairy products, seafood, or contaminated water and produce)	Brucellosis, *Campylobacter* infection, giardiasis, hepatitis A and E, listeriosis, traveler's diarrhea, enteric fever, trichinosis, viral gastroenteritis (ie, norovirus)
Sick contacts (both abroad and since returning to the US)	Routine viral or bacterial illnesses, Ebola infection, influenza, meningococcemia, tuberculosis
Fresh water exposure	Bacterial soft tissue infection (*Aeromonas* spp, atypical *Mycobacterium*), leptospirosis, schistosomiasis
Sexual encounters	Acute human immunodeficiency virus (HIV) infection; gonorrhea; hepatitis A, B, or C infection; primary herpesvirus 1 or 2 infection; syphilis; Zika virus infection
Insect bites	• Fleas: plague, murine typhus, rickettsioses • Flies: African sleeping sickness, leishmaniasis, sandfly fever • Lice: relapsing fever, rickettsioses • Reduviid bugs: Chagas disease • Mosquitoes: Chikungunya virus infection, dengue fever, filiarisis, Japanese encephalitis, West Nile virus infection, Zika virus infection • Ticks: African tick bite fever, babesiosis, Lyme disease, Q fever rickettsioses, tularemia
Animal bites	Cat-scratch disease, rat bite fever, rabies, simian herpesvirus B infection
Animal exposure (including exposure to urine, stool, or animal products; eg, infected carcasses or wool)	Anthrax, avian influenza, hantavirus infection, Hendra virus infection, infections from ectoparasites or endoparasites, Nipah virus infection, plague, psittacosis, toxoplasmosis
Body fluid exposures (tattoos, piercings, or medical procedures)	Acute HIV infection, babesiosis, cytomegalovirus infection, hepatitis B and C, malaria, multidrug-resistant bacteria, trypanosomiasis
Medical history (diseases associated with immunosuppression; eg, malignancy, asplenia, or immunodeficiency)	Cytomegalovirus infection, Epstein-Barr virus infection, fungal infection, mycobacterial infections
Vaccinations and prophylaxis (note: these interventions do not preclude infection with the pathogen prophylaxed against)	Malaria prophylaxis, travel-appropriate vaccines

Adapted from Refs.[50–52]

or other potential etiologic agents, polymerase chain reaction for Zika virus or other pathogens, chest radiographs, and cultures of the urine and stool. Patients with altered mental status may require head imaging and lumbar puncture. The most common and concerning causes of fever in a returning pediatric traveler are highlighted next.

Table 2
Tropical causes of fever based on geography

Location	Infection
Caribbean	Acute histoplasmosis, chikungunya, cholera, dengue fever, leptospirosis, malaria (Haiti, primarily *Plasmodium falciparum*)
Central America	Acute histoplasmosis, coccidioidomycosis, dengue fever, hepatitis A and B, malaria (primarily *P vivax*), tuberculosis
South America	Bartonellosis, dengue fever, malaria (primarily *P vivax*), enteric fever, leptospirosis, yellow fever
South Central Asia	Dengue fever, enteric fever, hepatitis B, Japanese encephalitis, malaria (primarily non-falciparum *Plasmodium* spp), tuberculosis
Southeast Asia	Chikungunya, cholera, dengue fever, hepatitis A, Japanese encephalitis, malaria (primarily non-falciparum *Plasmodium* spp), yellow fever
Sub-Saharan Africa	Acute schistosomiasis, enteric fever, filariasis, malaria (primarily *P falciparum*), meningococcus, rickettsioses, yellow fever

Adapted from Centers for Disease Control and Prevention. The yellow book: health information for international travel 2018. Philadelphia: Oxford University Press; 2017. p. 704. Available at: https://wwwnc.cdc.gov/travel/page/yellowbook-home. Accessed July 25, 2017; with permission.

Table 3
Incubation period for common tropical diseases causing

Disease	Incubation Period
Incubation of <14 d	
Acute HIV	7–21 d
Arboviral infections (ie, chikungunya and Zika viruses)	2–10 d
Dengue fever	4–8 d
Enteric fever	7–18 d
Leptospirosis	7–12 d
Influenza	1–3 d
Malaria	
P falciparum	6–30 d
P vivax	8 d–12 mo
Rickettsioses	3 d–3 wk
Incubation of 14 d to 6 wk	
Amebic liver abscess	Weeks–months
Hepatitis A	28–30 d
Hepatitis B infection	60–150 d
Rabies	Weeks–months
Schistosomiasis	28–60 d
Tuberculosis	Weeks for primary infection
Visceral leishmaniasis	2–10 mo

Adapted from Thwaites GE, Day NP. Approach to fever in the returning traveler. N Engl J Med 2017;376(6):548–60; and Centers for Disease Control and Prevention. The yellow book: health information for international travel 2018. Philadelphia: Oxford University Press; 2017. p. 704. Available at: https://wwwnc.cdc.gov/travel/page/yellowbook-home. Accessed July 25, 2017; with permission.

Malaria

Plasmodium falciparum malaria is one of the most common tropical infections. Approximately 15% to 20% of all imported malaria cases are diagnosed in the pediatric population in industrialized countries each year.[3] Malaria is transmitted via the nocturnal-feeding *Anopheles* genus of mosquito. Children who are VFRs are more likely to become infected with malaria than traditional tourists.[3] Nonimmune children are also susceptible to severe malaria from other malaria strains such as *Plasmodium vivax*[15] and many young patients can present with atypical symptoms such as abdominal pain and vomiting.[16] Older children may present with paroxysmal fever, fatigue, myalgias, headache, abdominal pain, back pain, hepatosplenomegaly, and hemolytic anemia. Additionally, severe malaria is more common in children after the first month of travel due to the incubation period of *P falciparum* (7–90 days), especially in those who visited sub-Saharan Africa.[17,18] Overall, sub-Saharan Africa is one of the most common geographic regions for acquisition, comprising 71.5% of cases according to a GeoSentinel study of travelers migrating or returning to Canada from 2004 to 2014.[19] Malaria should remain on the differential diagnosis for up to a year in an acutely ill, febrile child after travel to an endemic area where *P vivax* and *P ovale* strains are present.[17] Interestingly, 20% of malaria cases can be acquired during trips as short as 2 weeks with less utilization of pretravel services being a contributing factor.[19]

A minimum of 3 thick and thin blood smears must be performed before malaria can be excluded, preferably collected during febrile episodes. The specificity of blood smears is high but the sensitivity can be low depending on the experience of the individual interpreting the slides.[17] Rapid diagnostic tests that detect specific proteins or lactate dehydrogenase are alternatives for diagnosis at medical centers with limited experience in microbiologic evaluation for malaria.[20] The result should be confirmed, however, through the state public health department. In general, a febrile child without a localizing source or splenomegaly, thrombocytopenia, or indirect hyperbilirubinemia, in addition to exposure to an endemic area, should be presumptively approached as having malaria until an alternative diagnosis can be made.[21]

Treatment of malaria is well-established by the Centers for Disease Control and Prevention (CDC) guidelines. Children with acidosis, hypoglycemia, hyperparasitemia, end-organ dysfunction, and severe anemia meet the criteria for severe malaria and require prompt administration of parenteral medication. There is a growing body of evidence that artesunate may reduce mortality compared with quinidine and is becoming more common as first-line therapy in pediatric patients.[22,23] Artesunate must be obtained through the CDC Malaria Hotline (1–770–488–7788) because it is not routinely available in the United States.[24] Quinidine may be initiated until the medication arrives. Completion of therapy with an oral regimen for uncomplicated chloroquine-resistant *P falciparum*, such as atovaquone-proguanil, can be offered when the child is able to tolerate the medications and the parasite burden has decreased to less than 1%. Severe disease is less common in *P vivax* and *P ovale* and infection can be treated with chloroquine or hydroxychloroquine in most areas outside of Indonesia and Papua New Guinea.

Enteric fever (typhoid and paratyphoid)

Enteric fever accounts for 18% of the 3655 cases with life-threatening tropical diseases reported to GeoSentinel. Most recorded cases were from the Indian subcontinent and in VFRs.[1] Infection with *Salmonella typhi* and *Salmonella paratyphi* are clinically indistinguishable with fever, abdominal pain, nausea, vomiting, myalgias, and arthralgias. Diarrhea is greater than 2.5 times more common in infants than older children or adults,[25] although constipation can also be seen. Patients can exhibit a typhoid mask with dull features and confusion, as well as a stepladder fever progression with rising temperatures over time in untreated individuals. Relative bradycardia and rose spots are also classic signs.[25] Complications such as gastrointestinal bleeding are more common in young children who have been ill for 2 weeks or more.[1] Transmission is fecal-oral, and humans, especially adults, may be chronic carriers. Diagnosis of enteric fever is confirmed through cultures. The most sensitive sterile site is bone marrow (80%–95%). Blood culture has the highest yield during the first week of illness (70%), and stool cultures are more sensitive as the duration of illness increases.[26] Stool studies should be performed on all fellow travelers, and they must be monitored for signs of illness. Other abnormal laboratory findings include transaminitis and a normal or decreased white blood cell count.

The antimicrobial of choice for treatment varies based on the area in which the infection was acquired because multidrug resistance is increasing. Empiric treatment with ceftriaxone or fluoroquinolones is typically recommended. Strains in Latin America and the Caribbean can be susceptible to ampicillin and trimethoprim-sulfamethoxazole. South and Southeast Asian serovars more frequently require azithromycin or cefixime.[27,28] Children with multidrug-resistant strains have more complications such as myocarditis and shock than children infected with susceptible strains but case fatality is similar (1.0% vs 1.3%, respectively).[29] Relapse of infection can occur despite appropriate therapy, with the highest mortality in young children (6%).[29]

Dengue fever

Dengue remains an important cause of fever in travelers returning from all tropical regions except Africa.[30] The prevalence is rising, even in the United States, with 50 to 100 million global cases reported yearly and 22,000 deaths, primarily in children.[31] Risk factors are dissimilar from those for malaria because transmission occurs in urban areas during the daytime due to the vector *Aedes aegypti*, whereas malaria transmission is more common in rural areas from dusk to dawn with the *Anopheles* species mosquito.[32]

Some patients may be asymptomatic, whereas others have hemorrhagic fever and shock. The illness presents as 3 distinct phases: (1) febrile phase over 3 to 7 days characterized by myalgias, headache, retroorbital pain, and rash; (2) critical phase of 24 to 48 days with plasma leakage; and (3) convalescent phase.[32] A rising hemoglobin and gallbladder wall thickening due to increased vascular permeability suggests the development of severe dengue in children. Repeat infections with a different strain may lead to more severe disease.[31]

Serologies are most commonly used for diagnosis, although some rapid diagnostic tests are available. In cases in which infection is unclear, it may be helpful to repeat serologies 2 weeks after initial testing to monitor for an increase in titers. Other common laboratory findings include leukopenia and thrombocytopenia.[33]

Treatment consists of hydration and avoidance of salicylate-containing products to decrease the risk for bleeding.[32] Children who develop severe dengue with hemorrhage and shock may require blood products. No antivirals or vaccines are currently available.

Other causes of fever

In recent years, arboviral illnesses transmitted via infected *Aedes aegypti* mosquitos have caused epidemics of Zika virus and chikungunya in South America. A European study of travelers returning from Brazil in 2013 to 2016 reported that of the 29% of patients with travel-related complaints, 6% had dengue fever, 3% had chikungunya, and 3% had Zika virus infection.[34] The prevalence of yellow fever, which is seen throughout low-resource settings and shares the same vector, has remained stable.[35] These infections are difficult to distinguish clinically with fever, retroorbital pain, conjunctivitis, and myalgias. Knowledge on perinatal infection with Zika and the neuro-developmental sequelae of affected infants is rapidly evolving.[36] A Canadian study found that 5% of travelers developed neurologic complications such as Guillain-Barre syndrome with Zika, suggesting there is much to learn with this disease in non-perinatally acquired infections.[37] At this time, treatment is primarily supportive. Additional tropical diseases associated with fevers are outlined in **Table 4**.

Gastrointestinal Symptoms

Vomiting and diarrhea are common complaints in returning travelers. Up to 40% of children less than 2 years of age may develop diarrhea, with 15% requiring medical services.[38] Fevers, nausea, and vomiting can be seen with norovirus that occurs worldwide and is frequently associated with contaminated food and water on cruise ships.[39] Rotavirus, however, is one of the most frequent causes of diarrheal illnesses worldwide and is a common cause of infant mortality in low-resource settings.[5] The hepatitides present with a broad range of disease from mild abdominal pain and vomiting to fulminant liver failure, although serious complications are uncommon in pediatric travelers.[40]

Community-acquired *Clostridium difficile* is uncommon in children but infection should be considered if the patient received recent antimicrobials.[41] GeoSentinel data reported that 2% of patients diagnosed with *Clostridium difficile* after travel were 10 to 19 years of age.[42] There are many other causes of both febrile and nonfebrile gastrointestinal illness in children (**Table 5**).

Respiratory Symptoms

In the pediatric population, common respiratory infections may be seen on return from international trips including pharyngitis, sinusitis, otitis, and pneumonia from pathogens commonly seen in the United States, such as *Streptococcus pneumoniae* and rhinovirus.[4,43] Local epidemiology of infections can be helpful in diagnosis and management and is available through the CDC. In some tropical regions, influenza may occur throughout the year and should hence remain on the differential for patients who warrant treatment with oseltamivir.[44]

Mycobacterium tuberculosis is an important etiologic factor of lower respiratory tract disease worldwide and should be considered in children with risk factors or who do not recover with antimicrobials for bacterial pneumonia.[26] Of note, children younger than 3 years of age are more likely to present with miliary tuberculosis or neurologic involvement than adult patients. There are also many other less common causes of febrile respiratory tract infections (**Table 6**).

Urinary Symptoms

Children who present with dysuria, hematuria, and fevers may require urinalysis and culture to evaluate for urinary tract infection and/or pyelonephritis. Gross hematuria with the passage of clots in an afebrile child with exposure to freshwater in Africa, the Middle East, China, and Southeast Asia should be tested for the helminth parasite from the genus *Schistosoma* via serologies or microscopic identification of eggs in stool.[45] Praziquantel is the treatment of choice and may improve anemia and nutrition in some children.[46] Patients who may have early disease or a high parasite burden may require a repeat treatment.[45] Children who are at risk for sexual abuse and adolescents should undergo testing for sexually transmitted infections such as *Chlamydia trachomatis* and *Neisseria gonorrheae*.

Table 4
Tropical diseases associated with fever

Disease	Etiologic Pathogen	Geographic Regions	Vector or Exposure	Incubation Period	Presentation	Diagnosis	Management
Acute retroviral syndrome	HIV	Worldwide, highly prevalent in sub-Saharan Africa	Anal or vaginal sex, perinatal, needle stick, blood transfusion	1–3 wk	Arthralgia, fever, rash, lymphadenopathy, pharyngitis	HIV-1 RNA, p24 antigen, immunoassay for HIV-1 and HIV-2 antibodies (preferred)	Antiretroviral therapy, consider trimethoprim-sulfamethoxazole prophylaxis
Anthrax	*Bacillus anthracis*	Central and South America, sub-Saharan Africa, Central and Southwestern Asia, Eastern Europe	Ingestion or handling of contaminated meat, playing drums from contaminated hides, contaminated heroin in drug users	Cutaneous: 1–17 d Gastrointestinal: 1–7 d Injection: 1–4 d Inhalation: 7–60 d	Varies with infection type; black eschar, cough, fever, nausea and vomiting, meningeal signs, severe soft tissue infection, shock	Bacterial culture, RT-PCR	Combination antimicrobial therapy
Brucellosis	*Brucella* species	Central and South America, Africa, Middle East, Mediterranean basin, Eastern Europe	Unpasteurized dairy products, undercooked contaminated meat	2–4 wk	Fever, headache, malaise, myalgias, night sweats,	Culture of sterile site (blood or bone marrow), PCR	Combination antimicrobial therapy
Carrión's disease (Oroya fever)	*Bartonella bacilliformis, B rochalimae,* and *B ancashensis*	South America, especially Peru	Genus *Lutzomyia* (sandflies)	10–210 d	Fever, headache, myalgias, abdominal pain, anemia followed by nodular skin lesions	Bacterial culture	Antimicrobial therapy (aminoglycosides, tetracyclines, fluoroquinolones)

Disease	Agent	Distribution	Transmission	Incubation	Clinical features	Diagnosis	Treatment
Cat-scratch disease	B henselae	Worldwide	Scratches from infected cats or kittens	1–3 wk	Fever, lymphadenitis, follicular conjunctivitis, encephalitis	Culture, serologies, PCR	Usually self-limited, antimicrobials (macrolides)
Chikungunya[33]	Chikungunya virus	Africa, Asia, Central and South America, Pacific Islands	Aedes aegypti and Aedes albopictus mosquito	3–7 d	Fever, arthritis, headache, conjunctivitis, maculopapular rash, myalgias	Virus-specific IgM, PCR	Supportive care, nonsteroidal antiinflammatory drugs for joint pain
Ebola & Marburg virus diseases[40,41]	Ebola virus & Marburg virus	Africa	Body fluids Rousettus aegyptiacus (fruit bat), nonhuman primate contact, sex	2–21 d	Prodrome of fever, arthralgias, headache, myalgias followed by conjunctivitis, coagulopathy, profuse diarrhea, shock	Antigen detection, RT-PCR, serologies	Experimental immune therapies & antivirals, supportive care
Endemic typhus	Rickettsia typhi	Worldwide, especially Southeast Asia	Rodent fleas (eg, Xenopsylla cheopis)	7–14 d	Fever, headache, malaise, nausea and vomiting, rash	IgM and IgG ELISA, PCR	Antimicrobial therapy (chloramphenicol, doxycycline)
Epidemic typhus	R prowazekii	Central Africa, Asia, Central and South America	Pediculus humanus (human body louse)	7–14 d	Fever, headache, malaise, nausea and vomiting, rash	IgM and IgG ELISA, PCR	Antimicrobial therapy (doxycycline)
Japanese encephalitis	Japanese encephalitis virus	Asia, Western Pacific	Culex species mosquito	5–15 d	Febrile illness, aseptic meningitis, acute encephalitis	IgM ELISA	Supportive care

(continued on next page)

Table 4
(continued)

Disease	Etiologic Pathogen	Geographic Regions	Vector or Exposure	Incubation Period	Presentation	Diagnosis	Management
Lassa fever and other arenaviral infections	Argentine hemorrhagic fever, Lassa virus, Lujo virus, LCMV	Africa, Asia, Europe, North America, and South America	Rodent urine and feces	2–21 d	Fever, myalgia, arthralgia, headache, meningeal signs, retrosternal pain, coagulopathy, birth defects (Lassa and LCMV)	Cell culture, IgM ELISA, RT-PCR	Antimicrobial therapy (ribavirin for Lassa fever), supportive care
Leptospirosis	*Leptospira* species	Caribbean, sub-Saharan Africa, South America, Southeast Asia	Infected animal body fluid or urine, contaminated water, food, or soil	2–30 d	Fever, conjunctival suffusion, back pain, rash, diarrhea, vomiting, renal and liver failure	IgM and IgG ELISA, PCR	Antimicrobial therapy (penicillins, doxycycline)
Lyme disease	*Borrelia burgdorferi*	Europe, Northern to Central Asia	*Ixodes* ticks	3–30 d	Fever, cranial nerve palsy, erythema migrans, headache, malaise, myalgia, myocarditis, meningitis	2-tiered serologic testing (ELISA or IFA & Western blot)	Antimicrobial therapy (beta-lactams, doxycycline)
Murray Valley encephalitis	Murray Valley encephalitis virus	New Guinea, Northwestern or southeastern Australia	*Culex* mosquito	7–28 d	Fever, meningeal signs, seizures	IgM ELISA, neutralizing antibodies, RT-PCR	Supportive care
Plague	*Yersinia pestis*	Central and Southern Africa, Central Asia, Northeastern South America	*X cheopis* flea	1–6 d	Varies with infection type; fever, lymphadenitis, overwhelming pneumonia, sepsis with gangrene	Culture, serologies	Antimicrobial therapy (aminoglycoside, fluoroquinolone, tetracyclines)

Disease	Organism	Geography	Transmission	Incubation	Clinical features	Diagnosis	Treatment
Poliomyelitis	Enterovirus types 1,2,3	Sub-Saharan Africa, Middle East, South and Southeast Asia	Fecal-oral	7–21 d	Flaccid paralysis, respiratory failure	Cell culture, NAAT, PCR	Supportive care
Q fever	*Coxiella burnetii*	Africa, Middle East, Europe	Aerosolized birth fluids or feces from infected livestock	2–3 wk	Self-limiting respiratory illness, pneumonia, hepatitis, cardiac disease	Serial IgG IFA, PCR	Antimicrobial therapy (doxycycline, trimethoprim-sulfamethoxazole, fluoroquinolones)
Rabies	Rabies virus	Africa, Asia, Central and South America	Saliva from infected animal bite (especially bats)	Weeks–months	Prodrome of fever, pain, paresthesias followed by hydrophobia, delirium, seizures, death	Neutralizing antibodies, RT-PCR, IFA	Supportive care, experimental Milwaukee protocol
Rat lungworm	*Angiostrongylus cantonensis*	Caribbean, Asia, Pacific islands	Ingestion of infected snails & slugs or contaminated produce	1–3 wk	Fever, meningeal signs, paresthesias	Serum antibodies, PCR	Supportive care
Relapsing fever	*Borrelia recurrentis*	Sub-Saharan Africa	*Pediculus humanus* (human body louse)	4–14 d	Fever, headache, myalgia, arthralgia, rash	Microscopic evaluation of blood smear, IgM and IgG ELISA, PCR	Antimicrobial therapy (doxycycline)
Rickettsioses	Genera *Rickettsia, Orientia, Ehrlichia, Neorickettsia, Neoehrlichia, Anaplasma*	Africa, Europe, India, and Middle East	Ectoparasites (fleas, lice, mites and ticks)	7–14 d	Fever, headache, eschar (*R conorii*) at bite site, malaise, nausea and vomiting, rash maculopapular or petechial)	Clinical diagnosis, PCR, serologies, biopsy of eschar	Antimicrobial therapy (doxycycline)

(continued on next page)

Table 4
(continued)

Disease	Etiologic Pathogen	Geographic Regions	Vector or Exposure	Incubation Period	Presentation	Diagnosis	Management
RVF and other bunyaviral infections	RVF virus, CCHF, hantavirus	Africa, Eurasia, Middle East, North and South America	Aedes species mosquito, Hyalomma ticks, infected animal carcasses, rodent urine and feces	2–21 d	Fever, myalgia, arthralgia, headache, meningeal signs, vision loss (RVF), coagulopathy, renal failure (hantavirus), ecchymoses (CCHF)	Cell culture, IgM ELISA, RT-PCR	Antimicrobial therapy (ribavirin for CCHF), supportive care
Rubella	Rubella virus	Africa, Middle East, South and Southeast Asia	Person-to-person and droplet	14 d	Fever, conjunctivitis, lymphadenopathy, rash; congenital defects	Serologies, RT-PCR	Supportive care
Scrub typhus	Orientia tsutsugamushi	Asia, Pacific regions	Larval mite (chigger)	6–20 d	Fever, headache, malaise, nausea and vomiting, rash	IgM and IgG ELISA, PCR	Antimicrobial therapy (chloramphenicol, doxycycline)
Sleeping sickness	Trypanosoma brucei	Sub-Saharan, Central, and Western Africa	Glossina species (tsetse) fly	7–21 d	Fever, chancre at bite site, splenomegaly, renal failure, sleep cycle disruption	Microscopic examination of sterile sites or chancre-tissue biopsy	Antimicrobial therapy (suramin for early stage, eflornithine & nifurtimox for late stage)
Tetanus	Clostridium tetani	Worldwide, most common rurally	Contaminated wounds with dirt, excrement; punctures	10 d	Cranial nerve palsies, muscle spasms and rigidity, respiratory failure	Clinical diagnosis	Human tetanus immune globulin, tetanus toxoid, supportive care

Disease	Organism/Virus	Geographic location	Transmission	Incubation period	Clinical features	Diagnosis	Treatment
Tick-borne encephalitis[39]	Tick-borne encephalitis virus	Central and Eastern Europe and Northern Asia	Ixodes species ticks, ingestion of unpasteurized dairy products	4–28 d	Prodrome of febrile illness followed by aseptic meningitis, encephalitis, myelitis	IgM ELISA, RT-PCR	Supportive care
Toxoplasmosis	Toxoplasma gondii	Worldwide	Ingestion of undercooked meat or contaminated water, cat feces	5–23 d	Fever, lymphadenopathy, chorioretinitis, encephalitis or pneumonitis if immunocompromised; congenital syndrome	Serologies, ocular examination, computed tomography or MRI for intracranial lesions	Supportive care or antimicrobial therapy (pyrimethamine, sulfadiazine, leucovorin)
Yellow fever[39]	Yellow fever virus	Sub-Saharan Africa, South America	Aedes species mosquito	3–6 d	Fever, headache, back pain, nausea, vomiting, coagulopathy, shock	RT-PCR, IgM ELISA	Supportive care
Zika[35,36]	Zika virus	Africa, Asia, South and Central America	Aedes species mosquito, body fluids, sex	3–12 d	Fever, arthralgia, conjunctivitis, headache, rash; congenital syndrome	RT-PCR, serologies	Supportive care

Abbreviations: CCHF, Crimean-Congo hemorrhagic fever; ELISA, enzyme-linked immunoassay; Ig, immunoglobulin; IFA, immunofluorescence assay; LCMV, lymphocytic choriomeningitis; NAAT, nucleic acid amplification test; PCR, polymerase chain reaction; RT-PCR, real-time polymerase chain reaction; RVF, Rift Valley fever.

Adapted from Centers for Disease Control and Prevention. The yellow book: health information for international travel 2018. Philadelphia: Oxford University Press; 2017. p. 704. Available at: https://wwwnc.cdc.gov/travel/page/yellowbook-home. Accessed July 25, 2017; with permission.

Table 5
Tropical diseases associated with gastrointestinal symptoms

Disease	Etiologic Pathogen	Geographic Regions	Vector or Exposure	Incubation Period	Presentation	Diagnosis	Management
amebiasis	*Entamoeba histolytica*	Worldwide	Fecal-oral, contaminated food or water	Days–weeks	Abdominal cramps, watery or bloody diarrhea, weight loss, liver abscess with abdominal pain	Microscopic evaluation of stool, serologies	Antimicrobial therapy (metronidazole + iodoquinol or puromycin)
Campylobacteriosis	*Campylobacter jejuni, Campylobacter coli*	Worldwide	Contaminated foods (raw poultry) and water, unpasteurized milk, fecal-oral	2–4 d	Abdominal pain, fever, bloody diarrhea, nausea and vomiting, pseudoappendicitis, reactive arthritis, Guillain-Barre syndrome	Stool culture, darkfield microscopy, NAAT	Supportive care, antimicrobial therapies (fluoroquinolone, macrolide)
Chagas disease	*T cruzi*	Central and South America	Reduviid bug, contaminated food or water, blood transfusion	7 d	Chagoma (eg, Romaña sign), ventricular arrhythmias, megacolon, megaesophagus	Microscopic evaluation of blood smear, IgM ELISA, PCR (acute disease only)	Antimicrobial therapy (benznidazole, nifurtimox)
Cholera	*Vibrio cholerae* O-group 1 or O-group 139	Africa, Caribbean, Southeast Asia	Aquatic plants, brackish water, shellfish	5 d	Profuse, watery diarrhea, nausea and vomiting, muscle cramps, hypovolemic shock	Stool culture	Supportive care, antimicrobial therapy (azithromycin, doxycycline)
Cyclosporiasis	*Cyclospora cayetenensis*	Worldwide	Contaminated produce and water	2–14 d	Watery diarrhea, anorexia, weight loss, abdominal cramps, myalgias, vomiting	Microscopic evaluation of stool for oocysts	Antimicrobial therapy (trimethoprim-sulfamethoxazole)

Disease	Organism	Geographic distribution	Transmission	Incubation period	Clinical features	Diagnosis	Treatment
Echinococcosis	*Echinococcus* species	Eurasia, Central and South America, Africa	Contaminated dog feces, contaminated food or water	5–15 y	Hydatid cysts in liver and lungs, abdominal pain, liver failure	Imaging (ultrasound, computed tomography scan), serologies	Supportive care, surgical excision if cyst >10 cm, antimicrobial therapy (albendazole, praziquantel)
Traveler's diarrhea	Enterotoxigenic *Escherichia coli* (ETEC)	Worldwide	Fecal-oral, contaminated food or water	9 h–3 d	Abdominal pain, watery diarrhea	Clinical diagnosis, NAAT	Supportive care, antimicrobial therapy (ciprofloxacin, azithromycin)
Fascioliasis	*Fasciola hepatica* and *F gigantica*	South America, Middle East, Southeast Asia	Watercress or other aquatic plants, freshwater	6–12 wk	Intermittent, fever eosinophilia, abdominal pain, weight loss, urticaria, biliary colic, liver failure	Microscopic evaluation of stool, serologies, liver imaging	Antimicrobial therapy (triclabendazole)
Giardiasis	*Giardia intestinalis*	Worldwide	Fecal-oral, sexual contact, contaminated water	1–2 wk	Abdominal pain, anorexia, foul-smelling diarrhea, flatulence, nausea, reactive arthritis	Microscopic evaluation of stool, DFA	Antimicrobial therapy (metronidazole, tinidazole, nitazoxanide)
Peptic ulcer disease	*Helicobacter pylori*	Worldwide	Fecal-oral, oral-oral	Unknown	Epigastric pain, nausea and vomiting, anorexia, gastric cancer	Fecal antigen assay, urea breath test	Antimicrobial therapy (proton pump inhibitor + clarithromycin + amoxicillin)
Pinworm	*Enterobius vermicularis*	Worldwide	Fecal-oral, contaminated objects	1–2 mo	Perianal pruritus	Scotch tape test, microscopic evaluation of fingernails	Antimicrobial therapy (albendazole, pyrantel pamoate)

(continued on next page)

Table 5
(continued)

Disease	Etiologic Pathogen	Geographic Regions	Vector or Exposure	Incubation Period	Presentation	Diagnosis	Management
Sarcocystosis	*Sarcocystis* species	Worldwide, especially Southeast Asia	Undercooked beef or pork	2 wk	Fever, malaise, myalgia, headache, cough, arthralgia, nausea and vomiting, diarrhea, palpitations	Microscopic evaluation of stool, PCR, muscle biopsy	Antimicrobial therapy (trimethoprim-sulfamethoxazole)
Soil-transmitted helminths	*Ascaris lumbricoides* (roundworm), *Ancylostoma duodenale* (hookworm), *Necator americanus* (hookworm), *Trichuris trichiura* (whipworm)	Worldwide	Fecal-oral, skin penetration with contaminated soil (hookworms)	Variable	Abdominal pain, malnutrition, bowel obstruction, anemia, cough, chest pain	Microscopic evaluation of stool	Antimicrobial therapy (albendazole, mebendazole)
Strongyloidiasis	*Strongyloides stercoralis*	Worldwide	Auto-inoculation, skin penetration	Variable	Pruritic rash at penetration site, serpiginous rashes (larva currens), respiratory symptoms (Löffler-like pneumonitis), abdominal pain, diarrhea, severe disease if immuno-compromised	Microscopic evaluation of stool other body fluids if disseminated (eg, sputum, CSF)	Antimicrobial therapy (ivermectin, albendazole)

Disease	Organism	Geographic distribution	Source	Incubation period	Clinical features	Diagnosis	Treatment
Taeniasis	Taenia solium (pork) and T saginata or T asiatica (beef)	Central and South America, Africa, South and Southeast Asia	Undercooked contaminated pork or beef	8–10 wk for T solium, 10–14 wk for T saginata	Abdominal discomfort, weight loss, anorexia, perianal pruritus, insomnia, weakness	Microscopic evaluation of stool for eggs	Antimicrobial therapy (praziquantel, niclosamide unless symptomatic neurocysticercosis)
Visceral leishmaniasis	Leishmania donovani and L infantum-chagasi	South America, Central and Southwest Asia, East Africa	Phlebotomine sand fly, blood transfusions	Weeks–months	Fever, weight loss, hepatosplenomegaly, pancytopenia	Light-microscopic evaluation of specimens, culture, molecular methods	Antimicrobial therapy (amphotericin B, miltefosine)
Yersiniosis	Yersinia enterocolitica	Japan, Northern Europe	Undercooked contaminated pork, contaminated water, unpasteurized dairy	4–6 d	Fever, abdominal pain (pseudoappendicitis), bloody diarrhea, necrotizing enterocolitis in infants, reactive arthritis, erythema nodosum	Stool culture (or other body sits; eg, CSF, blood)	Supportive care, antimicrobial therapy if severe (trimethoprim-sulfamethoxazole, fluoroquinolones, aminoglycosides)

Abbreviations: CSF, cerebrospinal fluid; DFA, direct fluorescent antibody.

Adapted from Centers for Disease Control and Prevention. The yellow book: health information for international travel 2018. Philadelphia: Oxford University Press; 2017. p. 704. Available at: https://wwwnc.cdc.gov/travel/page/yellowbook-home. Accessed July 25, 2017; with permission.

Table 6
Tropical diseases associated with respiratory symptoms

Disease	Etiologic Pathogen	Geographic Regions	Vector or Exposure	Incubation Period	Presentation	Diagnosis	Management
Avian bird flu	H5N1 and H7N9 influenza A virus	East and Southeast Asia	Poultry	2–8 d	Fever, malaise, myalgia, headache, nasal congestion, cough, acute respiratory distress syndrome (ARDS)	RT-PCR	Supportive care
Diphtheria	*Corynebacterium diphtheriae*	Asia, South Pacific, Middle East, Eastern Europe, Caribbean	Person-to-person (oral or respiratory droplets), fomites	2–5 d	Fever, dysphagia, malaise, anorexia, pseudomembranes	Bacterial culture	Supportive care, equine diphtheria antitoxin (DAT), antimicrobial therapy (erythromycin, penicillin)
Coccidioidomycosis	*Coccidioides immitis* and *Coccidioides posadasii*	Central and South America	Inhalation of spores from soil	7–21 d	Fever, malaise, cough, headache, night sweats, myalgias, arthritis, rash	Culture, IgM and IgG ELISA, immunodiffusion and complement fixation	Supportive care, antimicrobial therapy if ill or at high risk of dissemination (amphotericin B, azoles)
Histoplasmosis	*Histoplasma capsulatum*	Worldwide, especially river valleys	Inhalation of spores from soil, bird droppings, bat guano	3–17 d	Fever, headache, cough, pleuritic chest pain, malaise	Culture, microscopic examination, PCR, EIA on serum or other samples, immunodiffusion complement fixation	Supportive care, antimicrobial therapy (azole for mild to moderate disease, amphotericin B for severe)

Disease	Organism	Geographic distribution	Transmission	Incubation period	Clinical features	Diagnosis	Treatment
Legionellosis (Legionnaire's disease and Pontiac fever)	*Legionella* species	Worldwide	Inhalation of freshwater aerosol	2–10 d	Fever, headache, myalgias, pneumonia, respiratory distress	Urine antigen assay, paired serologies, PCR	Antimicrobial therapy (fluoroquinolones, macrolides)
Melioidosis	*Burkholderia pseudomallei*	Central and Southeast Asia, northern Australia, South America	Subcutaneous inoculation, inhalation, ingestion; body fluids	1–21 d	Fever, cough, weight loss, pneumonia	Culture, indirect hemagglutination assay	Antimicrobial therapy (ceftazidime, meropenem)
Middle Eastern Respiratory Syndrome (MERS)	MERS coronavirus	North Africa, Middle East	Dromedary camel, person-to-person	2–14 d	Fever, cough, arthralgia, diarrhea, myalgia, acute respiratory failure, multiple organ dysfunction	RT-PCR	Supportive care
Pertussis (whooping cough)	*Bordetella pertussis*	Worldwide	Person-to-person (aerosolized respiratory droplets, respiratory secretions)	7–10 d	Paroxysmal cough, post-tussive vomiting, apnea in infants	Culture, serologies, PCR	Antimicrobial therapy (macrolides)

Adapted from Centers for Disease Control and Prevention. The yellow book: health information for international travel 2018. Philadelphia: Oxford University Press; 2017. p. 704. Available at: https://wwwnc.cdc.gov/travel/page/yellowbook-home. Accessed July 25, 2017; with permission

Table 7
Tropical diseases associated with dermatologic symptoms

Disease	Etiologic Pathogen	Geographic Regions	Vector or Exposure	Incubation Period	Presentation	Diagnosis	Management
B virus	*Macacine herpesvirus 1* or B virus	Worldwide	Bites, scratches, body fluids of infected macaque	3–30 d	Fever, headache, myalgias, vesicular lesions near exposure site with neuropathic pain, ascending encephalomyelitis	PCR, virus-specific antibodies	Supportive care, postexposure prophylaxis (valacyclovir), antimicrobial therapy (acyclovir, ganciclovir)
Cutaneous leishmaniasis	*Leishmania* species	Middle East, Southwest and Central Asia, North Africa, Southern Europe, Central and South America	Phlebotomine sand fly	Weeks–months	Papules that progress to ulcerated plaques, regional lymphadenopathy, and nodular lymphangitis	Light-microscopy evaluation of specimens, cultures, molecular methods	Antimicrobial therapy (miltefosine, amphotericin B)
Cutaneous larva migrans	*Ancylostoma* species (hookworms)	Caribbean, Africa, Asia, South America	Skin contact with contaminated sand	1–5 d	Serpiginous track on skin with pruritus and edema	Clinical	Supportive care, antimicrobial therapy if desired (albendazole, ivermectin)
Loiasis (African eye worm)	*Loa loa*	Central and West Africa	Genus *Chrysops* (deerflies)	7–12 d	Localized edema of extremities and joints (Calabar swelling), diffuse pruritus, eye pruritus and pain, and photophobia	Microscopic evaluation of adult worm from eye, microscopic evaluation of microfilariae on blood smear, serologies	Surgical excision of adult worms, antimicrobial therapy (diethylcarbamazine, albendazole)

	Organism	Geographic distribution	Transmission	Incubation	Clinical features	Diagnosis	Treatment
Lymphatic filariasis	Wuchereria bancrofti, Brugia malayi, and Brugia timori	Sub-Saharan Africa, Southern Asia, Pacific Islands, South America, Caribbean	Aedes, Culex, Anopheles, Mansonia mosquitoes	Years	Lymphatic dysfunction with affected limb edema and pain	Microscopic evaluation of peripheral blood smear, serologies	Antimicrobial therapy (diethylcarbamazine, doxycycline)
Myiasis	Maggots of Dermatobia hominis (human bot fly), Cochliomyia hominivorax (screw worm), and others	Central and South America, Africa, Caribbean	Bites of infected flies or egg laying on open wounds	1–2 wk	Localized skin nodule, pruritus, discharge from punctum	Clinical, serologies	Surgical excision of larvae
Rat-bite fever	Streptobacillus moniliformis and Streptobacillus minus	Worldwide	Bites, scratches, oral secretions of infected rats; unpasteurized milk or contaminated food or water	7–21 d	Relapsing fever, maculopapular or purpuric rash, migratory polyarthritis, lymphadenopathy	Culture, darkfield microscopy, stained peripheral blood smear	Antimicrobial therapy (penicillin G)
River blindness (onchocerciasis)	Onchocerca volvulus	Sub-Saharan Africa, Middle East, South America	Genus Simulium (blackflies)	Weeks – years	Pruritic, popular rash with subcutaneous nodules, lymphadenitis, ocular lesions, vision loss	Microscopic evaluation of skin shavings with microfilariae, histologic evaluation, serologies	Antimicrobial therapy (ivermectin + doxycycline)

(continued on next page)

Table 7
(continued)

Disease	Etiologic Pathogen	Geographic Regions	Vector or Exposure	Incubation Period	Presentation	Diagnosis	Management
Scabies	*Sarcoptes scabiei* var. *Hominis*	Worldwide	Prolonged skin-to-skin contact, fomites if crusted scabies	2–6 wk	Nocturnal pruritus, papulovesicular rash, crusts and scales if crusted scabies	Microscopic evaluation of skin scraping	Antimicrobial therapy (permethrin, ivermectin creams)
Strongyloidiasis	*Strongyloides stercoralis* (roundworm)	Worldwide	Skin penetration with contaminated soil	Unknown	Localized, pruritic, erythematous popular rash, pulmonary symptoms (Löffler-like pneumonitis), diarrhea, abdominal pain, eosinophilia, serpiginous urticarial rash (larva currens)	Microscopic evaluation of stool, peripheral blood eosinophilia if disseminated, serologies	Antimicrobial therapy (ivermectin, albendazole)
Tungiasis	*Tunga penetrans* (chigoe flea, jigger, sand flea)	Africa, South America	Skin penetration (especially walking barefoot)	1–2 d	Localized pruritus and pain with lesions and ulcerations with central black dot	Clinical	Extraction of flea using sterile needle

Adapted from Beeching N, Beadsworth M. Fever on return from abroad. In: Acute medicine–A practical guide to the management of medical emergencies. 5th edition. 2017. p. 207–14; and Centers for Disease Control and Prevention. The yellow book: health information for international travel 2018. Philadelphia: Oxford University Press; 2017. p. 704. Available at: https://wwwnc.cdc.gov/travel/page/yellowbook-home. Accessed July 25, 2017; with permission.

Dermatologic Symptoms

Rashes are a source of concern for parents without the context of travel and may be even more worrisome after going abroad. The differential diagnosis includes typical childhood illnesses, such as roseola or staphylococcal cellulitis, in addition to tropical infections. A study of Canadian travelers from 2009 to 2012 found that cutaneous larva migrans (13%) and skin and soft tissue infections (12.2%) were some of the most common infectious dermatologic complaints among tourists.[47]

In countries where vaccination rates are low, varicella zoster virus or rubella may cause disease, especially in young children who have not completed their immunization series. Measles remains an important risk, with tourists comprising 44% of the 94 cases reported to GeoSentinel from 2000 to 2014, and 13% of patients being younger than 18 years of age, although this may represent underreporting due to the surveillance system's primarily adult focus.[48] Petechiae on the extremities in an ill-appearing child may indicate a serious systemic process such as meningococcal or rickettsial infection. There are many other infections with primarily dermatologic manifestations that may not cause fevers (**Table 7**).[49]

SUMMARY

As the numbers of children who travel abroad continues to increase, clinicians need to remain up-to-date on potential etiologic factors for febrile illnesses on families' return home. After ruling out life-threatening disorders that can be acquired locally or internationally, physicians are able to develop a focused diagnosis and management plan best suited to the patient's clinical picture. There is a growing body of resources to assist clinicians, such as the CDC (www.cdc.gov/travel/) and GeoSentinel (www.istm.org/geosentinel) for data on epidemiology, geography, and other risk factors.

In the future, physicians will need to be prepared to deal with the global epidemic of antimicrobial drug resistance, evolving epidemics and pandemics caused by emerging pathogens, reemerging infections due to vaccine hesitancy or international conflicts, and medical tourism in both healthy and medically complex children.

REFERENCES

1. Cavagnaro CS, Brady K, Siegel C. Fever after international travel. Clin Pediatr Emerg Med 2008;9(4):250–7.
2. Bottieau E, Clerinx J, Schrooten W, et al. Etiology and outcome of fever after a stay in the tropics. Arch Intern Med 2006;166(15):1642–8.
3. Ladhani S, Aibara RJ, Riordan FA, et al. Imported malaria in children: a review of clinical studies. Lancet Infect Dis 2007;7(5):349–57.
4. Summer A, Stauffer WM. Evaluation of the sick child following travel to the tropics. Pediatr Ann 2008;37(12):821–6.
5. Tate JE, Burton AH, Boschi-Pinto C, et al. 2008 estimate of worldwide rotavirus-associated mortality in children younger than 5 years before the introduction of universal rotavirus vaccination programmes: a systematic review and meta-analysis. Lancet Infect Dis 2012;12(2):136–41.
6. World Tourism Organization. International tourist arrivals up 4% reach a record 1.2 billion in 2015. 2016. Available at: http://media.unwto.org/press-release/2016-01-18/international-tourist-arrivals-4-reach-record-12-billion-2015. Accessed July 25, 2017.

7. Freedman DO, Weld LH, Kozarsky PE, et al. Spectrum of disease and relation to place of exposure among ill returned travelers. N Engl J Med 2006;354(2): 119–30.

8. Leuthard D, Berger C, Staubli G, et al. Management of children with travel-related illness evaluated in a pediatric emergency room. Pediatr Infect Dis J 2015;34(12): 1279–82.

9. Wilson ME, Weld LH, Boggild A, et al. Fever in returned travelers: results from the GeoSentinel surveillance network. Clin Infect Dis 2007;44(12):1560–8.

10. Hill DR, Ericsson CD, Pearson RD, et al. The practice of travel medicine: guidelines by the infectious diseases society of america. Clin Infect Dis 2006;43(12): 1499–539.

11. Anwar E, Goldberg E, Fraser A, et al. Vaccines for preventing typhoid fever. Cochrane Database Syst Rev 2014;(1):CD001261.

12. Magwenzi MT, Gudza-Mugabe M, Mujuru HA, et al. Carriage of antibiotic-resistant Enterobacteriaceae in hospitalised children in tertiary hospitals in Harare, Zimbabwe. Antimicrob Resist Infect Control 2017;6:10, eCollection 2017.

13. Cousins S. Syrian crisis: health experts say more can be done. Lancet 2015; 385(9972):931–4.

14. Jensenius M, Davis X, von Sonnenburg F, et al. Multicenter GeoSentinel analysis of rickettsial diseases in international travelers, 1996-2008. Emerg Infect Dis 2009;15(11):1791–8.

15. Genton B, D'Acremont V, Rare L, et al. *Plasmodium vivax* and mixed infections are associated with severe malaria in children: a prospective cohort study from Papua New Guinea. PLoS Med 2008;5(6):e127.

16. Stauffer W, Fischer PR. Diagnosis and treatment of malaria in children. Clin Infect Dis 2003;37(10):1340–8.

17. Griffith KS, Lewis LS, Mali S, et al. Treatment of malaria in the United States: a systematic review. JAMA 2007;297(20):2264–77.

18. Boggild AK, Geduld J, Libman M, et al. Malaria in travellers returning or migrating to canada: surveillance report from CanTravNet surveillance data, 2004-2014. CMAJ Open 2016;4(3):E352–358.

19. Moody A. Rapid diagnostic tests for malaria parasites. Clin Microbiol Rev 2002; 15(1):66–78.

20. Taylor SM, Molyneux ME, Simel DL, et al. Does this patient have malaria? JAMA 2010;304(18):2048–56.

21. Dondorp A, Nosten F, Stepniewska K, et al. South East Asian Quinine Artesunate Malaria Trial (SEAQUAMAT) group. Artesunate versus quinine for treatment of severe falciparum malaria: a randomised trial. Lancet 2005;366(9487):717–25.

22. Dondorp AM, Fanello CI, Hendriksen IC, et al. Artesunate versus quinine in the treatment of severe falciparum malaria in African children (AQUAMAT): an open-label, randomised trial. Lancet 2010;376(9753):1647–57.

23. Centers for Disease Control and Prevention. Artesunate is available to treat severe malaria in the United States. 2012. Available at: https://www.cdc.gov/malaria/diagnosis_treatment/artesunate.html. Accessed July 25, 2017.

24. Britto C, Pollard AJ, Voysey M, et al. An appraisal of the clinical features of pediatric enteric fever: Systematic review and meta-analysis of the age-stratified disease occurrence. Clin Infect Dis 2017;64(11):1604–11.

25. Nield LS, Stauffer W, Kamat D. Evaluation and management of illness in a child after international travel. Pediatr Emerg Care 2005;21(3):184–95 [quiz:196–8].

26. Basnyat B, Maskey AP, Zimmerman MD, et al. Enteric (typhoid) fever in travelers. Clin Infect Dis 2005;41(10):1467–72.

27. Frenck RW Jr, Nakhla I, Sultan Y, et al. Azithromycin versus ceftriaxone for the treatment of uncomplicated typhoid fever in children. Clin Infect Dis 2000; 31(5):1134–8.
28. Azmatullah A, Qamar FN, Thaver D, et al. Systematic review of the global epidemiology, clinical and laboratory profile of enteric fever. J Glob Health 2015;5(2): 020407.
29. Schwartz E, Weld LH, Wilder-Smith A, et al. Seasonality, annual trends, and characteristics of dengue among ill returned travelers, 1997-2006. Emerg Infect Dis 2008;14(7):1081–8.
30. Centers for Disease Control and Prevention. Dengue 2014. Available at: https://www.cdc.gov/dengue/epidemiology/index.html. Accessed July 25, 2017.
31. Wilder-Smith A, Schwartz E. Dengue in travelers. N Engl J Med 2005;353(9): 924–32.
32. Gould EA, Solomon T. Pathogenic flaviviruses. Lancet 2008;371(9611):500–9.
33. Gautret P, Mockenhaupt F, Grobusch MP, et al. Arboviral and other illnesses in travellers returning from Brazil, June 2013 to May 2016: implications for the 2016 Olympic and Paralympic Games. Euro Surveill 2016;21(27). https://doi.org/10.2807/1560-7917.ES.2016.21.27.30278.
34. Barnett ED, Wilder-Smith A, Wilson ME. Yellow fever vaccines and international travelers. Expert Rev Vaccines 2008;7(5):579–87.
35. Hagmann SHF. Clinical impact of non-congenital Zika virus infection in infants and children. Curr Infect Dis Rep 2017;19(8):29.
36. Boggild AK, Geduld J, Libman M, et al. Surveillance report of Zika virus among Canadian travellers returning from the Americas. CMAJ 2017;189(9):E334–40.
37. Pitzinger B, Steffen R, Tschopp A. Incidence and clinical features of traveler's diarrhea in infants and children. Pediatr Infect Dis J 1991;10(10):719–23.
38. Ang JY, Mathur A. Traveler's diarrhea: updates for pediatricians. Pediatr Ann 2008;37(12):814–20.
39. Rendi-Wagner P, Korinek M, Mikolasek A, et al. Epidemiology of travel-associated and autochthonous hepatitis A in Austrian children, 1998 to 2005. J Trav Med 2007;14(4):248–53.
40. Cheng G, Li Z, Dai X, et al. Analysis of *Clostridium difficile* associated diarrhea in pediatric patients with antibiotic-associated diarrhea. Zhonghua Er Ke Za Zhi 2015;53(3):220–4.
41. Michal Stevens A, Esposito DH, Stoney RJ, et al. *Clostridium difficile* infection in returning travellers. J Trav Med 2017;24(3). https://doi.org/10.1093/jtm/taw099.
42. Barbosa F, Barnett ED, Gautret P, et al. Bordetella pertussis infections in travelers: data from the GeoSentinel global network. J Trav Med 2017;24(3). https://doi.org/10.1093/jtm/taw094.
43. Blanton L, Kniss K, Smith S, et al. Update: Influenza activity–united states and worldwide, may 24-september 5, 2015. MMWR Morb Mortal Wkly Rep 2015; 64(36):1011–6.
44. Clerinx J, Van Gompel A. Schistosomiasis in travellers and migrants. Travel Med Infect Dis 2011;9(1):6–24.
45. Stephenson LS, Latham MC, Kurz KM, et al. Single dose metrifonate or praziquantel treatment in Kenyan children. II. Effects on growth in relation to *Schistosoma haematobium* and hookworm egg counts. Am J Trop Med Hyg 1989;41(4): 445–53.
46. Stevens MS, Geduld J, Libman M, et al. Dermatoses among returned Canadian travellers and immigrants: Surveillance report based on CanTravNet data, 2009-2012. CMAJ Open 2015;3(1):E119–26.

47. Sotir MJ, Esposito DH, Barnett ED, et al. Measles in the 21st century, a continuing preventable risk to travelers: data from the GeoSentinel global network. Clin Infect Dis 2016;62(2):210–2.

48. Lederman ER, Weld LH, Elyazar IR, et al. Dermatologic conditions of the ill returned traveler: an analysis from the GeoSentinel surveillance network. Int J Infect Dis 2008;12(6):593–602.

49. Jensen K, Alvarado-Ramy F, Gonzalez-Martinez J, et al. B-virus and free-ranging macaques, Puerto Rico. Emerg Infect Dis 2004;10(3):494–6.

50. Beeching N, Beadsworth M. Fever on return from abroad. In: Acute medicine - A practical guide to the management of medical emergencies. 5th edition. Wiley; 2017. p. 207–14.

51. Thwaites GE, Day NP. Approach to fever in the returning traveler. N Engl J Med 2017;376(6):548–60.

52. Centers for Disease Control and Prevention. The yellow book: health information for international travel 2018. Philadelphia: Oxford University Press; 2017. p. 704. Available at: https://wwwnc.cdc.gov/travel/page/yellowbook-home. Accessed July 25, 2017.

Malaria in Children

Natasha M. Kafai, BS[a], Audrey R. Odom John, MD, PhD[b,c],*

KEYWORDS

- Malaria • Travel medicine • Fever • Diagnostics • Antiparasitic therapy
- Chemoprophylaxis

KEY POINTS

- Malaria is common worldwide and travel to malaria-endemic destinations is increasing.
- Travel history should be obtained for all children presenting with fever.
- Antigen-based malaria tests can provide rapid malaria diagnosis, although blood smears are still necessary.
- Treatment of malaria depends on severity of illness, species of malaria parasite, and epidemiologic likelihood of drug resistance.

INTRODUCTION

A century ago, malaria was a major public health threat in the United States, with ongoing transmission in 13 Southeastern states as late as the 1930s.[1] Although extensive efforts ultimately eliminated local malaria in North America, this mosquito-borne infection remains endemic throughout much of the world. Indeed, more than half of the children on our planet live in malaria-endemic countries. Despite continued success in malaria control, there are more than 200 million new infections each year and nearly half a million deaths, mostly in infants and children younger than 5 years old.[2] Importantly, in our increasingly global society, malaria and other imported infectious diseases remain of particular concern to the North American traveler, with nearly all American malaria cases acquired abroad.[3–6]

This article offers a brief overview of the *Plasmodium* parasite responsible for malaria, the epidemiology of infection, clinical features associated with uncomplicated

Disclosures: Research funding: NIH/NIAID (AI103280, AI123808), Bill and Melinda Gates Foundation, Children's Discovery Institute, and Dr A.R.O. John is a Burroughs Wellcome Fund Investigator in the Pathogenesis of Infectious Disease. Scientific advisory board member, Pluton Biosciences LLC (A.R.O. John).
a Medical Scientist Training Program, Washington University School of Medicine, 660 S. Euclid Avenue, Campus Box 8226, St Louis, MO 63110, USA; b Department of Pediatrics, Washington University School of Medicine, 660 South Euclid Avenue, Campus Box 8208, St Louis, MO 63110, USA; c Department of Molecular Microbiology, Washington University School of Medicine, 660 South Euclid Avenue, Campus Box 8208, St Louis, MO 63110, USA
* Corresponding author.
E-mail address: aodom@wustl.edu

Infect Dis Clin N Am 32 (2018) 189–200
https://doi.org/10.1016/j.idc.2017.10.008
0891-5520/18/© 2017 Elsevier Inc. All rights reserved.

id.theclinics.com

and severe malaria presentations, preventative measures for travelers, and current treatment strategies for childhood malaria infections.

DESCRIPTION OF THE PATHOGEN

Malaria is caused by infection with intracellular protozoan parasites of the genus *Plasmodium*, transmitted by the bite of a female *Anopheles* spp mosquito.[7,8] While feeding, the infected mosquito leaves behind sporozoites, the infectious motile form of the parasite. Sporozoites then migrate to the liver, asymptomatically invade hepatocytes, and amplify infection through the release of tens of thousands of daughter parasites. This release initiates the asexual erythrocytic replication stage of the parasite life cycle, the stage of parasite responsible for the malaria pathogenesis. Two species of *Plasmodium*, *P vivax* and *P ovale*, uniquely develop dormant parasite forms called hypnozoites, which may remain in the liver for months or years after primary infection before causing relapse and recurrent symptomatic disease.[9,10]

The clinical symptoms of malaria are due to cycles of asexual replication within red blood cells (**Fig. 1**). Fever is a hallmark symptom, triggered by erythrocyte rupture and parasite release every 2 to 3 days, depending on *Plasmodium* species.[7] Severe, life-threatening malaria may result from high parasite burdens, causing hemolysis and severe anemia, or from end-organ damage due to vascular adherence of infected erythrocytes and microocclusion.[11,12] Person-to-person transmission is mediated by mosquitoes, in which the sexual form of the parasite (gametocytes) infects a feeding mosquito to thus complete the parasite's complex life cycle.[7,8]

EPIDEMIOLOGY

More than half the world's population lives in areas where malaria transmission occurs, and the disease continues to cause a major public health burden to populations in areas of Africa, Asia, and Central and South America (**Fig. 2**).[2] In 2015, more than 200 million

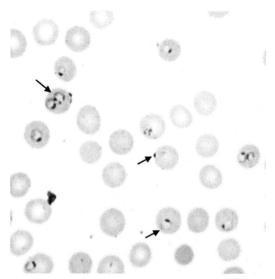

Fig. 1. Blood smear from patient with *P falciparum* malaria. Intraerythrocytic parasite forms are visible in nearly 20% of red blood cells, some of which are doubly-infected. Arrows: typical signet ring, headphones, and appliqué forms of the parasite. (*Courtesy of* Amruta Padhye MD, Columbia, MO.)

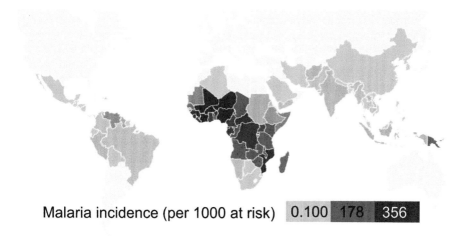

Malaria incidence (per 1000 at risk)   0.100 178 356

Fig. 2. Malaria incidence in 2015. Incidence of malaria per 1000 population at risk. Map created using OpenHeatMap (www.openheatmap.com). (*Data from* World Health Organization. World malaria report 2015. Geneva (Switzerland): World Health Organization; 2016. Available at: http://www.who.int/malaria/publications/world-malaria-report-2015/report/en/.)

cases of malaria were reported, resulting in nearly half a million deaths, an estimate 3 times higher than the number of people lost to armed conflicts that same year.[2,13] Most of malaria-associated deaths are caused by *P falciparum* species in sub-Saharan Africa, which kills about 1200 African children younger than the age of 5 years daily.[14]

Global malaria control efforts have focused on both mosquito vector control strategies and improved access to effective antimalarial therapies. There have been tremendous gains in the last decade; from 2000 to 2015, the incidence of malaria has dropped by 37%, and deaths have decreased by 60% globally.[2,15] However, drug resistance continues to hamper control efforts worldwide, with widespread resistance to the former first-line agents chloroquine and sulfadoxine-pyrimethamine.[16] The remarkable discovery of artemisinin by Nobel Laureate Youyou Tu ultimately led to development of rapidly parasiticidal artemisinin-based combination therapies (ACTs), powerful weapons in the face of rising resistance to older antimalarials.[17,18] Unfortunately, the emergence of artemisinin-resistant *P falciparum* in Southeast Asia, only a few years after ACT implementation, emphasizes the importance of sustaining control measures and the ongoing need for antimalarial development.[19,20]

Though malarial transmission remains possible in areas of the United States where anopheline mosquitoes are found, nearly all of the 1500 or so annual reported cases of malaria in the United States are infections acquired abroad.[3,5,21] Rare and unusual modes of transmission have also been reported, which include inadvertent airplane transport of mosquitos from endemic areas, congenital transmission, transfusion-associated malaria, and contaminated needles and syringes.[22–26]

CLINICAL FEATURES OF MALARIA

Uncomplicated malaria infection typically manifests as a nonspecific febrile illness, similar in presentation to influenza and other common viral infections.[27,28] Travelers with acute malaria most often present within 7 days to 3 months following an infected mosquito bite, and malaria should be suspected in any febrile traveler.[3] Malaria symptoms are highly variable, and may include chills, rigors, sweating, headaches, lethargy, myalgias, and cough. Gastrointestinal symptoms may be prominent, including nausea, emesis, diarrhea, and abdominal pain.[29] In addition to fever, physical findings may reflect end-organ involvement, including pallor, tachycardia, hepatosplenomegaly, jaundice, and increased respiratory rate, as well as, in the case of cerebral malaria, altered mental status.[30] The course of disease may be indolent or fulminant, and delays in or lack of treatment beyond 24 hours following onset of clinical symptoms may result in rapid progression to life-threatening, severe malarial disease.[31]

Children younger than 18 years of age tend to present sooner and are more likely to develop severe malaria. Of note, the classic cyclical fever patterns described for malaria may not be present in travelers and young children because parasite life cycles may not have synchronized by the time treatment is sought.[27,28] Unsurprisingly, travelers are more likely to present with severe malaria, compared with the semi-immune residents of endemic areas.[3,5] Additional risk factors for development of severe malaria include recent travel to *P falciparum*–endemic regions (especially sub-Saharan Africa), age older than 65 years or younger than 18 years, pregnancy, existing medical conditions, lack of malaria prophylaxis, and treatment delay.[5,30]

Severe malaria may manifest as 1 or more of the following syndromes[30,32]:

1. Cerebral malaria: Caused by parasite adherence to cerebral vasculature, symptoms may include altered mental status, coma, seizures, and evidence of increased intracranial pressure
2. Blackwater fever: Acute renal failure and hemoglobinuria caused by intravascular hemolysis
3. Severe anemia: Defined as hemoglobin less than 7 g/dL and caused by high parasite burden and hemolysis of infected erythrocytes
4. Acute respiratory distress syndrome
5. Hyperparasitemia: Typically defined as malaria parasite infection of greater than 5% of circulating red blood cells
6. Metabolic complications: Common abnormalities include severe metabolic acidosis and life-threatening hypoglycemia.

Although fever is an almost universal symptom of malaria, infections with different *Plasmodium* species may have somewhat variable clinical presentations (**Table 1**).

Table 1 Species of human malaria parasites		
Plasmodium Species	**Endemic Regions**	**Typical Drug Resistance**
P falciparum	• Sub-Saharan Africa • Haiti • Dominican Republic • Southeast Asia	• Chloroquine • Sulfadoxine-pyrimethamine • ACT therapies (in Southeast Asia)
P vivax	• Indian subcontinent • Central and South America • Southeast Asia	• Chloroquine (some areas)
P ovale	• Most cases reported in West Africa • May also be present in Asia	—
P malariae	Less common Wide global distribution	—
P knowlesi	Rare Cases in forested regions of Southeast Asia, associated with long-tailed macaques	—

Severe malaria is most often due to infection with *P falciparum*, which can reach higher parasite levels than other species.[8] *P falciparum* accounts for 80% of United States malaria cases seen in child travelers.[2] In contrast, *P vivax* and *P ovale* infections are rarely fatal but carry the risk of reactivation of dormant liver-stage parasites.[9,10] Chronic asymptomatic bloodstream infection may result from *P malariae* infection, which can also cause a nephrotic syndrome from immune complex deposition in the kidney.[33] Less often seen in travelers, *P knowlesi* is a zoonotic malaria parasite of long-tailed macaques, increasingly recognized as a cause of severe human infections that may be misdiagnosed as the less harmful *P malariae* species.[34]

MALARIA PREVENTION FOR TRAVELERS: AWARENESS AND BITES

Protective strategies against malaria infection are strongly recommended for all travelers to malaria-endemic regions. Because there is no approved vaccine for malaria, malaria prevention requires awareness of the risks of malaria infection, preventing mosquito bites and encouraging adherence to antimalarial chemoprophylactic regimens.[35]

A health care provider must first help to assess a traveler's risk of contracting malaria by determining the endemicity of a particular locale and the season of travel. Urban areas, air-conditioned locations, and geographic regions above 3300 m are typically free of malaria.[35] Clinicians who provide pretravel counseling should consult the most current and detailed information on health risks, including malaria, which may be found on the Centers for Disease Control and Prevention (CDC) Web site (www.CDC.gov/malaria), as well the World Health Organization Web site (http://www.who.int/malaria/travellers/en/). Parents and guardians are strongly cautioned against taking very young children to high endemicity areas, in part because it is challenging to provide a suitable preventative chemotherapeutic regimen that is approved for use in small infants (**Table 2**). Furthermore, malaria may be rapidly fatal in young pediatric patients, in whom early symptoms of *P falciparum* infection may go unrecognized.[36]

All species of malaria are mosquito-transmitted and, therefore, the first line of protection against infection is to prevent bites from *Anopheles* spp. Insect repellents containing DEET, picaridin, or IR3535 are recommended to protect exposed skin and should be reapplied every few hours in warmer climates. Protective clothing should be worn, with long sleeves and pants tucked into socks with appropriate footwear. A helpful tip is to treat clothing with repellent or long-lasting insecticides such as permethrin (readily available from online retailers), which lasts through several clothing washes. Finally, travelers are strongly recommended to use insecticide-treated mosquito bed nets with mesh sizes smaller than 1.5 mm, which are particularly effective against the night-feeding *A gambiae* vector.[36]

MALARIA PREVENTION FOR TRAVELERS: CHEMOPROPHYLAXIS

In addition to barrier protection, chemoprophylaxis should be offered to adults and children traveling to endemic malaria regions. Specific regimens are dictated by a traveler's risk of acquiring malaria and local antimalarial-resistance patterns, and providers are encouraged to follow country-specific recommendations from the CDC (https://www.cdc.gov/malaria/travelers/country_table/a.html). In the United States, approved malaria chemoprophylaxis options include atovaquone-proguanil, chloroquine, doxycycline, mefloquine, and primaquine (see **Table 2**).[37]

Most cases of *P falciparum* malaria infection result from inadequate adherence to prophylactic regimens or failure to take precautions against mosquitoes, with self-reported adherence rates in American military personnel of less than 50%.[38,39]

Table 2
Commonly used agents for antimalarial prophylaxis

	Treatment Recommendations	Contraindications	Target Population
Atovaquone-proguanil	Prevention and treatment of chloroquine-resistant *P falciparum*	Not recommended for pregnant or breastfeeding women, children <11 kg, or patients with impaired renal function	Last-minute travelers or travelers with short-term exposure to endemic regions Well-tolerated but may be more expensive than other options
Doxycycline	Can be used for prophylaxis but not treatment	Contraindicated in children <8 y old and pregnant women Gastrointestinal discomfort and sun sensitivity are common	Daily dosing, inexpensive option, suitable for last-minute travelers
Mefloquine	Effective against chloroquine-resistant parasites	Safe during pregnancy but not approved by the US Food and Drug Administration for children weighing <5 kg or younger than 6 mo Neuropsychiatric effects can be pronounced, contraindicated in patients with seizure disorders or cardiac conduction abnormalities	Weekly dosing regimen, preferred for long-term travelers
Primaquine	Recommended for prophylaxis in areas with *P vivax* malaria	Cannot be taken by pregnant or breast-feeding women Testing is necessary to exclude patients with glucose-6-phosphate dehydrogenase (G6PD) deficiency	Daily dosing
Chloroquine	Limited use due to widespread resistance	Safe for infants, young children, and pregnant women	Weekly dosing, must be started 1–2 wk before travel

Proper education about the risks of malaria and the efficacy of prevention methods has been shown to improve adherence to preventative measures, and this is particularly important with rising rates of international travel.[6,36] In summary, the ABCs of malaria prevention are as follows[36]:

A: Awareness of the risks of malaria. This can include understanding incubation periods, the possibility of delayed onset symptoms, and symptoms, especially fever.

B: Bites. Efforts to reduce the likelihood of mosquito bites.

C: Chemoprophylaxis. Using antimalarial drugs that target blood and liver-stage parasites to prevent progression of infection to disease.

D: Diagnosis. Prompt diagnosis and treatment is key to prevent complications of disease caused by malaria infection.

DIAGNOSIS OF MALARIA INFECTION

Because the symptoms of malaria can be highly variable, clinicians should maintain a high index of suspicion for all returning travelers presenting with fever. Clinicians should continue to consider routine pediatric infections, such as viral and bacterial respiratory tract infections, infectious diarrhea, and urinary tract infections. In patients with fever and altered mental status or seizure, cerebral malaria may mimic bacterial meningitis, which is of particular concern in young children who may not have completed routine vaccinations and in travelers returning from the Hajj or other parts of the meningitis belt of sub-Saharan Africa. Important additional considerations in travelers include typhoid fever (especially in children younger than 5 years) and dengue, both of which are common in malaria-endemic regions.[35] Clinicians should maintain awareness of any ongoing global infectious disease outbreaks, such as Ebola and severe acute respiratory syndrome (SARS), which may have immediate infection control implications.

When malaria is suspected, thick and thin blood films of peripheral blood should be examined.[31] Thick blood films provide for more sensitive detection of malaria parasites, whereas thin blood films permit speciation and quantification of parasitemia. Blood films should be repeated every 12 to 24 hours during the initial 72 hours of suspected malaria infection, regardless of whether parasites are observed.[37]

Lateral flow-based rapid diagnostic tests (RDTs) have recently become available to provide initial screening for malaria infection, especially for smaller facilities that may not have trained microscopists on staff at all times. Beginning in 2007, the US Food and Drug Administration (FDA) approved the BinaxNOW malaria RDT for use in commercial laboratories and hospitals. This antigen detection kit has high sensitivity and specificity for *P falciparum* and *P vivax* infection, with reduced sensitivity for *P ovale* and *P malariae*.[40,41] Because both false-positive and false-negative results have been reported with RDTs worldwide, suspected malaria should continue to be evaluated by blood smears, regardless of the results of rapid testing.[42–44]

Nucleic acid testing for malaria remains the gold standard, with the highest sensitivity and specificity[42,45]; however, such testing is unavailable at most North American facilities. Polymerase chain reaction testing for diagnostic confirmation and species identification is provided free-of-charge for referring facilities in the United States.[3]

TREATMENT OF MALARIA INFECTION

Single-agent (monotherapy) approaches to malaria treatment are a major contributor to drug resistance and are not recommended.[32] In general, antimalarial decision-making is based on severity of symptoms, parasite species, and likelihood of drug resistance (**Fig. 3**). Uncomplicated *P falciparum* (or unknown malaria species) infection is effectively treated with a 3-day regimen of ACT, which combines the fast-acting artemisinin derivative with a longer-acting antimalarial partner drug. In the United States, artemether-lumefantrine (Coartem), a single orally available ACT for treatment of uncomplicated malaria, is commercially available.[46]

P vivax, *P ovale*, *P malariae*, and *P knowlesi* infections acquired in chloroquine-susceptible endemic areas may be treated with chloroquine, otherwise treatment with an ACT is recommended.[31] Importantly, for radical cure and elimination of latent liver stages, *P vivax* and *P ovale* infections must additionally be treated with a 14-day

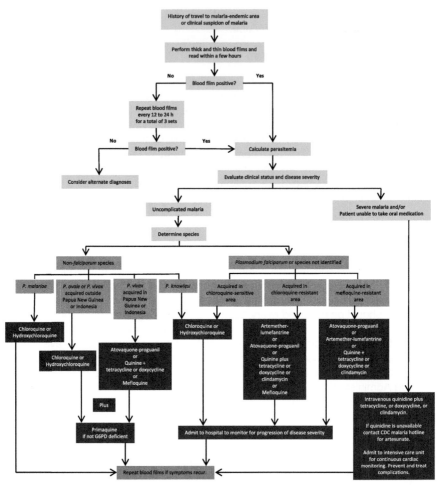

Fig. 3. Decision-tree for malaria treatment. G6PD, glucose 6-phosphatase. (*Courtesy of* CDC, Atlanta, GA. Available at: https://www.cdc.gov/malaria/resources/pdf/algorithm.pdf.)

course of primaquine to prevent future relapse. Note that patients must be evaluated for the presence of glucose 6-phosphatase (G6PD) deficiency before initiation of primaquine, which can precipitate hemolytic crisis.[37]

Patients with severe malaria will require intensive supportive care and parenteral treatment with intravenous antimalarial treatment. Worldwide, intravenous artesunate is strongly recommended because evidence suggests improved survival compared with quinine.[47] However, artesunate is not commercially available in the United States and, therefore, intravenous quinidine gluconate is the most commonly available treatment for severe malaria. Due to its arrhythmogenic cardiotoxicity, quinidine treatment requires cardiac telemetry and QTc monitoring.[31] As of 2007, intravenous artesunate, produced following Good Manufacturing Practices, has been made available on an emergency basis, through an investigational new drug protocol (FDA IND protocol # 76,725) for the treatment of severe malaria in the United States. Clinicians treating pediatric patients with severe malaria are encouraged to consult the CDC Malaria Hotline, which provides expert clinical advice and release of intravenous artesunate with severe malaria patients in whom quinidine is not appropriate.[48] Additional malaria treatment guidelines and dosing specifications can be found on the CDC Web site (https://www.cdc.gov/malaria/diagnosis_treatment/treatment.html). Monotherapy for malaria is not recommended and, therefore, all cases of severe malaria require a second agent, such as tetracycline, doxycycline, or clindamycin (intravenous or oral).[32,37] There is no consensus about the efficacy of exchange blood transfusion for severe disease.[32,49,50]

A few pediatric-specific treatment modifications may be necessary for treatment of malaria in children. Pyrimethamine should be avoided in the first few weeks of life because it competes with bilirubin and may aggravate neonatal hyperbilirubinemia. Data are limited on the safety and tolerability of primaquine in young infants, which is, therefore, contraindicated in children younger than 6 months of age, and tetracyclines are contraindicated for children younger than 8 years of age. Parenteral antimalarial treatment may be required for treatment of uncomplicated malaria in children with prominent gastrointestinal symptoms, until oral administration is possible.[32,37]

Best Practices

What is the current practice?

Pediatric malaria infection
  Best practice, guideline, and care path objectives
  - Counsel travelers to malaria-endemic regions on the ABCs of protective measures against infection, including limiting mosquito contact and chemoprophylaxis.
  - Consider malaria in the differential for any infant or child presenting with nonspecific febrile illness, particularly in returning travelers.
  - Rapid recognition and diagnosis of malaria infection is necessary to prevent disease progression.
  - Treatment of malaria depends on disease severity, *Plasmodium* species, and likelihood of antimalarial resistance.

What changes in current practice are likely to improve outcomes?

- Improve adherence to antimalarial regimens and other prevention techniques through proper traveler education.

- A travel history should be obtained for all pediatric patients presenting with fever or flu-like symptoms.

- Monotherapeutic regimens that promote development of drug resistance should be avoided.

Treatment recommendations
- Diagnosis depends on microscopic analysis of rapid antigen testing and thick and thin blood smears.
- Combination malaria treatment is based on disease severity, parasite species, and likelihood of drug resistance.
- For *P vivax* and *P ovale*, primaquine treatment (following G6PD testing) is necessary to prevent relapse from latent liver stages.

Summary

Properly informing travelers to malaria-endemic regions about preventative measures for infection is the most effective means of promoting adherence and preventing transmission. In the event of malaria infection, a high index of suspicion, rapid diagnosis, and immediate treatment is critical to prevent the morbidity and mortality associated with disease progression, particularly in pediatric patients.

REFERENCES

1. Bleakley H. Malaria eradication in the Americas: A retrospective analysis of childhood exposure. Am Econ J Appl Econ 2010;2(2):1–45.
2. World Health Organization. World malaria report 2016. Geneva (Switzerland): World Health Organization; 2016.
3. Mace KE, Arguin PM. Malaria surveillance—United States, 2014. MMWR Surveill Summ 2017;66:1–24.
4. Armed Forces Health Surveillance Branch. Update: malaria, US armed forces, 2015. MSMR 2016;23(1):2.
5. Hwang J, Cullen KA, Kachur SP, et al. Severe morbidity and mortality risk from malaria in the United States, 1985–2011. Open Forum Infectious Diseases 2014;1(1):ofu034.
6. World Tourism Organization. UNWTO World Tourism Highlights, 2015 edition. Madrid (Spain): World Tourism Organization; 2015. Available at: https://www.e-unwto.org/doi/book/10.18111/9789284416899.
7. Phillips MA, Burrows JN, Manyando C, et al. Malaria. Nat Rev Dis Primers 2017;3: 17050.
8. Cowman AF, Healer J, Marapana D, et al. Malaria: biology and disease. Cell 2016;167(3):610–24.
9. Markus MB. Malaria relapse. In: Mehlhorn H, editor. Encyclopedia of parasitology. Berlin: Springer-Verlag; 2016. p. 1–3.
10. Chu CS, White NJ. Management of relapsing *Plasmodium vivax* malaria. Expert Rev Anti Infect Ther 2016;14(10):885–900.
11. Dondorp AM, Kager PA, Vreeken J, et al. Abnormal blood flow and red blood cell deformability in severe malaria. Parasitol Today 2000;16(6):228–32.
12. Miller LH, Ackerman HC, Su XZ, et al. Malaria biology and disease pathogenesis: insights for new treatments. Nat Med 2013;19(2):156–67.
13. Studies IIfS. The IISS armed conflict survey: ACS, the Worldwide review of political, military and humanitarian trends in current conflicts. Routledge; 2015 . Available at: https://www.iiss.org/en/publications/acs/by%20year/armed-conflict-survey-2015-46e5.
14. Maitland K. Severe malaria in African children—the need for continuing investment. N Engl J Med 2016;375(25):2416–7.
15. Newby G, Bennett A, Larson E, et al. The path to eradication: a progress report on the malaria-eliminating countries. Lancet 2016;387(10029):1775–84.
16. Olliaro P. Drug resistance hampers our capacity to roll back malaria. Clin Infect Dis 2005;41(Supplement_4):S247–57.
17. Tu Y. Artemisinin—a gift from traditional Chinese medicine to the world (Nobel lecture). Angew Chem Int Ed 2015;55:2–19.
18. Bosman A, Mendis KN. A major transition in malaria treatment: the adoption and deployment of artemisinin-based combination therapies. Am J Trop Med Hyg 2007;77(6_Suppl):193–7.
19. Ashley EA, Dhorda M, Fairhurst RM, et al. Spread of artemisinin resistance in *Plasmodium falciparum* malaria. N Engl J Med 2014;371(5):411–23.
20. Woodrow CJ, White NJ. The clinical impact of artemisinin resistance in Southeast Asia and the potential for future spread. FEMS Microbiol Rev 2016;41(1):34–48.
21. Tatem AJ, Jia P, Ordanovich D, et al. The geography of imported malaria to non-endemic countries: a meta-analysis of nationally reported statistics. Lancet Infect Dis 2017;17(1):98–107.

22. Mier-y-Teran-Romero L, Tatem AJ, Johansson MA. Mosquitoes on a plane: Disinsection will not stop the spread of vector-borne pathogens, a simulation study. PLoS Negl Trop Dis 2017;11(7):e0005683.

23. Velasco E, Gomez-Barroso D, Varela C, et al. Non-imported malaria in non-endemic countries: a review of cases in Spain. Malar J 2017;16(1):260.

24. Lee EH, Adams EH, Madison-Antenucci S, et al. Healthcare-Associated Transmission of *Plasmodium falciparum* in New York City. Infect Control Hosp Epidemiol 2016;37(1):113–5.

25. Ruiz AIM, Bendicho AI, Fuster JL, et al. Unexplained Anemia in a young infant due to congenital malaria. Pediatr Infect Dis J 2016;35(4):468.

26. Holtzclaw A, Mrsic Z, Managbanag J, et al. Transfusion-transmitted malaria not preventable by current blood donor screening guidelines: a case report. Transfusion 2016;56(9):2221–4.

27. Oakley MS, Gerald N, McCutchan TF, et al. Clinical and molecular aspects of malaria fever. Trends Parasitol 2011;27(10):442–9.

28. Ladhani S, Aibara RJ, Riordan FAI, et al. Imported malaria in children: a review of clinical studies. Lancet Infect Dis 2007;7(5):349–57.

29. Gutman J, Guarner J. Pediatric malaria: 8-year case series in Atlanta, Georgia, and review of the literature. J Travel Med 2010;17(5):334–8.

30. Trampuz A, Jereb M, Muzlovic I, et al. Clinical review: severe malaria. Crit Care 2003;7(4):315.

31. Griffith KS, Lewis LS, Mali S, et al. Treatment of malaria in the United States: a systematic review. JAMA 2007;297(20):2264–77.

32. World Health Organization. Guidelines for the treatment of malaria. World Health Organization; 2015.

33. Collins WE, Jeffery GM. *Plasmodium malariae*: parasite and disease. Clin Microbiol Rev 2007;20(4):579–92.

34. Cox-Singh J, Davis TM, Lee K-S, et al. *Plasmodium knowlesi* malaria in humans is widely distributed and potentially life threatening. Clin Infect Dis 2008;46(2): 165–71.

35. Hahn WO, Pottinger PS. Malaria in the traveler: how to manage before departure and evaluate upon return. Med Clin North Am 2016;100(2):289–302.

36. World Health Organization. International travel and health: situation as on 1 January 2010. World Health Organization; 2010.

37. Kimberlin D, Brady M, Jackson M, et al. Red book. 2015 Report of the Committee on Infectious Diseases. Elk Grove Village (IL): American Academy of Pediatrics; 2015.

38. Itoh M, Arguin PM. A conversation about chemoprophylaxis. Travel Med Infect Dis 2016;14(5):434.

39. Kotwal RS, Wenzel RB, Sterling RA, et al. An outbreak of malaria in US army rangers returning from Afghanistan. JAMA 2005;293(2):212–6.

40. Wiese L, Bruun B, Bæk L, et al. Bedside diagnosis of imported malaria using the Binax Now malaria antigen detection test. Scand J Infect Dis 2006;38(11–12): 1063–8.

41. Stauffer WM, Cartwright CP, Olson DA, et al. Diagnostic performance of rapid diagnostic tests versus blood smears for malaria in US clinical practice. Clin Infect Dis 2009;49(6):908–13.

42. Bell D, Wongsrichanalai C, Barnwell JW. Ensuring quality and access for malaria diagnosis: how can it be achieved? Nat Rev Microbiol 2006;4(9):682.

43. Bell D, Peeling RW. WHO-Regional Office for the Western Pacific/TDR. Evaluation of rapid diagnostic tests: malaria. Nat Rev Microbiol 2006;4:S34–8.

44. Rubio J, Buhigas I, Subirats M, et al. Limited level of accuracy provided by available rapid diagnosis tests for malaria enhances the need for PCR-based reference laboratories. J Clin Microbiol 2001;39(7):2736–7.
45. Walk J, Schats R, Langenberg MC, et al. Diagnosis and treatment based on quantitative PCR after controlled human malaria infection. Malar J 2016; 15(1):398.
46. Gray AM, Arguin PM, Hamed K. Surveillance for the safety and effectiveness of artemether-lumefantrine in patients with uncomplicated *Plasmodium falciparum* malaria in the USA: a descriptive analysis. Malar J 2015;14(1):349.
47. Dondorp AM, Fanello CI, Hendriksen IC, et al. Artesunate versus quinine in the treatment of severe falciparum malaria in African children (AQUAMAT): an open-label, randomised trial. Lancet 2010;376(9753):1647–57.
48. Twomey PS, Smith BL, McDermott C, et al. Intravenous artesunate for the treatment of severe and complicated malaria in the United States: clinical use under an investigational new drug protocol intravenous artesunate for severe malaria. Ann Intern Med 2015;163(7):498–506.
49. Tan KR, Wiegand RE, Arguin PM. Exchange transfusion for severe malaria: evidence base and literature review. Clin Infect Dis 2013;57(7):923–8.
50. Shaz BH, Schwartz J, Winters JL, et al. American society for apheresis guidelines support use of red cell exchange transfusion for severe malaria with high parasitemia. Clin Infect Dis 2014;58(2):302–3.

Management of Ebola Virus Disease in Children

Indi Trehan, MD, MPH, DTM&H[a,b,c,*], Stephanie C. De Silva, MD[b]

KEYWORDS

- Children • Clinical management • Critical care • Diagnosis • Ebola • Pediatrics
- Screening • Therapy

KEY POINTS

- The care of children with Ebola should be standardized and include a reproducible, regimented treatment protocol.
- The major domains of care include fluid resuscitation, electrolyte repletion, empiric antimicrobial prophylaxis, and nutritional supplementation.
- Comprehensive care for children with Ebola is extremely challenging in resource-constrained tropical environments, especially when appropriate attention to infection prevention and the safety of health care providers limits patient contact.

INTRODUCTION

Long considered a disease with limited ability to spread across borders in epidemic fashion, Ebola virus grabbed the world's attention in an outbreak that stretched across the West African nations of Guinea, Sierra Leone, and Liberia in 2013 to 2016.[1] More than 11,300 people were confirmed to have died during this outbreak, although this quite likely underestimates the true burden of illness. In addition to reframing the medical community's understanding of this viral hemorrhagic fever,[2] the epidemic contributed to a massive disruption of health care services in already impoverished countries recovering from years of civil wars superimposed on pervasive, abject poverty.[3] It was only in the midst of the recent West African outbreak that the medical community remembered that some 6% to 14% of asymptomatic Liberians harbored Ebola antibodies in serosurveys dating back to 1970s.[4–6]

Given the size of this outbreak, the large number of reservoir mammals,[7,8] and the high rate of asymptomatic infection,[9] it is inevitable that future outbreaks, or at least sporadic cases, will emerge again, as has already been the case in the Democratic Republic of

No conflicts of interest.
[a] Lao Friends Hospital for Children, Luang Prabang, Lao PDR; [b] Department of Pediatrics, One Children's Place, Campus Box 8116, St Louis, MO 63110, USA; [c] Maforki Ebola Holding and Treatment Centre, Port Loko, Sierra Leone
* Corresponding author. Department of Pediatrics, One Children's Place, Campus Box 8116, St Louis, MO 63110.
E-mail address: indi@alum.berkeley.edu

Infect Dis Clin N Am 32 (2018) 201–214
https://doi.org/10.1016/j.idc.2017.10.010
0891-5520/18/© 2017 Elsevier Inc. All rights reserved.

Congo.[10] As with most illnesses, it is also unfortunately likely that children will suffer disproportionately, especially in areas where specialized pediatric care is relatively limited. Given the massive size of the recent West African outbreak, with thousands of health care workers involved in caring for Ebola suspects and cases in hundreds of centers, much was learned about how to deliver optimal care in austere settings under extremely harsh conditions.[11–13] In anticipation of future outbreaks, this article reviews the clinical management of children with, or suspected to have, Ebola virus disease.

Children usually constitute a disproportionately small number of cases in Ebola outbreaks.[14–17] Nevertheless, the large absolute number of cases seen and the specialized care required to optimally care for children infected (or suspected to be infected) with Ebola led to disproportionately high mortality rates ranging from 50% to 80%.[16,18–22] Beyond the individual cases of Ebola, an outbreak such as this devastates the entire system of pediatric health care for a generation to come,[23,24] leading to the disruption of immunization services,[25–27] measles epidemics,[28,29] breakdown of obstetric services,[30] and increased rates of acute malnutrition.[31]

ROUTES OF INFECTION

Infants born to mothers with Ebola rarely survive,[32] although novel experimental therapies may fortunately be challenging this dogma.[33] Thus, this article focuses on children infected via direct (horizontal) contact with infected body fluids, predominantly sweat, saliva, urine, stool, and blood. Children may also be infected via breast milk, including from asymptomatic survivors.[34,35]

PRINCIPLES OF CARE

Aggressive and comprehensive critical care, initiated early in the course of illness, has significant potential to decrease mortality for all Ebola patients.[13] This is especially worth emphasizing in children, in whom fluid shifts, electrolyte disturbances, underlying malnutrition,[36,37] and secondary infection can contribute to rapid and fatal decompensation.[38–41] The effectiveness of this aggressive approach was most prominently demonstrated at the Hastings Ebola treatment unit (ETU) in Sierra Leone, where the case-fatality rate approached 30% at a time when mortality rates in excess of 50% were the norm,[42] and in the very low mortality among evacuated infected expatriates. Nevertheless, such critical care is significantly hampered by the inability to fully examine patients and the need to adhere to strict infection prevention requirements for this extraordinarily contagious virus in resource-constrained, environmentally challenging settings.[43]

DIAGNOSIS AND ISOLATION CRITERIA

During an Ebola outbreak, clear criteria for ETU or holding center admission need to be established, based on the predominant manifestation of the particular Ebola strain responsible for that outbreak. For example, the Zaire strain responsible for the recent West African outbreak manifested primarily as a gastrointestinal illness, with profuse vomiting and diarrhea, rather than the prototypical hemorrhagic fever.

These criteria need to be highly sensitive to keep infected individuals isolated from the community, but this will inevitably make any suspect case definition less specific and contribute to a fair number of ETU admissions among those with other illness, such as malaria and viral gastroenteritis, that mimic Ebola. **Box 1** provides an overview of the clinical criteria used for ETU admission during the recent West African outbreak.[44]

The biggest challenge in tropical settings is the high degree of overlap that these criteria have to mimic many other acute childhood illnesses endemic in these settings,

---

Box 1
Clinical criteria used for Ebola suspect case identification during the 2013 to 2016 West African Ebola outbreak

Screening and Admission Criteria	Clinical Symptoms
• All patients: close contact with an Ebola case or suspected case within the prior 3 weeks	Abdominal pain
	Abnormal or unexplained bleeding
• Children <5 y of age: fever plus at least 1 clinical symptom	Anorexia
	Diarrhea
• Adults and children >5 y of age: fever plus at least 2 clinical symptoms	Difficulty breathing
	Difficulty swallowing
	Fatigue
	Headache
	Hiccups
	Nausea or vomiting

From World Health Organization. Interim guidance: clinical care for survivors of Ebola virus disease. Geneva (Switzerland): World Health Organization; 2016; with permission.

---

including malaria, measles,[29] gastroenteritis,[45] and other viral hemorrhagic fevers that may share a common geographic range.[46] This suspect case definition and similar criteria used in the field[22,47] was not in practice optimally sensitive or specific but still proved feasible to implement across the region in a diverse array of health centers. Ultimately, these criteria may indeed have been the best approach at the time, given the nature of the crisis. The major concern when operationalizing criteria that are too broad and nonspecific is the risk of nosocomial transmission in crowded ETUs, but, fortunately, this rate of nosocomial transmission was likely lower than originally feared.[48,49] Future developments in rapid point-of-care testing[50] can be anticipated to help with this triage process and decrease the spread of future outbreaks.[51]

PROGNOSTIC CRITERIA

Prediction rules and models have been developed to proactively identify children most at risk for mortality from Ebola.[20,52–55] From a practical standpoint, these may be useful in triaging which children to provide the most aggressive care to in the ETU if resources are limited. High viral load on admission, altered mental status, diarrhea, significant weakness, and bleeding have all been linked to higher mortality rates in children.

OVERVIEW OF CLINICAL CARE

Systematic, comprehensive care for children with Ebola (**Box 2**) includes a minimum empiric package of interventions for all patients, given that the ability to tailor therapies to individual patient circumstances can be quite limited by constraints on the amount of time and contact possible with each patient.

INITIAL ASSESSMENT AND MANAGEMENT

In addition to routine vital signs, nutritional status should be assessed on admission whenever possible by checking the child's weight and mid-upper arm circumference (MUAC). If the MUAC is below an age-adjusted threshold (**Table 1**), additional therapeutic feeding with F-100, ready-to-use therapeutic food (RUTF), or BP-100 biscuits, should be provided.

Box 2
Major elements in the management of children with suspected or confirmed Ebola virus disease in endemic settings

- Initial assessment and management
  - Routine vital signs
  - Nutritional assessment, including weight and mid-upper arm circumference
  - Assessment for dehydration and hemorrhage
  - Mental status evaluation
  - Obtain intravenous (IV) access, ideally securing 2 IV lines
  - Oral (preferred) or intramuscular vitamin K supplementation

- Fluid and electrolyte management
  - Oral rehydration solution for all children older than 6 months of age; consider also for younger infants
  - Ondansetron as needed for nausea and vomiting
  - Loperamide as needed for diarrhea
  - Intravenous fluids
    - Initial bolus of lactated Ringer with 5% dextrose
      - Reassess hydration status and repeat half boluses until euvolemic state achieved (as assessed by clinical examination or ultrasound examination)
    - Continued aggressive rehydration
    - Potassium and magnesium supplementation for those with significant diarrhea
  - Oral zinc daily

- Nutritional supplementation
  - F-100 formula or ready-to-use therapeutic food or BP-100 biscuits

- Empiric antimalarials
  - IV artesunate daily initially if vomiting
  - Complete treatment course with oral artemisinin combination therapy, preferably artesunate-amodiaquine

- Empiric antimicrobials
  - IV ceftriaxone or oral cefixime or ciprofloxacin
  - Consider metronidazole if particularly voluminous or bloody diarrhea

- Vitamin K
  - Consider additional doses for those with active bleeding

Dehydration should be corrected with fluid boluses. In anticipation of the need for significant fluid resuscitation, intravenous (IV) access should be obtained at the time of admission whenever possible. Due to the need for large volumes of fluid resuscitation, some providers also recommend that children with any recent vomiting, diarrhea, or evidence of moderate or severe dehydration should have 2 IV lines placed at admission. Intraosseous[56] or subcutaneous[57,58] rehydration can be considered as well for children in extremis. Bedside sonography can be helpful in obtaining access, as well as for assessing hydration status.[59]

A single dose of vitamin K should be provided to all patients at the time of admission because diminished hepatic function[60] may contribute to coagulopathy.[61] Oral administration is preferred over intramuscular administration, at a dose of 5 mg for children younger than 12 years of age, or 10 mg for older children.

FLUID RESUSCITATION

The Zaire strain of Ebola virus responsible for the 2013 to 2016 West African outbreak caused most morbidity and mortality due to profound gastroenteritis, and thus early and aggressive fluid and electrolyte resuscitation lay at the crux of

Table 1
Suggested age-adjusted thresholds for identifying acute malnutrition in Ebola treatment unit settings

Age	MUAC
<6 mo	<12.0 cm
6 mo–4 y	<12.5 cm
5 y	<13.1 cm
6 y	<13.6 cm
7 y	<14.2 cm
8 y	<14.8 cm
9 y	<15.3 cm
10 y	<15.9 cm
11 y	<16.5 cm
12 y	<17.0 cm
13 y	<17.6 cm
14 y	<18.2 cm
15 y	<18.7 cm
16 y	<19.3 cm
17 y	<19.9 cm
18 y	<20.4 cm
19 y	<21.0 cm

From Mramba L, Ngari M, Mwangome M, et al. A growth reference for mid upper arm circumference for age among school age children and adolescents, and validation for mortality: Growth curve construction and longitudinal cohort study. BMJ 2017;358:j3423; with permission.

care for Ebola patients. The major exception to this principle would be for children who have malaria or severe malnutrition because the risk of fluid overload and/or cardiovascular collapse in these patients has been associated with increased mortality.[62] The practical challenge to overcome is the severely limited amount of time that medical staff can be present at the bedside due to the heat and humidity of their own personal protective equipment. Encouraging oral rehydration in a child takes significant amount of time and IV lines generally need to be disconnected for safety when staff leave the bedside.

Oral Rehydration

Oral rehydration solution (ORS) should be provided liberally; intake may be increased if flavored solutions are available. In general, there need not be any limits placed on how much a child should drink and the child can determine their own intake based on their own thirst. Frightened and anxious children will need frequent positive reinforcement and encouragement for assisting in their own medical care by consuming as much ORS as possible (**Fig. 1**). Rehydration can be facilitated with adult Ebola survivors as bedside caretakers to assist with feeding and fluid intake when medical staff is not available. In general, fluids other than ORS, water, or therapeutic milk feeds should not be provided to children, especially those with added sugar because they may increase diarrhea.

Ondansetron may be helpful in increasing the intake of ORS.[63] Although controversial in patients who may have severe diarrhea due to a bacterial pathogen, the authors think there is a role for loperamide to decrease diarrheal fluid losses.[22,38,64] An initial

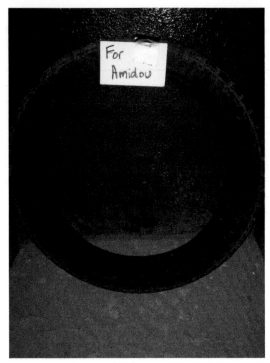

Fig. 1. A new bicycle tire requested by an Ebola patient in Sierra Leone, used by ETU staff as a reward to motivate the patient to drink as much oral rehydration solution as possible during his hospitalization.

dose of 2 mg can be used, with subsequent doses of 1 mg, increasing up to 8 mg per day. Caution is advised in the cases of bloody diarrhea because this may be a sign of bacterial enteritis. Loperamide should be discontinued if careful frequent abdominal examinations demonstrate signs of ileus. If concurrent epidemics of cholera or other bacterial pathogens are occurring, then loperamide may need to be withheld.

Parenteral Rehydration

Parenteral rehydration with lactated Ringer solution with 5% dextrose (D_5LR) will likely be needed for nearly all children because very few will be able to drink sufficient quantities of ORS to account for the large volumes of gastrointestinal losses. As a rule of thumb, children with only so-called dry symptoms at admission (without vomiting, diarrhea, or bleeding) should receive an initial bolus of 20 mL/kg of D_5LR in anticipation of impending fluid losses. Children with so-called wet symptoms should receive 40 mL/kg, unless the child has concomitant malaria or severe acute malnutrition, in which case the volume of the bolus may be limited to 20 mL/kg.

After the initial fluid bolus, hydration status should be frequently reassessed clinically using accepted local criteria, focusing on capillary refill, skin turgor, respiratory distress, and mental status.[65] Children who remain dehydrated should receive repeated boluses of half the volume as the initial bolus, reassessing hydration after each bolus and monitoring for an increase in heart rate or respiratory rate as signs of possible fluid overload.

Following this initial rehydration, children will require continued rehydration to correct for insensible losses due to fever, tachypnea, acidosis, and high ambient temperatures, even in the absence of ongoing gastrointestinal loss or bleeding. Dextrose should generally be included in these fluids, particularly in younger children and in those with anorexia. The specific volume of fluid provided to each child will need to be individualized, but, generally, children with dry symptoms and those with malaria or malnutrition may need 150 mL/kg/d for the first 10 kg of body weight, plus 75 mL/kg/d for the next 10 kg of body weight plus 40 mL/kg of remaining weight. Children with wet symptoms with significant concern for malaria or malnutrition may need an additional 50 to 100 mL of fluid for each loose stool or episode of vomiting, whenever it is possible to assess and record these events. Children with wet symptoms without obvious concern for malaria or malnutrition may be supplemented with up to 200 mL for each acute fluid loss.

ELECTROLYTE SUPPLEMENTATION

Glucose, potassium, and magnesium are all likely to be relatively deficient in children with profuse vomiting and diarrhea. If point-of-care electrolyte monitoring is available, this technology can augment individualized data-driven supplementation.[66]

Potassium

IV fluids for children with significant diarrhea should generally be supplemented with potassium, unless evidence of decreased urine output and concern for renal insufficiency or failure exist. If rapid bedside measurements of potassium are unavailable, empirically including 10 mEq/L of potassium to IV fluids when replacing stool losses is generally safe. Potassium-containing fluids should be infused by gravity rather than by rapid infusion, generally through a second IV line with nonpotassium-containing fluids infused at a more aggressive rate for resuscitation.

Magnesium

If available, magnesium supplementation of IV fluids is also advisable. However, if the systolic blood pressure is low or if the pulse pressure wide, resuscitation should begin without magnesium. For simplicity at the bedside, minimum systolic blood pressures at which magnesium is safe to administer are: 90 mm Hg for adolescents, 80 mm Hg for school-aged children, 70 mm Hg for toddlers, and 60 mm Hg for infants. Because rapid infusion of magnesium can lead to significant hypotension, these fluids should also be run over gravity rather than by rapid infusion. The typical dose of magnesium sulfate is 25 mg/kg, up to 100 mg/kg per day or a maximum of 2 g.

Zinc

Given the proven benefit of zinc in decreasing the duration and quantity of diarrhea due to a wide variety of infectious causes,[67] oral zinc supplementation should be provided to all children at a dose of 10 mg per day for children up to 6 months of age and 20 mg per day for older children.

ANTIMICROBIAL THERAPY
Empiric Antibacterials

In endemic areas, severe bacterial infections due to *Salmonella* species, *Streptococcus pneumoniae*, and other pathogens may complicate or mimic Ebola virus disease in children. Furthermore, given the limited diagnostics available in an ETU, it is generally impossible to distinguish between severe Ebola virus disease and bacterial sepsis. Furthermore, severe gastroenteritis and high rates of underlying malnutrition place children at high risk for bacterial translocation across a denuded gut mucosa, potentially leading to superimposed gram-negative sepsis[68] that can be difficult to recognize. Bowel edema and bacterial translocation are more likely to occur later in the course of the disease, during the period of most severe intestinal injury, potentially leading to an acute abdomen. It is thus prudent to empirically treat all children admitted to the ETU with broad-spectrum antibacterial therapy, particularly to cover enteric gram-negative pathogens.

Various options exist for such empiric coverage, including ceftriaxone, ciprofloxacin, amoxicillin-clavulanate, or another second-generation or third-generation cephalosporin. Some ETUs included metronidazole as part of their empiric regimen,[42] although many reserved this for cases when the abdominal examination became specifically concerning or if the child had particularly bloody or voluminous diarrhea. The balance between prudent antimicrobial stewardship concerns with empiric care for critically ill children with a very high mortality rate in a setting without most typical diagnostics is challenging; some units treated children throughout their hospitalization, whereas others provided a fixed duration based on time (generally 3–7 days) or symptom course.

Empiric Antimalarials

Future Ebola outbreaks will likely occur in settings also endemic for falciparum malaria. Some data suggested that coinfection with malaria correlated with a lower mortality rate among Ebola patients, even after controlling for confounders; this protection was higher among those with the highest level of parasitemia.[69] In contrast, other data found that coinfected patients had higher mortality rates.[70] Given that the clinical presentation of malaria overlaps significantly with suspected Ebola cases (see **Box 1**), empirically treating all children for malaria in an ETU is prudent even in the setting of a negative malaria test on admission. Children may become infected (or clinically manifest an incubating infection) while admitted in the ETU. Artemisinin-combination therapy (ACT) also provides short-term prophylaxis against malaria,[71] and can thus be useful when a new malaria infection may prove quite harmful to children suffering or recovering from Ebola. Therapy can begin with IV artesunate or intramuscular artemether if the child is not tolerating oral medications at the time of admission. All children should complete a 3-day course of ACT, either in the ETU or at home after discharge. Artesunate-amodiaquine has been associated with lower mortality in the context of an Ebola outbreak, compared with artemether-lumefantrine.[72]

NUTRITIONAL SUPPORT

Nutritional support is essential in the management of pediatric Ebola. Given the degree of anorexia, nausea, vomiting, sore throat, and abdominal pain children with Ebola suffer, it is important to provide complete energy-dense foods that can be eaten slowly throughout the day. These foods need to retain their taste and cleanliness while remaining at the bedside for many hours at a time, and be easy for weak patients to eat themselves or be fed quickly: RUTF and BP-100 biscuits are 2 examples.

One recommended approach is to provide all children able to tolerate solid or semi-solid foods with RUTF and/or BP-100 in ample quantities. Patients, caregivers, and staff should be educated that nutritional care will be optimized if all the intended therapeutic food is consumed daily. Intake goals are outlined in **Table 2**. Given their complete micronutrient and macronutrient content, these foods should be prioritized over

Table 2
Suggested minimum nutritional intake for children admitted to an Ebola treatment unit

Age	RUTF Sachets Per Day	BP-100 Biscuits Per Day
1–4 y	2–3	3–5
5–9 y	3–4	5–7
10–14 y	4–5	6–8
≥15 y female	4–5	6–8
≥15 y male	5–6	8–10

local diets in the acute phase. Young children may not be able to consume RUTF without some mixing with water; BP-100 can be crushed and mixed with water to make a porridge.

For children older than 6 months who are only able to tolerate liquids, F-75 or F-100 formula can be used because these provide much higher nutritional content than commercial infant formula or standard dairy milk.[73] F-100 is a more complete food than F-75 but has a higher osmotic load and may contribute to increased diarrhea in some children. These formulas will spoil if kept unrefrigerated and thus may need to be prepared multiple times daily. Children younger than 6 months of age should be provided with commercial infant formula. Nasogastric tubes may need to be used in children too weak to eat or drink on their own.

Children with acute malnutrition should be identified at the time of admission, most easily by MUAC thresholds (see **Table 1**) and by checking for bilateral pitting edema diagnostic for kwashiorkor. For simplicity, moderately and severely malnourished children can be treated identically.[74] Acutely malnourished children should consume only F-75, F-100, RUTF, or BP-100; breast milk (if appropriate from an infection prevention standpoint), water, and ReSoMal should be the only additional liquids they drink. Malnourished children will require particularly diligent attention to therapeutic feeding, including special arrangements to provide directly observed feedings around the clock. Malnourished children should all receive antibiotics,[75,76] even if antibiotics are not being used for all patients as previously described.

EXPERIMENTAL THERAPIES

Antiviral medications, monoclonal antibodies, serum from Ebola survivors, and other therapies were used and developed during the course of the West African outbreak.[77,78] Future outbreaks will potentially require these and additional novel therapeutics. The triple monoclonal antibody marketed as ZMapp seems particularly promising.[79]

DISCHARGE

Demonstration of virologic clearance on at least 2 tests 48 to 72 hours apart remains the mainstay of discharge criteria. The standard tests used in the West African outbreak relied on reverse-transcription polymerase chain reaction (RT-PCR) testing. Further developments in rapid testing can be expected[50] that will allow for significant improvements in testing at the time of screening and admission. Currently, patients should not be discharged unless RT-PCR testing is negative at least 72 hours since the onset of symptoms.[38]

Much is being learned about the lingering effects of Ebola following recovery; all patients will benefit from continued medical care following discharge.[80] For children, postdischarge nutritional supplementation is of particular importance in the short-term. The disruption of routine primary care services during an Ebola epidemic can be expected,[23,81] including disruptions in critical vaccinations,[82] and thus children discharged from an ETU should ideally be caught up on any vaccines they may have missed.

SUMMARY

Caring for children in an ETU requires the complex coordination of many aspects of care. Additional challenges exist in resource-limited settings where the direct provisions of care are further hampered by the need for staff to remain in PPE for prolonged periods of time and only being present at the bedside for relatively short stretches of time. Rigorous implementation of standardized treatment protocols will improve mortality rates. Particular attention to fluid resuscitation, electrolyte repletion, antimicrobial prophylaxis, and nutritional supplementation will be warranted to decrease mortality. It is hoped that new diagnostic and therapeutic technologies, including vaccination of contacts of Ebola cases, will be available during future outbreaks to further improve survival.

REFERENCES

1. Lo TQ, Marston BJ, Dahl BA, et al. Ebola: anatomy of an epidemic. Annu Rev Med 2017;68:359–70.
2. Baseler L, Chertow DS, Johnson KM, et al. The pathogenesis of Ebola virus disease. Ann Rev Pathol 2017;12:387–418.
3. Shoman H, Karafillakis E, Rawaf S. The link between the West African Ebola outbreak and health systems in Guinea, Liberia and Sierra Leone: a systematic review. Global Health 2017;13(1):1.
4. Knobloch J, Albiez EJ, Schmitz H. A serological survey on viral haemorrhagic fevers in Liberia. Ann Inst Pasteur Virol 1982;133(2):125–8.
5. Neppert J, Gohring S, Schneider W, et al. No evidence of LAV infection in the Republic of Liberia, West Africa, in the year 1973. Blut 1986;53(2):115–7.
6. Bower H, Glynn JR. A systematic review and meta-analysis of seroprevalence surveys of ebolavirus infection. Sci Data 2017;4:160133.
7. Leroy EM, Kumulungui B, Pourrut X, et al. Fruit bats as reservoirs of Ebola virus. Nature 2005;438(7068):575–6.
8. Jahrling PB, Geisbert TW, Dalgard DW, et al. Preliminary report: Isolation of Ebola virus from monkeys imported to USA. Lancet 1990;335(8688):502–5.
9. Glynn JR, Bower H, Johnson S, et al. Asymptomatic infection and unrecognised Ebola virus disease in Ebola-affected households in Sierra Leone: a cross-sectional study using a new non-invasive assay for antibodies to Ebola virus. Lancet Infect Dis 2017;17(6):645–53.
10. Green A. Ebola outbreak in the DR Congo. Lancet 2017;389(10084):2092.
11. Rojek A, Horby P, Dunning J. Insights from clinical research completed during the west Africa Ebola virus disease epidemic. Lancet Infect Dis 2017;17(9):e280–92.
12. Duraffour S, Malvy D, Sissoko D. How to treat Ebola virus infections? A lesson from the field. Curr Opin Virol 2017;24:9–15.
13. Lamontagne F, Fowler RA, Adhikari NK, et al. Evidence-based guidelines for supportive care of patients with Ebola virus disease. Lancet 2017. [Epub ahead of print].

14. Dean NE, Halloran ME, Yang Y, et al. Transmissibility and pathogenicity of Ebola virus: a systematic review and meta-analysis of household secondary attack rate and asymptomatic infection. Clin Infect Dis 2016;62(10):1277–86.

15. Glynn JR. Age-specific incidence of Ebola virus disease. Lancet 2015;386(9992): 432.

16. WHO Ebola Response Team, Agua-Agum J, Ariyarajah A, Blake IM, et al. Ebola virus disease among children in West Africa. N Engl J Med 2015;372(13):1274–7.

17. Bower H, Johnson S, Bangura MS, et al. Exposure-specific and age-specific attack rates for Ebola virus disease in Ebola-affected households, Sierra Leone. Emerg Infect Dis 2016;22(8):1403–11.

18. Fitzgerald F, Awonuga W, Shah T, et al. Ebola response in Sierra Leone: the impact on children. J Infect 2016;72(Suppl):S6–12.

19. Fitzgerald F, Naveed A, Wing K, et al. Ebola virus disease in children, Sierra Leone, 2014-2015. Emerg Infect Dis 2016;22(10):1769–77.

20. Cherif MS, Koonrungsesomboon N, Kasse D, et al. Ebola virus disease in children during the 2014-2015 epidemic in Guinea: a nationwide cohort study. Eur J Pediatr 2017;176(6):791–6.

21. Damkjaer M, Rudolf F, Mishra S, et al. Clinical features and outcome of Ebola virus disease in pediatric patients: a retrospective case series. J Pediatr 2017; 182(3):378–81.e1.

22. Smit MA, Michelow IC, Glavis-Bloom J, et al. Characteristics and outcomes of pediatric patients with Ebola virus disease admitted to treatment units in Liberia and Sierra Leone: a retrospective cohort study. Clin Infect Dis 2017;64(3):243–9.

23. Delamou A, El Ayadi AM, Sidibe S, et al. Effect of Ebola virus disease on maternal and child health services in Guinea: a retrospective observational cohort study. Lancet Glob Health 2017;5(4):e448–57.

24. Hermans V, Zachariah R, Woldeyohannes D, et al. Offering general pediatric care during the hard times of the 2014 Ebola outbreak: looking back at how many came and how well they fared at a Medecins Sans Frontieres referral hospital in rural Sierra Leone. BMC Pediatr 2017;17(1):34.

25. Sun X, Samba TT, Yao J, et al. Impact of the Ebola outbreak on routine immunization in western area, Sierra Leone - a field survey from an Ebola epidemic area. BMC Public Health 2017;17(1):363.

26. Wesseh CS, Najjemba R, Edwards JK, et al. Did the Ebola outbreak disrupt immunisation services? A case study from Liberia. Public Health Action 2017; 7(Suppl 1):S82–7.

27. Camara BS, Delamou AM, Diro E, et al. Influence of the 2014-2015 Ebola outbreak on the vaccination of children in a rural district of Guinea. Public Health Action 2017;7(2):161–7.

28. Sesay T, Denisiuk O, Shringarpure KK, et al. Paediatric care in relation to the 2014-2015 Ebola outbreak and general reporting of deaths in Sierra Leone. Public Health Action 2017;7(Suppl 1):S34–9.

29. Colavita F, Biava M, Castilletti C, et al. Measles cases during Ebola outbreak, West Africa, 2013-2106. Emerg Infect Dis 2017;23(6):1035–7.

30. Jones SA, Gopalakrishnan S, Ameh CA, et al. 'Women and babies are dying but not of Ebola': The effect of the Ebola virus epidemic on the availability, uptake and outcomes of maternal and newborn health services in Sierra Leone. BMJ Glob Health 2016;1(3):e000065.

31. Kamara MH, Najjemba R, van Griensven J, et al. Increase in acute malnutrition in children following the 2014-2015 Ebola outbreak in rural Sierra Leone. Public Health Action 2017;7(Suppl 1):S27–33.

32. Nelson JM, Griese SE, Goodman AB, et al. Live neonates born to mothers with Ebola virus disease: a review of the literature. J Perinatol 2016;36(6):411–4.

33. Dornemann J, Burzio C, Ronsse A, et al. First newborn baby to receive experimental therapies survives Ebola virus disease. J Infect Dis 2017;215(2):171–4.

34. Vetter P, Fischer WA 2nd, Schibler M, et al. Ebola virus shedding and transmission: review of current evidence. J Infect Dis 2016;214(suppl 3):S177–84.

35. Sissoko D, Keita M, Diallo B, et al. Ebola virus persistence in breast milk after no reported illness: a likely source of virus transmission from mother to child. Clin Infect Dis 2017;64(4):513–6.

36. WHO/UNICEF/WFP. Interim guideline: nutritional care of children and adults with Ebola virus disease in treatment centres. Geneva (Switzerland): World Health Organization; 2014.

37. Iannotti LL, Trehan I, Clitheroe KL, et al. Diagnosis and treatment of severely malnourished children with diarrhoea. J Paediatr Child Health 2015;51(4):387–95.

38. Chertow DS, Kleine C, Edwards JK, et al. Ebola virus disease in West Africa–clinical manifestations and management. N Engl J Med 2014;371(22):2054–7.

39. Eriksson CO, Uyeki TM, Christian MD, et al. Care of the child with Ebola virus disease. Pediatr Crit Care Med 2015;16(2):97–103.

40. Fowler RA, Fletcher T, Fischer WA 2nd, et al. Caring for critically ill patients with ebola virus disease. Perspectives from West Africa. Am J Respir Crit Care Med 2014;190(7):733–7.

41. Trehan I, Kelly T, Marsh RH, et al. Moving towards a more aggressive and comprehensive model of care for children with Ebola. J Pediatr 2016;170:28–33.e1–7.

42. Ansumana R, Jacobsen KH, Sahr F, et al. Ebola in Freetown area, Sierra Leone–a case study of 581 patients. N Engl J Med 2015;372(6):587–8.

43. Sprecher A, Van Herp M, Rollin PE. Clinical management of Ebola virus disease patients in low-resource settings. Curr Top Microbiol Immunol 2017. [Epub ahead of print].

44. World Health Organization. Clinical management of patients with viral haemorrhagic fever: a pocket guide for front line health workers. Geneva (Switzerland): World Health Organization; 2016.

45. Fitzgerald F, Wing K, Naveed A, et al. Refining the paediatric Ebola case definition: a study of children in Sierra Leone with suspected Ebola virus disease. Lancet 2017;389:S19.

46. MacDermott NE, De S, Herberg JA. Viral haemorrhagic fever in children. Arch Dis Child 2016;101(5):461–8.

47. World Health Organization. Manual for the care and management of patients in Ebola care units/community care centres: interim emergency guidance. Geneva (Switzerland): World Health Organization; 2015.

48. Haidar G, Philips NJ, Shields RK, et al. Ceftolozane-tazobactam for the treatment of multidrug-resistant pseudomonas aeruginosa infections: clinical effectiveness and evolution of resistance. Clin Infect Dis 2017;65(1):110–20.

49. Arkell P, Youkee D, Brown CS, et al. Quantifying the risk of nosocomial infection within Ebola holding units: A retrospective cohort study of negative patients discharged from five Ebola holding units in Western Area, Sierra Leone. Trop Med Int Health 2017;22(1):32–40.

50. Broadhurst MJ, Brooks TJ, Pollock NR. Diagnosis of Ebola virus disease: past, present, and future. Clin Microbiol Rev 2016;29(4):773–93.

51. Dhillon RS, Srikrishna D, Garry RF, et al. Ebola control: rapid diagnostic testing. Lancet Infect Dis 2015;15(2):147–8.

52. Barry M, Toure A, Traore FA, et al. Clinical predictors of mortality in patients with Ebola virus disease. Clin Infect Dis 2015;60(12):1821–4.
53. Shah T, Greig J, van der Plas LM, et al. Inpatient signs and symptoms and factors associated with death in children aged 5 years and younger admitted to two Ebola management centres in Sierra Leone, 2014: A retrospective cohort study. Lancet Glob Health 2016;4(7):e495–501.
54. Crowe SJ, Maenner MJ, Kuah S, et al. Prognostic indicators for Ebola patient survival. Emerg Infect Dis 2016;22(2):217–23.
55. Hartley MA, Young A, Tran AM, et al. Predicting Ebola severity: a clinical prioritization score for Ebola virus disease. PLoS Negl Trop Dis 2017;11(2):e0005265.
56. Paterson ML, Callahan CW. The use of intraosseous fluid resuscitation in a pediatric patient with Ebola virus disease. J Emerg Med 2015;49(6):962–4.
57. Rouhani S, Meloney L, Ahn R, et al. Alternative rehydration methods: a systematic review and lessons for resource-limited care. Pediatrics 2011;127(3):e748–57.
58. Spandorfer PR. Subcutaneous rehydration: updating a traditional technique. Pediatr Emerg Care 2011;27(3):230–6.
59. Shah S, Price D, Bukham G, et al. The partners in health manual of ultrasound for resource-limited settings. Boston: Partners In Health; 2011.
60. Lyon GM, Mehta AK, Varkey JB, et al. Clinical care of two patients with Ebola virus disease in the United States. N Engl J Med 2014;371(25):2402–9.
61. Liddell AM, Davey RT Jr, Mehta AK, et al. Characteristics and clinical management of a cluster of 3 patients with Ebola virus disease, including the first domestically acquired cases in the United States. Ann Intern Med 2015;163(2):81–90.
62. Maitland K, Kiguli S, Opoka RO, et al. Mortality after fluid bolus in African children with severe infection. N Engl J Med 2011;364(26):2483–95.
63. Tomasik E, Ziolkowska E, Kolodziej M, et al. Systematic review with meta-analysis: Ondansetron for vomiting in children with acute gastroenteritis. Aliment Pharmacol Ther 2016;44(5):438–46.
64. Chertow DS, Uyeki TM, DuPont HL. Loperamide therapy for voluminous diarrhea in Ebola virus disease. J Infect Dis 2015;211(7):1036–7.
65. Levine AC, Glavis-Bloom J, Modi P, et al. External validation of the DHAKA score and comparison with the current imci algorithm for the assessment of dehydration in children with diarrhoea: a prospective cohort study. Lancet Glob Health 2016; 4(10):e744–51.
66. Palich R, Gala JL, Petitjean F, et al. A 6-year-old child with severe Ebola virus disease: laboratory-guided clinical care in an Ebola treatment center in Guinea. PLoS Negl Trop Dis 2016;10(3):e0004393.
67. Lazzerini M, Wanzira H. Oral zinc for treating diarrhoea in children. Cochrane Database Syst Rev 2016;(12):CD005436.
68. Kreuels B, Wichmann D, Emmerich P, et al. A case of severe Ebola virus infection complicated by gram-negative septicemia. N Engl J Med 2014;371(25): 2394–401.
69. Rosenke K, Adjemian J, Munster VJ, et al. Plasmodium parasitemia associated with increased survival in Ebola virus-infected patients. Clin Infect Dis 2016; 63(8):1026–33.
70. Waxman M, Aluisio AR, Rege S, et al. Characteristics and survival of patients with Ebola virus infection, malaria, or both in Sierra Leone: A retrospective cohort study. Lancet Infect Dis 2017;17(6):654–60.
71. Nosten F, White NJ. Artemisinin-based combination treatment of falciparum malaria. Am J Trop Med Hyg 2007;77(6 Suppl):181–92.

72. Gignoux E, Azman AS, de Smet M, et al. Effect of artesunate-amodiaquine on mortality related to Ebola virus disease. N Engl J Med 2016;374(1):23–32.

73. World Health Organization. Management of severe malnutrition: a manual for physicians and other senior health workers. Geneva (Switzerland): World Health Organization; 1999.

74. Trehan I, Manary MJ. Management of severe acute malnutrition in low-income and middle-income countries. Arch Dis Child 2015;100(3):283–7.

75. Trehan I, Goldbach HS, LaGrone LN, et al. Antibiotics as part of the management of severe acute malnutrition. N Engl J Med 2013;368(5):425–35.

76. Isanaka S, Langendorf C, Berthe F, et al. Routine amoxicillin for uncomplicated severe acute malnutrition in children. N Engl J Med 2016;374(5):444–53.

77. Mendoza EJ, Qiu X, Kobinger GP. Progression of Ebola therapeutics during the 2014-2015 outbreak. Trends Mol Med 2016;22(2):164–73.

78. Uyeki TM, Mehta AK, Davey RT Jr, et al. Clinical management of Ebola virus disease in the United States and Europe. N Engl J Med 2016;374(7):636–46.

79. PREVAIL II Writing Group, Multi-National PREVAIL II Study Team, Davey RT Jr, Dodd L, Proschan MA, et al. A randomized, controlled trial of ZMapp for Ebola virus infection. N Engl J Med 2016;375(15):1448–56.

80. World Health Organization. Interim guidance: clinical care for survivors of Ebola virus disease. Geneva (Switzerland): World Health Organization; 2016.

81. Walker NF, Whitty CJ. Tackling emerging infections: clinical and public health lessons from the West African Ebola virus disease outbreak, 2014-2015. Clin Med (Lond) 2015;15(5):457–60.

82. Takahashi S, Metcalf CJ, Ferrari MJ, et al. Reduced vaccination and the risk of measles and other childhood infections post-Ebola. Science 2015;347(6227): 1240–2.

Zika Virus Infection in Children

David Taylor Hendrixson, MD*, Jason G. Newland, MD, MEd

KEYWORDS

- Arthropod-borne disease • Congenital infection • *Flavivirus* • Microcephaly
- Vertical transmission • Zika virus

KEY POINTS

- Zika virus is a mosquito-borne *Flavivirus* associated with symptomatic and asymptomatic infection in infants and children.
- Vertical transmission of Zika virus can occur, resulting in congenital infection with mild-to-severe neurologic manifestations.
- All infants born to mothers with possible Zika virus infection should be evaluated and tested for Zika virus and other causes of congenital infections.
- Supportive care is the mainstay management of disease in older infants and children, but infants with congenital infection require close follow-up.

INTRODUCTION

Zika virus is an arthropod-borne *Flavivirus* that was first described in 1947 in rhesus monkeys and in 1952 in humans in a forested region of Uganda.[1] Since then, Zika virus has been reported as a cause of sporadic febrile illnesses throughout Africa and Asia.[2–7] In 2007, the first recognized large outbreak of Zika virus was documented on the Yap islands of Micronesia. Infected patients had rash, fever, and conjunctivitis.[4] It was estimated that up to 73% of residents older than 3 years of age had been infected with the virus during the outbreak.[4] Zika virus was not detected in the Western hemisphere until 2014 when it was identified during an outbreak on Easter Island.[8] Beginning in March 2015, reports of Zika virus transmission in Brazil emerged.[9,10] Zika virus transmission has now been reported throughout South America, Central America, the Caribbean, and parts of the United States (**Fig. 1**).[10] **Fig. 2** depicts countries with known Zika transmission. Zika virus is an emerging pathogen, causing both asymptomatic and symptomatic infection, and research is ongoing to better understand transmission, pathogenesis, and optimal management of this virus.

Department of Pediatrics, Division of Infectious Diseases, Washington University in St. Louis, St. Louis Children's Hospital, Campus Box 8116, 1 Children's Place, St Louis, MO 63110, USA
* Corresponding author.
E-mail address: dthendrixson@wustl.edu

Infect Dis Clin N Am 32 (2018) 215–224
https://doi.org/10.1016/j.idc.2017.10.003
0891-5520/18/© 2017 Elsevier Inc. All rights reserved.
id.theclinics.com

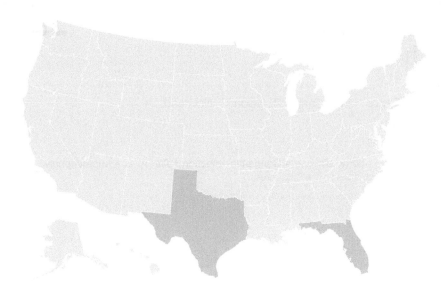

Fig. 1. States with reported Zika transmission.

TRANSMISSION
Arthropod Vectors

The primary vector for Zika virus transmission is the mosquito. *Aedes africanus* was first implicated in transmission when Zika virus was initially described.[1] The Asian tiger mosquito, *Aedes albopictus*, was confirmed as a vector for transmission in 2007 during an epidemic in Gabon. *Aedes hensilli* was the presumed vector during the Yap Islands outbreak in 2007; however, only laboratory infection has been documented.[4,11] Zika virus has been isolated from *Aedes aegypti*, implicating it in the

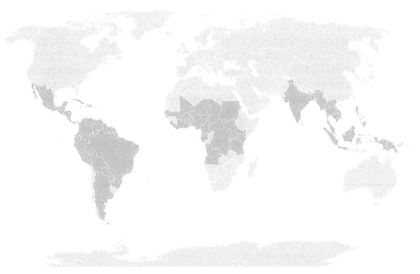

Fig. 2. Countries and territories with Zika transmission risk.

transmission of the virus in North America.[12] *A aegypti* is pervasive in most Zika-endemic regions and is the primary vector for transmission. Research into the role of other mosquitos in transmission is ongoing.

Sexual Transmission

Human-to-human transmission of Zika virus is documented to occur via both horizontal and vertical routes. Sexual transmission between both male and female infected sexual partners is reported. Sexual transmission was first suspected in 2008 when the wife of an American scientist who had traveled to Senegal became sick with an illness compatible with Zika virus.[13] The virus was never isolated from any samples, but serologic testing ultimately found the likely etiology was Zika virus. Numerous cases of male-to-female transmission were reported during the most recent outbreak.[14] Male-to-male sexual transmission was first reported in January 2016 and female-to-male sexual transmission is also documented.[15,16] Zika virus shedding persists in the semen for as long as 141 days (much longer than in the blood or urine) suggesting the possibility of sexual transmission for months after symptomatic resolution.[17] Zika virus shedding has been demonstrated in vaginal secretions for up 14 days.[18]

Other Modes of Transmission

Reports exist of nonsexual human-to-human transmission of Zika virus.[19] The route of transmission in these cases remains unclear, although acquisition of the virus may occur via tears, saliva, or urine when a patient has a high viral load.

Zika virus RNA can be detected in body fluids other than semen and vaginal secretions. Viral RNA has been isolated from urine, saliva, and tears.[20] Shedding of the virus from the conjunctiva and in the tears can occur up to 30 days after infection.[21] Persistence of the viral shedding in the urine and saliva has been found up to 91 days after symptom onset.[21] Given the prolonged shedding of virus in body fluids and risk for exposure, further understanding of transmission via these routes is needed.

Vertical Transmission

Vertical transmission of Zika virus from mother to fetus can also occur. Acquisition of the virus can occur before pregnancy or at any time during pregnancy. A risk of virus transmission to the fetus remains at any time during the pregnancy when maternal viremia is present. Zika virus causes placental infection and is found to infect the basal decidua and chorionic villi, allowing for both placental and paraplacental routes of transmission.[22] Zika virus RNA has been detected in the amniotic fluid of infected mothers with symptomatic fetuses.[23,24] Zika antigen and RNA can be detected in the placenta and brain tissues of miscarried fetuses or infants who died shortly after birth.[25,26]

Perinatal transmission has been reported in 2 infants in French Polynesia.[27] In both of these cases, the mothers had symptomatic infection within a few days of delivery, and although both infants were confirmed to be infected, they had no apparent clinical disease. The route of transmission is unknown. Zika virus has also been detected in breast milk, although no cases of infection acquired through this route are reported.[28]

Transfusion-Associated Transmission

As with other *Flaviviruses*, Zika virus can be transmitted via transfusions of infected blood products. The risk for transfusion-associated transmission was first recognized during the outbreak in French Polynesia where 3% of asymptomatic blood donors were positive for Zika virus[29]; however, no transfusion-associated infections were identified during this outbreak. Three probable transfusion-associated transmissions, all associated with platelet transfusion, have now been reported.[30,31] Screening of blood donations in the United States began in Puerto Rico in February 2016. Initial prevalence of Zika virus–positive donations was 0.3%,[32] but this increased to a prevalence of 1.8% by July 2016.[33] In August 2016, the US Food and Drug Administration (FDA) issued guidance instructing that all donated units in the U.S. blood supply be screened for Zika virus.[34] As of October 2017, the FDA has approved the use of the cobas Zika, a qualitative polymerase chain reaction (PCR) based test, for screening of blood products in the United States.[35] Zika virus has now been identified in blood products donated by persons residing in areas of the United States with and without local transmission.[36,37]

CLINICAL MANIFESTATIONS
Congenital Infection

Zika virus can cause asymptomatic-to-severe congenital infections. Symptomatic congenital infections can occur with maternal infection at any time during the pregnancy, although infection earlier in gestation is associated with higher rates of adverse outcomes.[38,39] Rates of adverse outcomes do not differ between fetuses or infants born to symptomatic or asymptomatic mothers.

Abnormalities may be detected in utero by ultrasonography or MRI. The major ultrasound findings include ventriculomegaly, cerebral calcifications, posterior fossa abnormalities, and arthrogyposis.[38,40] A range of abnormalities on fetal MRI can be present including subependymal pseudocysts, polymicrogyria, and absent or hypoplastic corpus callosum.[41]

In Brazil, 63% of Zika-infected infants had at least 1 abnormal neurologic finding at birth.[38] The United States Zika Pregnancy Registry, however, only documented neurologic defects in 6% to 11% of fetuses and infants.[39] Microcephaly was one of the first abnormalities reported in infants with congenital Zika virus infection and appears to be one of the most common manifestations in symptomatic infants.[42,43] Currently, there is not a complete understanding of the mechanisms leading to the neurologic manifestations; however, experimental models suggest that Zika virus causes microcephaly and neurologic abnormalities by targeting cortical progenitor cells, inducing cellular death and altering brain development.[44,45] Severe microcephaly is observed in the fetal brain disruption sequence, which also includes, overlapping cranial sutures, prominent occipital bone, and redundant scalp skin.[46] Findings found on brain imaging in these infants include abnormalities of the corpus callosum, cortical malformations, cerebral atrophy, hydrocephaly, intracranial calcifications, and ventriculomegaly.[39] These abnormalities can be present even in the absence of microcephaly. In a cohort of 70 infants from Brazil with microcephaly and evidence of Zika virus infection, sensorineural hearing loss was present in 5.8%.[47] It remains unknown if Zika virus–associated hearing loss is progressive, similar to congenital cytomegalovirus and other common congenital infections. In addition to neurologic abnormalities, arthrogryposis has been reported in small numbers of congenitally infected infants.[48] A recent study reported higher rates of congenital heart disease in infants with congenital Zika virus infection when compared with rates in the general population, although the true relationship of these anomalies with Zika virus is unknown.[49]

Data on long-term outcomes of infants with congenital Zika virus are lacking, but those infants with severe neurologic abnormalities are likely to have significant impairment. Congenital Zika virus infection can result in death of the fetus or infant. Death in a cohort of Brazilian infants is reported to occur in 4% to 6% of infants born with confirmed or probable Zika virus infection, although the cause of death was not documented or available.[50]

Postnatal Infection in Children Younger than 18 Years

The incubation period for Zika virus is estimated to be between 3 and 14 days with 50% of patients experiencing onset of symptoms within 1 week.[51] Macular or papular rash was the most common symptom found in up to 90% of patients during the outbreak on Yap Island.[4] Fever, arthritis or arthralgia, nonpurulent conjunctivitis, myalgia, headache, and retro-orbital pain are also reported in a substantial number of patients.[4] Most reports of clinical manifestations have been in cohorts of mainly adults, although 2 cases series of Zika virus infection in children have been published.[52,53] Both series identified rash, fever, conjunctivitis, and arthralgia to be the most common signs and symptoms. In the series of children from the United States, rash was the most common sign, present in 82% of children.[53] Fever was the second most common sign, occurring in 55% of children.[53] Neither series reported any neurologic manifestations. Neurologic complications have occurred in temporal relationship to Zika virus infection and include Guillain-Barré syndrome,[54,55] acute myelitis,[56] and meningoencephalitis.[57,58] Death from Zika virus infection outside of the newborn period seems to be rare but has occurred in both children and adults and is typically associated with severe thrombocytopenia.[19,59,60]

DIAGNOSIS

Zika virus RNA can be detected in clinical specimens including blood, semen, saliva, tears, and urine by real time reverse transcriptase PCR (RT-PCR). Additionally, testing for Zika virus IgM is available using enzyme-linked immunosorbent assay (ELISA). Plaque reduction neutralization test (PRNT) should be performed to exclude false-positive Zika virus IgM results as cross-reactivity between Flavivirus IgM antibodies can occur.[61] Testing for Zika virus is available through the health department and Centers for Disease Control and Prevention (CDC) and some commercial laboratories, although tests have not been FDA approved.

Congenital Infection

As with other congenital infections, the diagnosis of congenital Zika virus infection can be difficult. The CDC recommends that laboratory testing for congenital Zika virus be performed for all infants of mothers with confirmed Zika virus infection and infants with findings suggestive of congenital infection with an appropriate epidemiologic link, such as travel or residence in an area of endemic transmission.[62] Maternal infection is confirmed when a clinical specimen is positive for Zika virus RNA by RT-PCR or identification of Zika virus IgM with confirmatory neutralizing antibody titer for Zika virus.[61] Testing in the infant should include Zika virus RT-PCR of serum and urine and Zika virus IgM ELISA on the serum.[62] Testing for both Zika virus RNA and Zika virus IgM can be performed on cerebrospinal fluid if the specimen is available. Testing of cord blood is not recommended because of the risk of contamination with maternal blood.[63] To distinguish between congenital, perinatal, and postnatal infection, the CDC recommends initiation of testing within the first 2 days of life.[62] Congenital Zika virus infection is confirmed when Zika virus RNA is detected in infant specimens within the first 2 days of life, regardless of the result of IgM testing.[62] Infants with positive Zika virus IgM by ELISA but negative RT-PCR for Zika virus RNA are classified as having probable congenital Zika virus infection.[62] If results of both RT-PCR and IgM for Zika virus are negative but clinical concern remains high, the CDC suggests that PRNT at 18 months can be performed, although positive results would not distinguish between congenital or postnatal infection.[62]

Postnatal Infection in Children Younger Than 18 Years

Acute Zika virus infection should be suspected in individuals with an epidemiologic risk factor and 2 or more of the following clinical manifestations: arthralgia, conjunctivitis, fever, or rash.[64,65] Testing should include evaluation of serum andurine for Zika virus RNA by RT-PCR. Cerebrospinal fluid can be tested but should not be obtained solely for this purpose. If symptoms have been present for at least 4 days, and Zika virus RNA is not detected in clinical specimens, Zika virus IgM by ELISA and PRNT should be sent.[64] Acute Zika virus infection is confirmed if either Zika virus RNA or a positive Zika virus IgM with neutralizing antibodies is detected.

CLINICAL EVALUATION

Infants born to mothers with suspected or confirmed Zika virus infection should be thoroughly evaluated by physical examination for appropriate head circumference, neurologic abnormalities, and any other abnormal findings. In addition to testing for Zika virus and other etiologies of congenital infections, a complete blood count and complete metabolic panel should be obtained.[62] The CDC recommends that all infected infants have an ophthalmologic examination, hearing test, and a postnatal head ultrasound scan with further neuroimaging if indicated before discharge from the hospital.[62] Older infants and children with postnatal acquisition of Zika virus do not require any further routine evaluation.

MANAGEMENT

The CDC has made recommendations for the long-term management of infants with congenital Zika virus infection. Neurologic examination should be performed by the primary pediatrician at 1 and 2 months of life with referral to the neurology department for any abnormalities. An ophthalmologic examination should occur within the first month of life and again at age 3 months if the initial examination was normal. Auditory brainstem response audiometry should also be performed before 1 month of life and again at the age of 4 to 6 months, as hearing loss may be progressive. Those infants with abnormal brain development may require endocrinologist consultation for evaluation of hypothalamic-pituitary function. Developmental monitoring with standardized screening tools should occur at routine visits with appropriate referral to specialists as indicated.

The management of symptomatic Zika virus infection in infants and children with postnatal disease acquisition is supportive. Nonsteroidal anti-inflammatory agents and acetaminophen may be used for symptomatic relief.

PREVENTION

The primary prevention strategy against Zika virus infection is avoidance of travel to areas with transmission of the disease. If traveling to or residing in an area with Zika transmission, adherence to mosquito prevention measures, including the use of repellants and protective clothing is recommended. DEET-containing repellants are effective and safe for use on children older than 2 months of age and pregnant women.[66,67] Clothing can also be treated with permethrin, a synthetic compound toxic to insects.

Prevention of congenital infection relies largely on the strategies described above. The CDC recommends that pregnant women avoid all travel to areas with Zika transmission.[68] Additionally, condoms should be used for any sexual encounters with individuals who have traveled or reside in a Zika endemic area.

SUMMARY

Regions at risk for Zika virus transmission have increased over the last several years to include many countries of South and Central America, the Caribbean, and parts of the United States. As transmission is occurring more widely, more information about the clinical manifestations has been described. Zika virus is now known to cause both symptomatic and asymptomatic congenital infection. Congenital infection can result in severe manifestations, most notably neurologic abnormalities. Outside of the newborn period, Zika virus typically results in a self-limited illness, although complications have been described. Because the emergence of this pathogen as a cause of congenital infection has only recently been described, further research regarding the transmission, pathogenesis, treatment, and prevention is needed.

REFERENCES

1. Dick GW, Kitchen SF, Haddow AJ. Zika virus. I. Isolations and serological specificity. Trans R Soc Trop Med Hyg 1952;46(5):509–20.
2. Alera MT, Hermann L, Tac-An IA, et al. Zika virus infection, Philippines, 2012. Emerg Infect Dis 2015;21(4):722–4.
3. Buathong R, Hermann L, Thaisomboonsuk B, et al. Detection of Zika virus infection in Thailand, 2012-2014. Am J Trop Med Hyg 2015;93(2):380–3.
4. Duffy MR, Chen TH, Hancock WT, et al. Zika virus outbreak on Yap Island, Federated States of Micronesia. N Engl J Med 2009;360(24):2536–43.
5. Fagbami AH. Zika virus infections in Nigeria: virological and seroepidemiological investigations in Oyo State. J Hyg 1979;83(2):213–9.
6. Heang V, Yasuda CY, Sovann L, et al. Zika virus infection, Cambodia, 2010. Emerg Infect Dis 2012;18(2):349–51.
7. Olson JG, Ksiazek TG, Suhandiman, et al. Zika virus, a cause of fever in Central Java, Indonesia. Trans R Soc Trop Med Hyg 1981;75(3):389–93.
8. Tognarelli J, Ulloa S, Villagra E, et al. A report on the outbreak of Zika virus on Easter Island, South Pacific, 2014. Arch Virol 2016;161(3):665–8.
9. Zanluca C, Melo VC, Mosimann AL, et al. First report of autochthonous transmission of Zika virus in Brazil. Mem Inst Oswaldo Cruz 2015;110(4):569–72.
10. Campos GS, Bandeira AC, Sardi SI. Zika virus outbreak, Bahia, Brazil. Emerg Infect Dis 2015;21(10):1885–6.
11. Ledermann JP, Guillaumot L, Yug L, et al. Aedes hensilli as a potential vector of Chikungunya and Zika viruses. PLoS Negl Trop Dis 2014;8(10):e3188.
12. Guerbois M, Fernandez-Salas I, Azar SR, et al. Outbreak of Zika virus infection, Chiapas State, Mexico, 2015, and first confirmed transmission by aedes aegypti mosquitoes in the Americas. J Infect Dis 2016;214(9):1349–56.
13. Foy BD, Kobylinski KC, Chilson Foy JL, et al. Probable non-vector-borne transmission of Zika virus, Colorado, USA. Emerg Infect Dis 2011;17(5):880–2.
14. Hills SL, Russell K, Hennessey M, et al. Transmission of Zika virus through sexual contact with travelers to areas of ongoing transmission - continental United States, 2016. MMWR Morb Mortal Wkly Rep 2016;65(8):215–6.

15. Deckard DT, Chung WM, Brooks JT, et al. Male-to-male sexual transmission of Zika virus–Texas, January 2016. MMWR Morb Mortal Wkly Rep 2016;65(14): 372–4.

16. Davidson A, Slavinski S, Komoto K, et al. Suspected female-to-male sexual transmission of Zika virus - New York City, 2016. MMWR Morb Mortal Wkly Rep 2016; 65(28):716–7.

17. Mansuy JM, Suberbielle E, Chapuy-Regaud S, et al. Zika virus in semen and spermatozoa. Lancet Infect Dis 2016;16(10):1106–7.

18. Murray KO, Gorchakov R, Carlson AR, et al. Prolonged detection of Zika virus in vaginal secretions and whole blood. Emerg Infect Dis 2017;23(1):99–101.

19. Swaminathan S, Schlaberg R, Lewis J, et al. Fatal Zika virus infection with secondary nonsexual transmission. N Engl J Med 2016;375(19):1907–9.

20. Paz-Bailey G, Rosenberg ES, Doyle K, et al. Persistence of Zika virus in body fluids - preliminary report. N Engl J Med 2017. [Epub ahead of print].

21. Tan JJL, Balne PK, Leo YS, et al. Persistence of Zika virus in conjunctival fluid of convalescence patients. Sci Rep 2017;7(1):11194.

22. Tabata T, Petitt M, Puerta-Guardo H, et al. Zika virus targets different primary human placental cells, suggesting two routes for vertical transmission. Cell Host Microbe 2016;20(2):155–66.

23. Calvet G, Aguiar RS, Melo AS, et al. Detection and sequencing of Zika virus from amniotic fluid of fetuses with microcephaly in Brazil: a case study. Lancet Infect Dis 2016;16(6):653–60.

24. Oliveira Melo AS, Malinger G, Ximenes R, et al. Zika virus intrauterine infection causes fetal brain abnormality and microcephaly: tip of the iceberg? Ultrasound Obstet Gynecol 2016;47(1):6–7.

25. Martines RB, Bhatnagar J, Keating MK, et al. Notes from the field: evidence of Zika virus infection in brain and placental tissues from two congenitally infected newborns and two fetal losses–Brazil, 2015. MMWR Morb Mortal Wkly Rep 2016;65(6):159–60.

26. Meaney-Delman D, Hills SL, Williams C, et al. Zika virus infection among U.S. pregnant travelers - August 2015-February 2016. MMWR Morb Mortal Wkly Rep 2016;65(8):211–4.

27. Besnard M, Lastere S, Teissier A, et al. Evidence of perinatal transmission of Zika virus, French polynesia, December 2013 and February 2014. Euro Surveill 2014; 19(13) [pii:20751].

28. Dupont-Rouzeyrol M, Biron A, O'Connor O, et al. Infectious Zika viral particles in breastmilk. Lancet 2016;387(10023):1051.

29. Musso D, Nhan T, Robin E, et al. Potential for Zika virus transmission through blood transfusion demonstrated during an outbreak in French Polynesia, November 2013 to February 2014. Euro Surveill 2014;19(14) [pii:20761].

30. Barjas-Castro ML, Angerami RN, Cunha MS, et al. Probable transfusion-transmitted Zika virus in Brazil. Transfusion 2016;56(7):1684–8.

31. Motta IJ, Spencer BR, Cordeiro da Silva SG, et al. Evidence for transmission of Zika virus by platelet transfusion. N Engl J Med 2016;375(11):1101–3.

32. Kuehnert MJ, Basavaraju SV, Moseley RR, et al. Screening of blood donations for Zika virus infection - Puerto Rico, April 3-June 11, 2016. MMWR Morb Mortal Wkly Rep 2016;65(24):627–8.

33. Adams L, Bello-Pagan M, Lozier M, et al. Update: ongoing Zika virus transmission - Puerto Rico, November 1, 2015-July 7, 2016. MMWR Morb Mortal Wkly Rep 2016;65(30):774–9.

34. United States Food and Drug Administration. Guidance for industry: revised recommendations for reducing the risk of Zika virus transmission by blood and blood components. Silver Spring (MD): CBER Office of Communication, Outreach, and Development; 2016.

35. United States Food and Drug Administration. cobas Zika BL 125653/0 approval letter. In: Center for Biologics Evaluation and Research, editor. U.S. Food and Drug Administration; 2017.

36. Galel SA, Williamson PC, Busch MP, et al. First Zika-positive donations in the continental United States. Transfusion 2017;57(3pt2):762–9.

37. Williamson PC, Linnen JM, Kessler DA, et al. First cases of Zika virus-infected US blood donors outside states with areas of active transmission. Transfusion 2017; 57(3pt2):770–8.

38. Brasil P, Pereira JP Jr, Moreira ME, et al. Zika virus infection in pregnant women in Rio de Janeiro. N Engl J Med 2016;375(24):2321–34.

39. Honein MA, Dawson AL, Petersen EE, et al. Birth defects among fetuses and infants of US women with evidence of possible Zika virus infection during pregnancy. JAMA 2017;317(1):59–68.

40. Sarno M, Aquino M, Pimentel K, et al. Progressive lesions of Central Nervous System in microcephalic fetuses with suspected congenital Zika virus syndrome. Ultrasound Obstet Gynecol 2016. [Epub ahead of print].

41. Guillemette-Artur P, Besnard M, Eyrolle-Guignot D, et al. Prenatal brain MRI of fetuses with Zika virus infection. Pediatr Radiol 2016;46(7):1032–9.

42. Schuler-Faccini L, Ribeiro EM, Feitosa IM, et al. Possible association between Zika virus infection and microcephaly - Brazil, 2015. MMWR Morb Mortal Wkly Rep 2016;65(3):59–62.

43. de Araujo TV, Rodrigues LC, de Alencar Ximenes RA, et al. Association between Zika virus infection and microcephaly in Brazil, January to May, 2016: preliminary report of a case-control study. Lancet Infect Dis 2016;16(12):1356–63.

44. Cugola FR, Fernandes IR, Russo FB, et al. The Brazilian Zika virus strain causes birth defects in experimental models. Nature 2016;534(7606):267–71.

45. Garcez PP, Loiola EC, Madeiro da Costa R, et al. Zika virus impairs growth in human neurospheres and brain organoids. Science 2016;352(6287):816–8.

46. Moore CA, Staples JE, Dobyns WB, et al. Characterizing the pattern of anomalies in congenital Zika syndrome for pediatric clinicians. JAMA Pediatr 2017;171(3): 288–95.

47. Leal MC, Muniz LF, Ferreira TS, et al. Hearing loss in infants with microcephaly and evidence of congenital Zika virus infection - Brazil, November 2015-May 2016. MMWR Morb Mortal Wkly Rep 2016;65(34):917–9.

48. van der Linden V, Filho EL, Lins OG, et al. Congenital Zika syndrome with arthrogryposis: retrospective case series study. BMJ 2016;354:i3899.

49. Cavalcanti DD, Alves LV, Furtado GJ, et al. Echocardiographic findings in infants with presumed congenital Zika syndrome: retrospective case series study. PLoS One 2017;12(4):e0175065.

50. França GVA, Schuler-Faccini L, Oliveira WK, et al. Congenital Zika virus syndrome in Brazil: a case series of the first 1501 livebirths with complete investigation. Lancet 2016;388(10047):891–7.

51. Krow-Lucal ER, Biggerstaff BJ, Staples JE. Estimated incubation period for zika virus disease. Emerg Infect Dis 2017;23(5):841–5.

52. Li J, Chong CY, Tan NW, et al. Characteristics of Zika virus disease in children: clinical, hematological and virological findings from an outbreak in Singapore. Clin Infect Dis 2017;64(10):1445–8.

53. Goodman AB, Dziuban EJ, Powell K, et al. Characteristics of children aged <18 years with Zika virus disease acquired postnatally - U.S. states, January 2015-July 2016. MMWR Morb Mortal Wkly Rep 2016;65(39):1082–5.
54. Cao-Lormeau VM, Blake A, Mons S, et al. Guillain-Barre syndrome outbreak associated with Zika virus infection in French Polynesia: a case-control study. Lancet 2016;387(10027):1531–9.
55. Parra B, Lizarazo J, Jimenez-Arango JA, et al. Guillain-Barre syndrome associated with Zika virus infection in Colombia. N Engl J Med 2016;375(16):1513–23.
56. Mecharles S, Herrmann C, Poullain P, et al. Acute myelitis due to Zika virus infection. Lancet 2016;387(10026):1481.
57. Carteaux G, Maquart M, Bedet A, et al. Zika virus associated with meningoencephalitis. N Engl J Med 2016;374(16):1595–6.
58. Schwartzmann PV, Ramalho LN, Neder L, et al. Zika virus meningoencephalitis in an immunocompromised patient. Mayo Clin Proc 2017;92(3):460–6.
59. Arzuza-Ortega L, Polo A, Perez-Tatis G, et al. Fatal sickle cell disease and Zika virus infection in girl from Colombia. Emerg Infect Dis 2016;22(5):925–7.
60. Sharp TM, Munoz-Jordan J, Perez-Padilla J, et al. Zika virus infection associated with severe thrombocytopenia. Clin Infect Dis 2016;63(9):1198–201.
61. Rabe IB, Staples JE, Villanueva J, et al. Interim guidance for interpretation of Zika virus antibody test results. MMWR Morb Mortal Wkly Rep 2016;65(21):543–6.
62. Russell K, Oliver SE, Lewis L, et al. Update: interim guidance for the evaluation and management of infants with possible congenital Zika virus infection - United States, August 2016. MMWR Morb Mortal Wkly Rep 2016;65(33):870–8.
63. Masuzaki H, Miura K, Miura S, et al. Labor increases maternal DNA contamination in cord blood. Clin Chem 2004;50(9):1709–11.
64. Fleming-Dutra KE, Nelson JM, Fischer M, et al. Update: interim guidelines for health care providers caring for infants and children with possible Zika virus infection–United States, February 2016. MMWR Morb Mortal Wkly Rep 2016; 65(7):182–7.
65. Adebanjo T, Godfred-Cato S, Viens L, et al. Update: interim guidance for the diagnosis, evaluation, and management of infants with possible congenital Zika virus infection - United States, October 2017. MMWR Morb Mortal Wkly Rep 2017;66(41):1089–99.
66. Koren G, Matsui D, Bailey B. DEET-based insect repellents: safety implications for children and pregnant and lactating women. CMAJ 2003;169(3):209–12.
67. Wylie BJ, Hauptman M, Woolf AD, et al. Insect repellants during pregnancy in the era of the Zika virus. Obstet Gynecol 2016;128(5):1111–5.
68. Oduyebo T, Polen KD, Walke HT, et al. Update: interim guidance for health care providers caring for pregnant women with possible Zika virus exposure - United States (including U.S. Territories), July 2017. MMWR Morb Mortal Wkly Rep 2017; 66(29):781–93.

Infections in Children on Biologics

Lara Danziger-Isakov, MD, MPH

KEYWORDS

- Pediatrics • Infectious disease • Biologics • Opportunistic infection

KEY POINTS

- Biologics represent a wide range of products that often target immune system pathways resulting in unintended consequences, including infectious events.
- Tumor necrosis factor-α inhibitors in pediatric patients may have a differential infection risk based on the agent and underlying condition being treated.
- Emerging data on infections specific to biologic administration in pediatrics will be essential to determine the risks of these agents in the future.

INTRODUCTION

According to the US Food and Drug Administration, biologics represent a wide range of products, including vaccines, blood components, allergenics, somatic cells, gene therapy, tissues, and recombinant therapeutic proteins (**Table 1**).[1] In the past decade, there has been an explosion of biologics, specifically recombinant therapeutic proteins, developed and approved to treat a broad range of immunologically mediated pediatric diseases, including rheumatologic diseases and inflammatory bowel disease (IBD), whereas other biologic products target pathways to disrupt cancer cell replication. Biologics aim to modify targeted pathways to interfere with the immunologic aberration creating the clinical disease either through dampening or upregulating responses (**Fig. 1**). However, alteration of the pathways results in selective deficits in the immune system potentially increasing the risk of infection. Risk for infection varies based not only on the biologic target but also on the intensity of dosing as evidenced by a recent meta-analysis of primarily adult studies that reported increased risk for infection in patients with rheumatoid arthritis (RA) who received standard or high-dose biologics compared with low-dose or traditional medications for the disease.[2] Although much has been reported in the adult literature regarding increased

Disclosures: No relationships to report.
Division of Infectious Diseases, Cincinnati Children's Hospital Medical Center, 3333 Burnet Avenue, MLC 7017, Cincinnati, OH 45229, USA
E-mail address: Lara.Danziger-Isakov@cchmc.org

Infect Dis Clin N Am 32 (2018) 225–236
https://doi.org/10.1016/j.idc.2017.10.004
id.theclinics.com

Table 1
Biologics and associated infectious events

Target	Agent	Pediatric Indications	Associated Infections in Pediatrics
TNF-α	—	—	URI, pneumonia, abscesses, varicella zoster, histoplasmosis
	Infliximab	CD, UC	Listeria meningitis, cutaneous blastomycosis,
	Adalimumab	JIA, CD, UC	*Mycobacterium avium*
	Etanercept	Polyarticular JIA, psoriasis	Purpura fulminans
IL-1	Anakinra	NOMID and CAPS, systemic JIA	Visceral leishmaniasis, varicella, labial herpes, URI
	Canakinumab	JIA, FMF, hyperimmunoglobulin D, TRAPS	URI, nasopharyngitis
IL-2	Basiliximab	Organ transplant rejection prophylaxis	—
IL-6	Tocilizumab	Polyarticular and systemic JIA	URI, pneumonia, bronchitis, cellulitis, varicella
IL-12/23	Ustekinumab	UC	—
CD28 blockade	Abatacept	JIA	—
a-4 Integrin	Vedolizumab	Off-label: refractory inflammatory bowel disease	URI, cellulitis
JAK	Tofacitinib	Off-label: GVHD, JAK/STAT pathway mutations, alopecia areata	Viral infection (BK, CMV, adenovirus), bacterial infection
CD20	Rituximab	Off-label: PTLD, EBV-related HLH, glomerular diseases, CNS-inflammatory diseases, Burkitt lymphoma	Viral infection (varicella, CMV, adenovirus), pneumonia, empyema, mastoiditis, *Salmonella enteritis*, candidiasis

Abbreviations: CAPS, cryopyrin-associated periodic syndromes; CD, Crohn disease; CMV, cytomegalovirus; CNS, central nervous system; EBV, Epstein-Barr virus; FMF, familial Mediterranean fever; GVHD, graft-versus-host disease; HLH, hemophagocytic lymphohistiocytosis; JAK, Janus kinase; JIA, juvenile idiopathic arthritis; NOMID, neonatal-onset multisystem inflammatory disease; PTLD, posttransplant lymphoproliferative disease; STAT, signal transducers and activators of transcription; TRAPS, tumor necrosis factor receptor associated periodic syndrome; UC, ulcerative colitis; URI, upper respiratory infection.

infectious risk with these biologics, pediatric data are limited; but inference from prior experiences may be taken.

BIOLOGIC TARGETS AND ASSOCIATED INFECTIONS
Tumor Necrosis Factor-α Inhibitors

Tumor necrosis factor (TNF)-α, a cell-signaling protein produced acutely by macrophages and monocytes, activates the vascular endothelium and increases vascular permeability. TNF-α inhibitors block the signaling to reduce acute inflammation in patients with RA, juvenile idiopathic arthritis (JIA), various types of psoriasis, and IBD, such as Crohn disease (CD) and ulcerative colitis (UC). Infliximab (CD), adalimumab (CD, JIA), and etanercept (JIA, plaque psoriasis) currently have approved indications

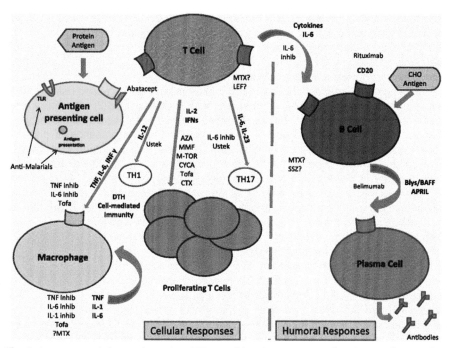

Fig. 1. Immunomodulatory therapies. AZA, azathioprine; BAFF, B-cell activating factor; Blys, B lymphocyte stimulator; CHO, carbohydrate; CTX, cyclophosphamide; CYCA, cyclosporine A; DTH, delayed-type hypersensitivity; IL, interleukin; INF, interferon; inhib, inhibitor; LEF, leflunomide; MMF, mycophenolate mofetil; M-TOR, mammalian target of rapamycin; MTX, methotrexate; SSZ, sulfasalazine; TLR, toll-like receptor; TNF, tumor necrosis factor; Tofa, tofacitinib; Ustek, ustekinumab. (*From* McMahan ZH, Bingham III CO. Effects of biological and non-biological immunomodulatory therapies on the immunogenicity of vaccines in patients with rheumatic diseases. Arthritis Res Ther 2104:16(6):506; with permission.)

in pediatrics, with certolizumab and golimumab approved in adults. Exact reasons for the differential risk of infection among these agents is uncertain; however, in vitro experiments indicate that infliximab suppresses cellular responses to mycobacteria and suppresses more gene expression by lymphocytes compared with etanercept.[3] Reports from adult patients indicated an increased risk of serious infections with the use of TNF-α inhibitors, including reactivation of tuberculosis.[4,5] Preinitiation screening for tuberculosis (TB) as well as endemic fungi and hepatitis B virus (HBV) infection is recommended with these agents. The differential risk for infection clinically may occur based on the agent used, with infliximab and adalimumab associated with an increased risk of infection events in adult patients with psoriasis.[6]

The predominant reporting of TNF-α–associated infectious events in pediatric patients stem from individual case reports and case series. Events include a variety of bacterial infections, such as *Streptococcus pyogenes* purpura fulminans in an 8 year old with JIA on etanercept[7] and listeria meningitis in a 17 year old with UC on infliximab.[8] Occult infections that can be difficult to distinguish from underlying inflammatory disease processes have also been reported, including at least one systemic *Mycobacterium avium* complex infection in a 13 year old with CD[9] and endemic fungal infections, such as histoplasmosis in 5 patients with IBD.[10] Furthermore, cutaneous blastomycosis was reported in a 9 year old with JIA treated with infliximab and methotrexate.[11]

Pediatric patients receiving TNF-α inhibitors have been explored as part of larger studies to interrogate several specific questions related to infectious risk. Cohorts of pediatric patients receiving approved TNF-α inhibitors indicate upper respiratory tract infections, pneumonia, gastrointestinal abscesses, cellulitis, and varicella zoster virus reactivation as common infections during therapy.[12–14]

Assessing if pediatric patients on TNF-α inhibitors have an increased risk of infection compared with (1) patients without immunologic disease and (2) with similar disease with and without TNF-α inhibitor therapy yield mixed results. Comparisons with patients without immune-mediated disease indicate that the presence of disease alone may increase the risk for infection. For example, a study comparing Taiwanese children with and without JIA found that children with JIA developed TB at twice the rate of children without JIA.[15] However, only 7.4% of the 1495 children with JIA received a TNF-α inhibitor, and the rate of TB was not increased for this subset compared with children without JIA. Similarly, pediatric patients with JIA in the United States in the early 2000s had increased rates of hospitalizations for bacterial infections compared with children with attention-deficit/hyperactivity disorder; but among patients with JIA, high-dose steroid use was most strongly associated with infectious events regardless of TNF-α inhibitor administration, predominantly etanercept, or methotrexate use.[16] A Spanish study also found latent TB rates in patients on TNF-α inhibitors similar to that in local population screening studies[17] but did not explore the rates among all patients with immunologic disease as in the Taiwanese cohort. Pooled analysis of pediatric patients with IBD show both pediatric patients on steroids and adult patients receiving TNF-α inhibitors develop infection at twice the rate of pediatric patients on TNF-α inhibitors indicating that the role of TNF-α inhibitors in the risk for infection may vary in pediatric compared with adult patients.[18]

A more recent study by Becker and Horneff[19] reported that etanercept and adalimumab were associated with an increased risk of serious infection compared with methotrexate for patients with JIA in the German Biologic Registry for Pediatric Rheumatology. Increased risk of herpes zoster infections with etanercept compared with methotrexate for the treatment of JIA has also been reported.[13] Reactivation of Epstein-Barr virus (EBV) occurred in 1 of 136 patients on infliximab for CD in a Polish cohort,[20] whereas Hradsky and colleagues[21] reported increased EBV viral loads with infliximab dosing without increases in cytomegalovirus (CMV) or BK viral loads. Therefore, the association between TNF-α inhibitor therapy and the risk for infectious complications in pediatric patients seems less clear than in adults for whom it is associated with increased risk of infection. Additional population studies will be needed to assess the risk in this population based on age, agents used, and underlying disease, especially as treatment options change.

TNF-α inhibitors' impact on vaccine responses have been explored in the literature as well. Moses and colleagues[22] evaluated HBV vaccine responses in pediatric patients with IBD on infliximab finding that 44% did not have evidence of sero-protection from HBV vaccination. HBV booster vaccination resulted in sero-response in 76%, although nonresponse was associated with more frequent infliximab administration. These results highlight the gaps in knowledge around vaccination responses and other infectious events with the use of TNF-α inhibitors specifically in pediatric patients. A recent systematic review including pediatric studies of both measles and varicella vaccination suggested that events were limited; however, too few patients have been evaluated to deviate from the recommendation that live virus vaccination be deferred while on significant immunosuppressive therapy, such as TNF-α inhibitors.[23]

Interleukin Inhibitors

Interleukins are a diverse group of cytokines involved in signaling between cells as part of the inflammatory cascade. Defects in either interleukin production or response to interleukins have been implicated in both autoimmune diseases and immunodeficiency syndromes. In response, biologics targeted against various interleukins have been developed to treat a variety of diseases. Similar to TNF-α inhibitors, reports of infections have followed the introduction of these biologics, although fewer reports exist compared with the more commonly used TNF-α inhibitors.

Interleukin-1 inhibitors

Interleukin-1 (IL-1) mediates macrophage and T-cell activation with systemic development of fever. Anakinra acts by blocking the receptor for IL-1 competitively inhibiting IL-1 action and is currently approved for the treatment of neonatal-onset multisystem inflammatory disease and cryopyrin-associated periodic syndromes. Additionally, off-label pediatric uses include treatment of systemic JIA.[24] In adults, infectious events, including TB, pneumonia, cellulitis, and sepsis, have been reported.[25,26] A study that included 20 pediatric patients with systemic JIA treated over a mean of 7 years (range 1–16 years) revealed the following infectious events in the cohort: visceral leishmaniasis (1), varicella (1), labial herpes simplex virus (HSV) (1), and upper respiratory infection (2),[27] with similar events reported in the 15 adults also followed as part of the study. Canakinumab, another IL-1 inhibitor, binds to IL-1β preventing it from attaching to the cellular receptor. Canakinumab has multiple pediatric indications, including the treatment of JIA, familial Mediterranean fever, hyperimmunoglobulin D syndrome, and TNF receptor–associated periodic syndrome. In 2 trials evaluating canakinumab therapy for JIA, serious infections occurred in 5% or less of patients with similar rates in patients on canakinumab or placebo.[28] Interestingly, in these studies and an additional report, several patients experienced the development of macrophage-activating syndrome (MAS); but rates of MAS were not different in patients on canakinumab compared with placebo.[28,29] As clinicians continue to explore the repertoire of biologics and the immune dysregulation that these biologic agents target, it is certain that we will discover more about the underlying risk for infectious and noninfectious events.

Interleukin-6 inhibitors

Interleukin-6 (IL-6) modulates T- and B-cell growth and differentiation and stimulates acute-phase protein production. Tocilizumab, an IL-6 receptor blocker, is the most commonly used agent in this category with pediatric indications to treat JIA, systemic and polyarticular. In adults, tocilizumab use is associated with an increased risk of infection when administered after rituximab or in conjunction with steroids or leflunomide in patients with RA.[30] Further, tocilizumab therapy for RA has been associated with HBV reactivation in Chinese patients with chronic HBV not on HBV prophylaxis[31] and CMV hepatitis and gastritis in Japan.[32] The pediatric experience is equally limited. Of 6 pediatric patients with JIA with primary varicella while on tocilizumab, none experienced severe disease, but one patient developed MAS with elevated IL-6 levels.[33] Brunner and colleagues[34] reported a more comprehensive evaluation of infectious events with tocilizumab therapy for 270 pediatric patients with JIA. Severe infections secondary to pneumonia, bronchitis, and cellulitis occurred in 2% of patients, although nearly 14% of patients on therapy experienced an adverse event, including upper respiratory infections, pharyngitis, and cough.

Interleukin-2 inhibitors

Interleukin (IL-2) promotes T-cell proliferation, and IL-2 receptor blockers have been predominantly used in solid organ transplantation to disrupt T-cell proliferation early after organ implantation. Basiliximab is approved for prophylaxis against renal transplant rejection in children, although it is commonly used in other pediatric solid organ transplant recipients. The use of basiliximab has not been associated with an increased risk of infection in pediatric kidney transplant recipients.[35] Further, basiliximab induction compared with steroids was associated with decreased infection and acute rejection events in a cohort of pediatric liver transplant recipients.[36] Either the limited duration of use during the peri-transplant period or the immunologic impact of alternative immunosuppression for solid organ transplantation may account for the lack of infectious events, as both studies compared basiliximab use with other immunosuppressive regimens. Therefore, basiliximab does not seem to increase therisk of infection after solid organ transplantation any more than routine immunosuppression.

Interleukins 12, 17, and 23

Interleukin (IL-12) is produced by macrophages and dendritic cells and promotes both natural killer cell activation and T-cell differentiation via interferon (INF)-γ production. IL-23 stimulates proliferation of Th17 cells through INF-γ, while IL-17 is produced by Th17 cells to stimulate proinflammatory cytokines impacting endothelia, epithelia and fibroblasts. Ustekinumab (IL-12/23 receptor blocker) has orphan drug status for the treatment of pediatric ulcerative colitis. Other medications in this group have adult indications, including secukinumab (IL-17A antibody) for psoriasis, psoriatic arthritis, ankylosing spondylitis, brodalumab (IL-17 receptor A antibody) for psoriasis, and the most-recently approved ixekizumab (IL-17A antibody) and gesulkumab (IL-23 antibody) for psoriasis. As medications blocking these pathways are just emerging, information regarding infection-related side effects is limited and predominantly reports on adult patients with psoriasis. Similar to other agents, reports of nasopharyngitis and upper respiratory infections predominate occurring in 4% to 17% each in clinical trials for secukinumab, gesulkumab, and ixekizumab[37-40] with little differences in rates among the different agents evaluated. Case reports of bacterial infections in adults include *Staphylococcus aureus* bacteremia with ustekinumab[41] and staphylococcal endophthalmitis and osteomyelitis with secukinumab.[42] Pediatric reports of infectious events do not yet appear in the literature, but these agents seem to have limited infectious complications in adults to date.

Noninterleukin Targets

Several other immunologic targets that are not directly related to interleukins have been developed to combat immune-mediated diseases. Abatacept, a CTLA4-Ig, interrupts T-cell activation through binding costimulators preventing interaction of antigen-presenting cells with CD28 expressed by T cells. Abatacept is approved to treat JIA in pediatric patients, although no reports of associated infections appear in the literature. In adults, one case report of HBV reactivation has been reported.[43]

Natalizumab (multiple sclerosis, CD) and vedolizumab (UC, CD) interrupt memory T-cell migration across the endothelium by blocking $\alpha 4$ integrins. Neither is approved for use in pediatrics to date. Although no reports of pediatric events appear in the literature for natalizumab, adult data indicate an increased risk of progressive multifocal leukoencephalopathy (PML) with natalizumab.[44] Vedolizumab does not seem to have an increased infectious risk compared with other IBD biologic therapies in adults, but a statistically insignificant increase in enteric infections occurred in vedolizumab-exposed patients compared with controls.[45] An increased risk of surgical site infection with perioperative vedolizumab administration was also reported in this analysis.[45] Vedolizumab has been evaluated in a limited number of pediatric patients with IBD who had failed TNF-α inhibitors. One study reported no infectious complications in 52 subjects, whereas a smaller study of 21 patients described 2 skin infections and 5 upper respiratory infections in the cohort.[46,47] No episodes of PML were described in either study, although based on events reported in adults, a significantly larger cohort would be needed to exclude an association with PML.

Janus kinase (JAK) inhibitors interrupt intracellular signaling after cytokine binding before initiation of gene transcription. Tofacitinib (JAK1/2 inhibitor) and ruxolitinib (JAK3 inhibitor) are approved in adults to treat RA and myelofibrosis, respectively. While neither is approved for pediatric use, off-label uses include graft-versus-host disease (GVHD) after hematopoietic stem cell transplantation, in patients with identified JAK/signal transducers and activators of transcription pathway mutations, as part of cancer chemotherapy regimens and for alopecia areata.[48–51] Adult studies indicate an increased risk for viral infections, including CMV and BK virus, in a cohort of kidney transplant recipients[52] and herpes zoster in RA.[53] A recent study reports that tofacitinib use incurs a 2-fold increased risk of herpes zoster compared with other biologic agents in adults, highlighting the potential for a differential risk in a population determined by the biologic target rather than the underlying disease process.[54] Additional adult studies report an increased risk for TB, especially in high-prevalence areas and esophageal candidiasis.[55] Pediatric studies again are limited, but emerging data from the treatment of 11 pediatric patients with GVHD indicate that viral infections were common during the treatment period, including adenovirus (n = 2), BK (n = 3), and EBV (n = 2).[48] Furthermore, 6 of 11 developed a bacterial infection. Teasing out the risk related specifically to tofacitinib in this study is difficult, as most patients received concomitant therapy with other various biologics stressing the difficulty that will exist assigning infectious risk to specific biologic agents, as these medications are used in combination to treat refractory diseases.

Additional agents are directed specifically at cell-surface markers to eliminate specific types of cells. Rituximab, ofatumumab, and ocrelizumab target CD20 on B cells depleting this compartment of the immune system. Rituximab has been most widely administered with reports of administration for posttransplant lymphoproliferative disease, EBV-related hemophagocytic lymphohistiocytosis, glomerular diseases, central nervous system inflammatory diseases, and Burkitt lymphoma. Secondary to the depletion of CD20+ B cells, immunoglobulin production decreases leaving a significant proportion of patients with hypogammaglobinemia and, therefore, at risk for a variety of infections that depend on the humoral arm of the immune system suggesting the potential for the evaluation of hypogammaglobulinemia after rituximab administration and appropriate immunoglobulin replacement. Eight of 18 pediatric kidney transplant recipients receiving rituximab developed an assortment of serious infections, including bacterial sepsis, CMV, varicella, acute pyelonephritis, and BK nephropathy.[56] A study of 144 pediatric patients with a central nervous system–inflammatory condition reported 11 (8%) developed severe infectious events, including 2 deaths (CMV colitis, staphylococcal toxic shock syndrome) during rituximab administration.[57] Other nonfatal infections included CMV retinitis, shock, pneumonia, empyema, mastoiditis, and *Salmonella* enteritis. The largest assessment of rituximab in pediatrics evaluated discharge diagnosis codes at pediatric hospitals in the United States, assessing infection events in 2246 pediatric patients receiving rituximab.[58] In this study, 4.9% of patients had bacteremia, whereas 6.1% of patients were diagnosed with sepsis ranging from 2.4% in patients with autoimmune disease to 12.2% in patients with primary immunodeficiency. Other infections included viral infections (CMV 2.4%; adenovirus 2.2%; HSV/varicella zoster virus 1.5%) and fungal infections (candidiasis 1.5%; aspergillosis <1.0%; pneumocystis pneumonia <1.0%). Rituximab is also associated with impairment of vaccine response. Seasonal influenza, pneumococcal, and *Haemophilus influenza* type b (HIB) antibody responses to vaccination in adult patients on rituximab are decreased.[59–61] In addition, one study found that T-cell responses to pneumococcal and HIB vaccines were reduced in parallel with reductions in the B-cell compartment with effects lasting for up to 6 months indicating that the effects of rituximab are not limited to B cells alone but affect the costimulatory effect of B cells.[59] Therefore, the timing and type of vaccines administered to pediatric patients who have received rituximab therapy should be carefully considered to ensure adequate responses and decrease the risk for vaccine-associated complication, especially with live-viral vaccination.

SUMMARY

Biologic agents target specific pathways to treat immune-mediated diseases, and the use of biologics has expanded exponentially. Pediatric use continues to develop with new indications and emergence of new targets. Epidemiologic data reporting infection-related complications of biologics in pediatric patients are limited, but current data suggest that differences in types of pathogens exist relative to the pathways targeted by the agents. Further reporting of infectious events associated with the administration of biologics is key to a more comprehensive understanding of the consequences of these agents.

ACKNOWLEDGMENTS

The author acknowledges Grant Paulsen, MD for his careful review of this article.

REFERENCES

1. Administration USFaD. What are "biologics" questions and answers. 2017. Available at: https://www.fda.gov/AboutFDA/CentersOffices/OfficeofMedicalProducts andTobacco/CBER/ucm133077.htm. Accessed August 25, 2017.
2. Singh JA, Cameron C, Noorbaloochi S, et al. Risk of serious infection in biological treatment of patients with rheumatoid arthritis: a systematic review and meta-analysis. Lancet 2015;386(9990):258–65.
3. Gottlieb AB. Tumor necrosis factor blockade: mechanism of action. J Investig Dermatol Symp Proc 2007;12(1):1–4.
4. Medina-Gil C, Dehesa L, Vega A, et al. Prevalence of latent tuberculosis infection in patients with moderate to severe psoriasis taking biologic therapies in a dermatologic private practice in Miami, Florida. Int J Dermatol 2015;54(7): 846–52.
5. Keane J, Gershon S, Wise RP, et al. Tuberculosis associated with infliximab, a tumor necrosis factor alpha-neutralizing agent. N Engl J Med 2001;345(15): 1098–104.
6. Kalb RE, Fiorentino DF, Lebwohl MG, et al. Risk of serious infection with biologic and systemic treatment of psoriasis: results from the psoriasis longitudinal assessment and registry (PSOLAR). JAMA Dermatol 2015;151(9):961–9.
7. Renaud C, Ovetchkine P, Bortolozzi P, et al. Fatal group A Streptococcus purpura fulminans in a child receiving TNF-alpha blocker. Eur J Pediatr 2011;170(5): 657–60.

8. Chuang MH, Singh J, Ashouri N, et al. Listeria meningitis after infliximab treatment of ulcerative colitis. J Pediatr Gastroenterol Nutr 2010;50(3):337–9.

9. Jordan N, Waghmare A, Abi-Ghanem AS, et al. Systemic Mycobacterium avium complex infection during antitumor necrosis factor-alpha therapy in pediatric Crohn disease. J Pediatr Gastroenterol Nutr 2012;54(2):294–6.

10. Dotson JL, Crandall W, Mousa H, et al. Presentation and outcome of histoplasmosis in pediatric inflammatory bowel disease patients treated with antitumor necrosis factor alpha therapy: a case series. Inflamm Bowel Dis 2011;17(1):56–61.

11. Smith RJ, Boos MD, Burnham JM, et al. Atypical cutaneous blastomycosis in a child with juvenile idiopathic arthritis on infliximab. Pediatrics 2015;136(5):e1386–1389.

12. Hyams J, Crandall W, Kugathasan S, et al. Induction and maintenance infliximab therapy for the treatment of moderate-to-severe Crohn's disease in children. Gastroenterology 2007;132(3):863–73 [quiz: 1165–6].

13. Nimmrich S, Horneff G. Incidence of herpes zoster infections in juvenile idiopathic arthritis patients. Rheumatol Int 2015;35(3):465–70.

14. Paller AS, Siegfried EC, Pariser DM, et al. Long-term safety and efficacy of etanercept in children and adolescents with plaque psoriasis. J Am Acad Dermatol 2016;74(2):280–7.e1-3.

15. Hsin YC, Zhuang LZ, Yeh KW, et al. Risk of tuberculosis in children with juvenile idiopathic arthritis: a nationwide population-based study in Taiwan. PLoS One 2015;10(6):e0128768.

16. Beukelman T, Xie F, Chen L, et al. Rates of hospitalized bacterial infection associated with juvenile idiopathic arthritis and its treatment. Arthritis Rheum 2012;64(8):2773–80.

17. Calzada-Hernandez J, Anton-Lopez J, Bou-Torrent R, et al. Tuberculosis in pediatric patients treated with anti-TNFalpha drugs: a cohort study. Pediatr Rheumatol Online J 2015;13:54.

18. Dulai PS, Thompson KD, Blunt HB, et al. Risks of serious infection or lymphoma with anti-tumor necrosis factor therapy for pediatric inflammatory bowel disease: a systematic review. Clin Gastroenterol Hepatol 2014;12(9):1443–51 [quiz: e88–9].

19. Becker I, Horneff G. Risk of serious infection in juvenile idiopathic arthritis patients associated with tumor necrosis factor inhibitors and disease activity in the German biologics in pediatric rheumatology registry. Arthritis Care Res 2017;69(4):552–60.

20. Iwanczak BM, Ryzko J, Jankowski P, et al. Evaluation of the infliximab therapy of severe form of pediatric Crohn's disease in Poland: retrospective, multicenter studies. Adv Clin Exp Med 2017;26(1):51–6.

21. Hradsky O, Copova I, Zarubova K, et al. Seroprevalence of Epstein-Barr virus, cytomegalovirus, and polyomaviruses in children with inflammatory bowel disease. Dig Dis Sci 2015;60(11):3399–407.

22. Moses J, Alkhouri N, Shannon A, et al. Hepatitis B immunity and response to booster vaccination in children with inflammatory bowel disease treated with infliximab. Am J Gastroenterol 2012;107(1):133–8.

23. Croce E, Hatz C, Jonker EF, et al. Safety of live vaccinations on immunosuppressive therapy in patients with immune-mediated inflammatory diseases, solid organ transplantation or after bone-marrow transplantation - a systematic review of randomized trials, observational studies and case reports. Vaccine 2017;35(9):1216–26.

24. DeWitt EM, Kimura Y, Beukelman T, et al. Consensus treatment plans for new-onset systemic juvenile idiopathic arthritis. Arthritis Care Res 2012;64(7): 1001–10.
25. Cabral VP, Andrade CA, Passos SR, et al. Severe infection in patients with rheumatoid arthritis taking anakinra, rituximab, or abatacept: a systematic review of observational studies. Rev Bras Reumatol 2016;56(6):543–50.
26. Migkos MP, Somarakis GA, Markatseli TE, et al. Tuberculous pyomyositis in a rheumatoid arthritis patient treated with anakinra. Clin Exp Rheumatol 2015; 33(5):734–6.
27. Lequerre T, Quartier P, Rosellini D, et al. Interleukin-1 receptor antagonist (anakinra) treatment in patients with systemic-onset juvenile idiopathic arthritis or adult onset still disease: preliminary experience in France. Ann Rheum Dis 2008;67(3):302–8.
28. Ruperto N, Brunner HI, Quartier P, et al. Two randomized trials of canakinumab in systemic juvenile idiopathic arthritis. N Engl J Med 2012;367(25):2396–406.
29. Grom AA, Ilowite NT, Pascual V, et al. Rate and clinical presentation of macrophage activation syndrome in patients with systemic juvenile idiopathic arthritis treated with canakinumab. Arthritis Rheumatol 2016;68(1):218–28.
30. Lang VR, Englbrecht M, Rech J, et al. Risk of infections in rheumatoid arthritis patients treated with tocilizumab. Rheumatology 2012;51(5):852–7.
31. Chen LF, Mo YQ, Jing J, et al. Short-course tocilizumab increases risk of hepatitis B virus reactivation in patients with rheumatoid arthritis: a prospective clinical observation. Int J Rheum Dis 2017;20(7):859–69.
32. Komura T, Ohta H, Nakai R, et al. Cytomegalovirus reactivation induced acute hepatitis and gastric erosions in a patient with rheumatoid arthritis under treatment with an anti-IL-6 receptor antibody. Intern Med 2016;55(14):1923–7.
33. Nozawa T, Nishimura K, Ohara A, et al. Primary varicella infection in children with systemic juvenile idiopathic arthritis under tocilizumab therapy. Mod Rheumatol 2016. [Epub ahead of print].
34. Brunner HI, Ruperto N, Zuber Z, et al. Efficacy and safety of tocilizumab in patients with polyarticular-course juvenile idiopathic arthritis: results from a phase 3, randomised, double-blind withdrawal trial. Ann Rheum Dis 2015;74(6):1110–7.
35. Ojogho O, Sahney S, Cutler D, et al. Mycophenolate mofetil in pediatric renal transplantation: non-induction vs. induction with basiliximab. Pediatr Transplant 2005;9(1):80–3.
36. Spada M, Petz W, Bertani A, et al. Randomized trial of basiliximab induction versus steroid therapy in pediatric liver allograft recipients under tacrolimus immunosuppression. Am J Transplant 2006;6(8):1913–21.
37. Kavanaugh A, Mease PJ, Reimold AM, et al. Secukinumab for long-term treatment of psoriatic arthritis: a two-year follow-up from a phase III, randomized, double-blind placebo-controlled study. Arthritis Care Res 2017;69(3):347–55.
38. McInnes IB, Mease PJ, Kirkham B, et al. Secukinumab, a human anti-interleukin-17A monoclonal antibody, in patients with psoriatic arthritis (FUTURE 2): a randomised, double-blind, placebo-controlled, phase 3 trial. Lancet 2015;386(9999): 1137–46.
39. Langley RG, Tsai TF, Flavin S, et al. Efficacy and safety of guselkumab in patients with psoriasis who have an inadequate response to ustekinumab: results of the randomized, double-blind, Phase 3 NAVIGATE trial. Br J Dermatol 2017 [Epub ahead of print].
40. Kazemi T, Farahnik B, Koo J, et al. Emerging targeted therapies for plaque psoriasis - impact of ixekizumab. Clin Cosmet Investig Dermatol 2017;10:133–9.

41. Joost I, Steinfurt J, Meyer PT, et al. Staphylococcus aureus bacteremia with iliac artery endarteritis in a patient receiving ustekinumab. BMC Infect Dis 2016;16(1): 586.

42. Martinez CE, Allen JB, Davidorf FH, et al. Endogenous endophthalmitis and osteomyelitis associated with interleukin 17 inhibitor treatment for psoriasis in a patient with diabetes. BMJ case Rep 2017;2017 [pii:bcr-2017-219296].

43. Talotta R, Atzeni F, Sarzi Puttini P. Reactivation of occult hepatitis B virus infection under treatment with abatacept: a case report. BMC Pharmacol Toxicol 2016;17:17.

44. Butzkueven H, Kappos L, Pellegrini F, et al. Efficacy and safety of natalizumab in multiple sclerosis: interim observational programme results. J Neurol Neurosurg Psychiatry 2014;85(11):1190–7.

45. Bye WA, Jairath V, Travis SPL. Systematic review: the safety of vedolizumab for the treatment of inflammatory bowel disease. Aliment Pharmacol Ther 2017; 46(1):3–15.

46. Singh N, Rabizadeh S, Jossen J, et al. Multi-center experience of vedolizumab effectiveness in pediatric inflammatory bowel disease. Inflamm Bowel Dis 2016;22(9):2121–6.

47. Conrad MA, Stein RE, Maxwell EC, et al. Vedolizumab therapy in severe pediatric inflammatory bowel disease. Inflamm Bowel Dis 2016;22(10):2425–31.

48. Khandelwal P, Teusink-Cross A, Davies SM, et al. Ruxolitinib as salvage therapy in steroid-refractory acute graft-versus-host disease in pediatric hematopoietic stem cell transplant patients. Biol Blood Marrow Transplant 2017;23(7):1122–7.

49. Mayfield JR, Czuchlewski DR, Gale JM, et al. Integration of ruxolitinib into dose-intensified therapy targeted against a novel JAK2 F694L mutation in B-precursor acute lymphoblastic leukemia. Pediatr Blood Cancer 2017. [Epub ahead of print].

50. Baris S, Alroqi F, Kiykim A, et al. Severe early-onset combined immunodeficiency due to heterozygous gain-of-function mutations in STAT1. J Clin Immunol 2016; 36(7):641–8.

51. Craiglow BG, Liu LY, King BA. Tofacitinib for the treatment of alopecia areata and variants in adolescents. J Am Acad Dermatol 2017;76(1):29–32.

52. Busque S, Leventhal J, Brennan DC, et al. Calcineurin-inhibitor-free immunosuppression based on the JAK inhibitor CP-690,550: a pilot study in de novo kidney allograft recipients. Am J Transplant 2009;9(8):1936–45.

53. Iwamoto N, Tsuji S, Takatani A, et al. Efficacy and safety at 24 weeks of daily clinical use of tofacitinib in patients with rheumatoid arthritis. PLoS One 2017;12(5): e0177057.

54. Curtis JR, Xie F, Yun H, et al. Real-world comparative risks of herpes virus infections in tofacitinib and biologic-treated patients with rheumatoid arthritis. Ann Rheum Dis 2016;75(10):1843–7.

55. Winthrop KL, Park SH, Gul A, et al. Tuberculosis and other opportunistic infections in tofacitinib-treated patients with rheumatoid arthritis. Ann Rheum Dis 2016;75(6):1133–8.

56. Gulleroglu K, Baskin E, Moray G, et al. Rituximab therapy and infection risk in pediatric renal transplant patients. Exp Clin Transplant 2016;14(2):172–5.

57. Dale RC, Brilot F, Duffy LV, et al. Utility and safety of rituximab in pediatric autoimmune and inflammatory CNS disease. Neurology 2014;83(2):142–50.

58. Kavcic M, Fisher BT, Seif AE, et al. Leveraging administrative data to monitor rituximab use in 2875 patients at 42 freestanding children's hospitals across the United States. J Pediatr 2013;162(6):1252–8, 1258.e1.

59. Nazi I, Kelton JG, Larche M, et al. The effect of rituximab on vaccine responses in patients with immune thrombocytopenia. Blood 2013;122(11):1946–53.
60. Crnkic Kapetanovic M, Saxne T, Jonsson G, et al. Rituximab and abatacept but not tocilizumab impair antibody response to pneumococcal conjugate vaccine in patients with rheumatoid arthritis. Arthritis Res Ther 2013;15(5): R171.
61. Berglund A, Willen L, Grodeberg L, et al. The response to vaccination against influenza A(H1N1) 2009, seasonal influenza and Streptococcus pneumoniae in adult outpatients with ongoing treatment for cancer with and without rituximab. Acta Oncol 2014;53(9):1212–20.

Overview of Infections Complicating Pediatric Hematopoietic Cell Transplantation

Monica I. Ardura, DO, MSCS

KEYWORDS

- Infection • Hematopoietic cell transplantation • Immunocompromised children

KEY POINTS

- Despite improvements in supportive care, infections remain a significant cause of morbidity and mortality both early and late after hematopoietic cell transplantation.
- The complex interplay of host, transplant, and pathogen-related factors determine the risk of infectious complications after hematopoietic cell transplantation.
- Knowledge of the epidemiology and risk factors for infection at each phase after hematopoietic cell transplantation is needed to develop a differential diagnosis and institute optimal diagnostics and therapies.
- Prevention of infection and timely immune reconstitution are key to successful hematopoietic cell transplantation outcomes and are influenced by pretransplant, transplant, and posttransplant factors.

INTRODUCTION

Advances in hematopoietic cell transplantation (HCT) and refinements in supportive care strategies have led to an increasing number of HCT with improved outcomes in recent years in both adults and children.[1] However, infections remain an important cause of morbidity and mortality after HCT.[2] This article provides an overview of the epidemiology and risk factors for infections complicating HCT in children.

THE RISK FOR INFECTION IN CHILDREN AFTER HEMATOPOIETIC CELL TRANSPLANTATION

HCT is used to treat malignant (eg, leukemias, myelodysplastic syndromes, and high-risk solid tumors) and nonmalignant diseases (eg, hemoglobinopathies,

The author has no commercial financial conflicts of interest to disclose.
Pediatric Infectious Diseases, Host Defense Program, The Ohio State University, Nationwide Children's Hospital, 700 Children's Drive, C5C-J5428, Columbus, OH 43205, USA
E-mail address: monica.ardura@nationwidechildrens.org

Infect Dis Clin N Am 32 (2018) 237–252
https://doi.org/10.1016/j.idc.2017.11.003
0891-5520/18/© 2017 Elsevier Inc. All rights reserved.

id.theclinics.com

bone marrow failure syndromes, inborn errors of metabolism, and primary immuno-deficiencies). Possible HCT graft cell sources include bone marrow, peripheral blood stem cells, and umbilical cord blood (UCB). The recipient's immune system is altered or ablated by an immunosuppressive conditioning regimen, which may include a combination of chemotherapy, immunotherapy, and irradia-tion, given 4 to 10 days before intravenous infusion of the hematopoietic cell (HC) graft source (day 0) from either the patient's own previously harvested HC (autologous) or HC from a distinct donor (allogeneic; syngeneic if from twin donor). Immune reconstitution after HCT generally is heralded first by neutro-phil engraftment, followed by monocyte and natural killer cell recovery, platelet recovery, and over the subsequent months, by B- and T-cell recovery, first with normalization of numbers, followed by qualitative immune recovery (**Fig. 1**). Many factors affect the success and tempo of immune reconstitution after HCT, including the HC source and presence of graft-versus-host disease (GVHD). For example, in allogeneic HCT recipients without evidence of GVHD, lymphocyte class switching can be seen as early as 6 to 8 months after HCT. Conversely, in patients with GHVD requiring ongoing or augmented immunosuppression, immune dysregu-lation of the phagocytic, humoral, and cellular arms of the immune system is ongoing and leads to an overall increased risk of infection. Reconstitution of distinct immune cell subsets has been associated not only with risk of infection, but also to HCT outcomes including development of GVHD, relapse, and overall survival.[3]

The risk of infectious complications, type of pathogen, and timing of infections after HCT varies according to type of HCT, with pretransplant, transplant, and post-transplant factors contributing to this risk (**Fig. 2, Table 1**). Infections after HCT may represent infections derived from a patient's microbial flora, reactivation of latent infection, or primary infection, the latter more frequently observed in children than adults. In addition, noninfectious HCT complications such as engraftment syn-drome, hepatic venoocclusive disease (or sinusoidal obstruction syndrome), GVHD, and transplant-associated thrombotic microangiopathy may mimic infections and further confound the post-HCT period. Knowledge of the epidemiology and risk

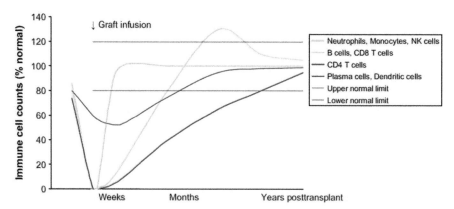

Fig. 1. General timing of immune reconstitution after myeloablative hematopoietic cell transplantation. (*From* Tomblyn M, Chiller T, Einsele H, et al. Guidelines for preventing infec-tious complications among hematopoietic cell transplantation recipients: a global perspec-tive. Biol Blood Marrow Transplant 2009;15(10):1150; with permission.)

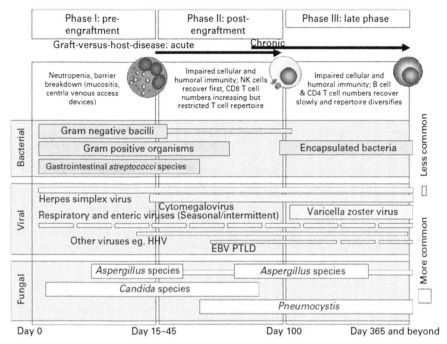

Fig. 2. Timing of infections after hematopoietic cell transplantation. (*From* Mackall C, Fry T, Gress R, et al. Background to hematopoietic cell transplantation, including post transplant immune recovery. Bone Marrow Transplant 2009;44(8):461; with permission.)

factors associated with infection at distinct time points after HCT is crucial to optimally assess a patient's risk for infection and allow for timely diagnostic and therapeutic management.

INFECTIONS BEFORE HEMATOPOIETIC CELL TRANSPLANTATION

The pretransplant infectious diseases consultation is an important component of the HCT process. One goal is to evaluate for possible acute infections in both the donor (which may be a contraindication to HC donation) and in the recipient (which may require additional therapy before HCT). The identification of possible latent infections may require therapy or surveillance. Pretransplant infectious diseases screening, including pathogen-specific testing and additional testing based on epidemiologic exposures, is required[4–6] (**Table 2**). In addition, because serologic testing in infants younger than 12 to 15 months of age and in patients with underlying primary immunodeficiency disorders may be unreliable, screening using polymerase chain reaction assays should be considered for certain pathogens (eg, cytomegalovirus [CMV] polymerase chain reaction in urine).

The pre-HCT consultation includes review of a HCT candidate's history of past infections and colonization, possible allergies, and awareness of local epidemiologic and susceptibility data, to inform recommendations for empirical antimicrobials after HCT when the patient develops fever and neutropenia without an obvious primary source. In addition to pre-HCT colonization or infections, conditioning and GVHD prevention and treatment strategies, will also guide recommendations for antimicrobial

Table 1
Transplant factors and risk for infectious diseases

Timing	Variable	Infection Risk
Pretransplant	Underlying disease	Higher with AML, AA, relapsed ALL.
	Comorbidities: organ dysfunction, splenectomy, iron overload	Higher risk of bacterial and fungal pathogens.
	CMV status	Highest risk if CMV serostatus D±/R+.
Transplant	Transplant type	Higher with allogeneic transplantation owing to risk of graft failure, GVHD, and more delayed B and T cell IR.
	Donor-recipient HLA match	Higher with URD or MUD compared with MSD owing to risk of GVHD, requiring more immunosuppression, prolonged neutropenia, and delayed IR.
	Conditioning regimen	Higher incidence of early infections with MA regimens (ATG and alemtuzumab) owing to greater amount of host tissue injury, including mucositis and severity/duration of neutropenia.
	HC graft source	Higher in UCB > BM > PBSC owing to delay in neutrophil engraftment and T-cell IR. Higher infectious risk weighed against lower GVHD risk.
	T cell depletion (CD34+ graft manipulation or use of ATG, alemtuzumab)	Higher owing to longer time to engraftment, B- and T-cell IR. Greater risk of fungal and viral infections, offset by decreased incidence of GVHD.
Posttransplant	GVHD	Higher risk with grades III–IV aGVHD and cGVHD due to GVHD therapy depressing cell-mediated immune response.

Abbreviations: AA, aplastic anemia; aGVHD, acute graft-versus-host disease; ALL, acute lymphoblastic leukemia; AML, acute myeloid leukemia; ATG, antithymocyte globulin; BM, bone marrow; cGVHD, chronic graft-versus-host disease; CMV, cytomegalovirus; D, donor; GVHD, graft-versus-host disease; HC, hematopoietic cells; IR, immune reconstitution; MA, myeloablative; MSD, matched sibling donor; MUD, matched unrelated donor; PBSC, peripheral blood stem cells; R, recipient; UCB, umbilical cord blood; URD, unrelated donor.

prophylaxis. It is recommended that HCT candidates not already immunosuppressed receive age-appropriate vaccinations before the start of conditioning regimens (if the interval to start is $\geq$2 weeks for inactivated vaccines and $\geq$4 weeks for live vaccines).[7] Ensuring that all household contacts are up-to-date with age-appropriate vaccines is imperative. Preparing the patient and family for possible infections early and late after HCT is an important component of the pre-HCT consultation and should include education on safe living practices and the development of strategies to mitigate individual risks for infection after HCT.[8]

It is recommended that patients with active bacterial infections be treated appropriately to eliminate the organism pre-HCT. Similarly, active fungal infections, such as hepatosplenic candidiasis or invasive pulmonary aspergillosis, are not absolute contraindications to proceeding with HCT.[9,10] In general, HCT may proceed once the candidate has a favorable response to antifungal therapy.[11] Upon completion of treatment, secondary antifungal prophylaxis should be considered during periods of immunosuppression to prevent relapse of infection.[12] However, decisions

Table 2
Infectious disease screening of potential donors and recipients before HCT

Evaluate for:	Possible Testing	Donor	Candidate
CMV	CMV IgG or CMV total, CMV PCR[a]	x	x
EBV	EBV VCA IgM, VCA IgG, EBNA	x	x
HBV	HBsAg, anti-HBs, anti-HBc, HBV NAT	x	x
HCV	Anti-HCV, HCV NAT	x	x
HIV	Anti-HIV 1/2 assay, HIV NAT	x	x
HSV 1/2 antibodies	Anti-HIV 1/anti-HIV2	—	x
HTLV I/II	Anti-HTLV I/II	x	x
Syphilis	RPR or syphilis antibody	x	x
Toxoplasma gondii	*Toxoplasma* serology, PCR	x	x
VZV	VZV IgG	x	x
WNV	WNV serology, WNV NAT	x	
Additional screening depending on epidemiologic exposures/risk or local requirements			
Chagas	*Trypanosoma cruzi* antibodies	x	x
Dimorphic fungi			
Histoplasma	*Histoplasma* serology, antigens	—	x
Coccidiodes	*Coccidioides* antibodies	—	x
Malaria	Malaria screen, blood smear, PCR	x	x
Strongyloides	*Strongyloides stercoralis* antibodies, stool ova, and parasites	x	x
Tuberculosis	Risk factor assessment, TST, IGRA	x	x
Vaccinia	Risk factor assessment	x	—
Zika virus	Risk factor assessment, Zika PCR	x	—

Abbreviations: anti-HBc, antibody to hepatitis B core antigen; anti-HBs, antibody to hepatitis B surface antigen; CMV, cytomegalovirus; EBNA, Epstein–Barr Virus Nuclear Antigen; EBV, Epstein–Barr virus; HBsAg, hepatitis B surface antigen; HBV, hepatitis B virus; HCT, hematopoietic cell transplantation; HCV, hepatitis C virus; HIV, human immunodeficiency virus; HSV, herpes simplex virus; HTLV, human T-cell leukemia virus; NAT, nucleic acid amplification test; PCR, polymerase chain reaction; TST, tuberculin skin test; VCA, viral capsid antigen; VZV, varicella zoster virus; WNV, West Nile virus.
[a] CMV PCR detection in urine should be considered.

regarding the optimal timing of HCT for an individual patient should weigh the risk of progressive infection during periods of augmented immunosuppression against the risk of complications from underlying malignancy if antineoplastic treatment or HCT is delayed.

Viral infections preceding HCT may also complicate management. CMV infection remains one of the most important viral infections in HCT. CMV infection preceding HCT is associated with an increased risk of reactivation and death after myeloablative HCT.[13] In a small retrospective study, children with CMV before HCT had a high incidence of recurrence after HCT, leading to a 50% all-cause mortality rate.[14] As such, in patients with documented CMV disease before HCT, HCT should be delayed until the candidate is adequately treated and, after HCT, secondary CMV prophylaxis (eg, with foscarnet until neutrophil engraftment) and systematic viral monitoring should be performed.[4]

Community respiratory viral infections are common in children and every effort should be made to prevent their transmission in HCT candidates.[15] Detection of respiratory viruses in children immediately before HCT poses unique challenges.

Although the usefulness of viral screening before HCT has not been adequately studied, the detection of respiratory viruses in nasal specimens from patients before HCT, even if asymptomatic, has been associated with higher overall mortality at day 100 compared with patients without viral detection before HCT.[16] Currently, it is recommended that HCT candidates with respiratory symptoms should postpone starting conditioning until symptoms resolve, given the concern for possible progression to lower respiratory tract infection during immunosuppression.[4,15,17] The risk of progression varies by virus detected, but lymphopenia (absolute lymphocyte count of <100–300/mm^3) at the time of viral infection is an established risk factor for disease progression, severity, and mortality. For patients with documented influenza infection, neuraminidase inhibitors should be promptly initiated. For other community respiratory viruses, there are limited data and a lack of controlled trials confirming the efficacy of antiviral therapies. In high-risk HCT candidates and recipients with respiratory syncytial virus infection, limited data from retrospective studies have suggested that ribavirin reduced the risk of progression to lower respiratory tract infection and improved outcomes in patients with respiratory syncytial virus pneumonia.

TIMING OF INFECTION AFTER HEMATOPOIETIC CELL TRANSPLANTATION

The timing of infections after HCT has traditionally been divided into 3 phases: preengraftment (where neutrophil engraftment is defined as an absolute neutrophil count of >500 cells/μL on 2 consecutive days, generally occurring between days 0 and 30), postengraftment (from neutrophil engraftment to approximately days 31 through 100), and late post-HCT (day ≥100). In general, recipients of granulocyte colony stimulating factor–mobilized peripheral blood stem cells have neutrophil engraftment approximately 2 weeks after HCT and before bone marrow or UCB recipients. UCB transplants generally carry a smaller stem cell dose and lack antigen-specific memory T cells. As such, these patients have a longer time to neutrophil engraftment (~4 weeks) and T- and B-cell immune reconstitution respectively than patients receiving bone marrow or peripheral blood stem cells, putting them at increased risk of infections. The timing of infections will also be affected by antimicrobial prophylaxis strategies and the use of medications to prevent and treat GVHD. Thus, clinicians should have a heightened clinical suspicion, given that bacterial, viral, and fungal infections may occur during all phases after HCT.

INFECTIONS OCCURRING BEFORE NEUTROPHIL ENGRAFTMENT

In the preengraftment period, infections are generally related to complications of prolonged and severe neutropenia and disruption to the normal host immune barriers (eg, presence of mucositis, indwelling catheters). It follows that bloodstream infections (BSI) occur most frequently during this time, although incidences and microbiologic epidemiology in pediatric HCT vary widely by geographic location and underlying HCT factors.[18,19] Preengraftment BSI has been associated with engraftment failure, development of acute GVHD, and increased mortality.[20] BSI can be secondary to an infection at another site or from a primary BSI arising from the central venous catheter or from bacterial translocation across nonintact oral and gastrointestinal mucosa. The importance of skin and oral care should be emphasized during this period. In addition, adherence to insertion and maintenance bundles for the prevention of catheter-related BSI should be followed.

In 2013, the Centers for Disease Control and Prevention modified the central line-associated BSI definition to include mucosal barrier injury laboratory-confirmed BSIs (MBI-LCBI). This distinction is important for identifying risk factors and optimal prevention strategies because, unlike central line-associated BSI, MBI-LCBI rates are not impacted by improvements in catheter care. In a retrospective review of 100 children with microbiologically proven BSI events during their first year after HCT, 46% of patients had at least 1 BSI before neutrophil engraftment with the majority being MBI-LCBI.[21] These MBI-LCBI were associated with a significant burden on the healthcare system and an increase in 1 year nonrelapse mortality when compared with children with non–MBI central line-associated BSI.

Prophylaxis strategies have been used in an effort to prevent or reduce bacterial infections in high-risk HCT patients with neutropenia. Despite the frequent use of intravenous immunoglobulin in clinical practice, a recent metaanalysis of 30 randomized, controlled trials using intravenous immunoglobulin prophylaxis in HCT recipients did not demonstrate an effect on all-cause mortality or infection-related outcomes, but noted a trend for increased risk of hepatic venoocclusive disease.[22]

The use of prophylactic antibiotics in HCT recipients has been evaluated in multiple studies. The largest prospective, controlled trial included 760 adult patients with cancer and HCT recipients with chemotherapy induced neutropenia, who were randomized to receive either levofloxacin or placebo from the start of chemotherapy until the resolution of neutropenia.[23] Subjects who received levofloxacin had significantly lower rates of fever during periods of neutropenia and of microbiologically proven infections when compared with patients who received placebo. However, there were no differences in mortality in either group. These results have led to current guidelines recommending consideration of fluoroquinolone prophylaxis in adult HCT recipients with continued neutropenia.[4,24] Similar recommendations are not currently endorsed in the pediatric-specific guidelines.[25] Thus, we eagerly await data from the Children's Oncology Group ACCL0934 randomized, phase III trial that will evaluate the clinical efficacy of levofloxacin for the prevention of bacteremia in children with underlying acute leukemia and undergoing HCT (clinicaltrials.org # NCT01371656).

The use of fluoroquinolone prophylaxis must also be weighed against the emergence of bacterial resistance and impact on other infections such as *Clostridium difficile*. Contemporary studies in HCT recipients in whom fluoroquinolone prophylaxis was frequently used demonstrate a decreased incidence of total number of BSI over time, but note an increased incidence of BSI caused by fluoroquinolone-resistant Gram-negative bacteria and resistant enterococci.[18,26]

Less commonly, invasive fungal infections can occur during the preengraftment phase. Antifungal prophylaxis during this period significantly decreased all-cause mortality in HCT recipients.[27] Fluconazole prophylaxis during the preengraftment period decreases the incidence of invasive candidiasis and fungal-related mortality. The optimal duration of fluconazole prophylaxis is not known, but prophylaxis until day 75 after HCT was associated with overall improved survival.[28] Prospective surveillance for invasive fungal infections in HCT recipients in the United States from 2001 to 2006 noted that invasive aspergillosis has surpassed invasive candidiasis as the most frequent invasive fungal infections among adult and pediatric HCT recipients, likely reflecting in part the application of fluconazole as standard prophylaxis; with the mold infections occurring later after HCT.[29] Mold-active prophylaxis may be considered in the highest risk patients (eg, myeloablative HCT for acute myeloid leukemia, relapsed acute lymphoblastic leukemia, with grades 2–4 GVHD); however, a survival benefit has not been demonstrated in patients receiving mold-active prophylaxis compared with those receiving fluconazole.[4,29,30] The choice of antifungal prophylaxis should also take into account risk for specific infections (eg, posaconazole if at risk for or with a prior history of infection with *Mucorales* spp) and possible drug interactions with medications received during conditioning (eg, vincristine, high-dose cyclophosphamide) and for GVHD prevention.

Concomitant use of azole antifungals and certain immunosuppressants (eg, calcineurin and mammalian target of rapamycin inhibitors) will affect therapeutic drug levels of the immunosuppressants and require dose adjustment or modification of therapy. When azoles are contraindicated, micafungin prophylaxis may be considered for candidiasis prevention during preengraftment.[4]

Viral reactivation occurs during this early time period. Herpes simplex virus infection may present as mucositis and fever. Herpes simplex virus prophylaxis with acyclovir or valacyclovir should be offered to seropositive patients from conditioning and until engraftment, resolution of mucositis, or day 30, whichever is longer. BK virus–associated hemorrhagic cystitis can occur after the direct toxicity of the conditioning regimen on bladder epithelium. The chemotherapy-induced cystitis allows for reactivation of the BK polyomavirus in the urothelial and renal tubular epithelial cells. BK viruria may frequently be detected after HCT (in 60%–80% of patients), without hemorrhagic cystitis. However, BK viremia after HCT has been associated with the development of hemorrhagic cystitis, renal impairment, and, rarely, BK virus-associated nephropathy.[31] Treatment regimens for BK virus-associated hemorrhagic cystitis and nephropathy are not well-established and reduction in immunosuppression is generally not possible this early after HCT.[32]

INFECTIONS OCCURRING AFTER NEUTROPHIL ENGRAFTMENT

During the postengraftment period, BSI may continue to occur. Risk factors for postengraftment bacteremia include ongoing neutropenia, renal or hepatic dysfunction, and the presence of GVHD. In a multicenter US study evaluating the impact of BSI on transplant-related mortality in 395 children after HCT, lack of neutrophil engraftment and the development of a BSI with enteric bacteria after the onset of acute GVHD were predictors of transplant-related mortality.[33] Rates of gram-positive and gram-negative resistance to antimicrobials were reported: 38% of enterococci were resistant to vancomycin and 8% to 20% of gram-negative bacteria were resistant to cefepime and piperacillin/tazobactam. Having a BSI with resistant bacteria was not associated with increased transplant-related mortality as has been demonstrated in adult studies.[18,19]

GVHD is a common transplant-related complication that may occur around the time of neutrophil engraftment, affecting the skin, liver, and gastrointestinal tract. The importance of gut microbiota diversity, infections, and immune regulation in HCT outcomes and development of GVHD is an evolving area of investigation.[34] Allo-HCT recipients receiving broad spectrum antibiotics with anaerobic coverage (eg, imipenem-cilastatin or piperacillin-tazobactam) were found to have more microbiota gastrointestinal injury and an increased incidence and severity of GVHD and GVHD-associated mortality.[35]

After neutrophil engraftment, infections are primarily related to ongoing profound defects in cellular immunity from the conditioning regimen and prophylaxis measures against the development of GVHD. During this period, the reactivation of viruses predominates. CMV infection remains the most common viral infection associated with significant morbidity and mortality after HCT.[36,37] HCT recipients at risk for post-HCT disease include all CMV-seropositive recipients (CMV R+) and CMV-negative recipients (CMV R–) with a CMV-positive donor (CMV D+), mismatched or unrelated donor source in allo-HCT, and patients with GVHD. Two strategies are equally effective at preventing CMV after HCT: (1) universal primary CMV antiviral prophylaxis to all patients at risk from time of engraftment to day 100 and (2) viral surveillance with preemptive antiviral treatment. Many centers that routinely use sensitive polymerase chain reaction–based assays for CMV detection apply the preemptive strategy, avoiding possible bone marrow suppression and renal toxicities associated with prolonged antiviral therapy.[38,39] However, there is no single endorsed strategy or validated viral load threshold to inform starting therapy. It is important to note that CMV DNAemia may be absent despite end-organ disease of the gastrointestinal tract, eye, and central nervous system; thus, any concerning symptoms in these areas warrant additional diagnostic evaluation.

Ganciclovir is primarily used for preemptive and targeted CMV therapy after engraftment. The effectiveness and safety profiles of newer antivirals such as letermovir and maribavir for CMV prevention or treatment require further study in children.[25,40,41] Cell therapies using adoptive transfer of CMV-specific cytotoxic T cells to reconstitute viral immunity after HCT have successfully been used in experimental clinical trials in children.[42] Monitoring of CMV-specific cell-mediated immunity after transplantation may allow for earlier and more targeted clinical interventions based on an individual's specific immune parameters. The quantification of surrogate markers of CMV-specific cell-mediated immunity in HCT recipients has been evaluated to predict risk for CMV and requires further validation and assessment in children.[43]

The absence of CD4 T-cell reconstitution has been found to predict reactivation of certain viruses (adenovirus [AdV], Epstein–Barr virus).[44] Incidence rates of AdV infection in HCT are between 3% and 47%, with the higher rates occurring in pediatric patients. AdV can cause a wide spectrum of clinical manifestations in HCT recipients varying from asymptomatic shedding to invasive localized and disseminated disease associated with mortality rates of 26% to 80%. The optimal management is unknown, but reduction or withdrawal of immunosuppression may prevent progression, if clinically feasible. There is no treatment for AdV infection that has been approved by the US Food and Drug Administration, although intravenous cidofovir may be used in patients with risk factors for AdV disease severity. Risk factors include receipt of UCB, T-cell depletion, young age, presence of GVHD, ongoing immunosuppression (eg, oral corticosteroids or lymphocyte proliferation inhibitor), and high AdV DNAemia in plasma.[45] Brincidofovir, a lipid conjugate of cidofovir, offers higher intracellular levels of active drug and less nephrotoxicity when compared with cidofovir and has good oral bioavailability. A phase II, randomized, placebo-controlled trial in pediatric and adult allo-HCT recipients with asymptomatic AdV DNAemia was performed where subjects were stratified by absolute lymphocyte count (<300 cells/mm^3) and then randomized to receive placebo or preemptive oral brincidofovir at distinct doses for 6 to 12 weeks, and followed for 4 weeks.[46] There were no differences in the proportion of subjects experiencing progression to probable or proven AdV disease or increasing AdV DNAemia (increase in $\geq$1 log$_{10}$ copies/mL) among treatment groups, although resolution of DNAemia occurred more frequently and quickly in the treatment arm. There was no evidence of myelotoxicity or nephrotoxicity, but gastrointestinal-related events (eg, diarrhea and diagnosis of GVHD of the gastrointestinal tract) occurred more frequently in the patients treated with brincidofovir.

After engraftment and extending late post-HCT, Epstein–Barr virus associated post-transplant lymphoproliferative disorder (PTLD) may occur. Quantitative Epstein–Barr virus viral load monitoring is recommended in HCT recipients at high risk, including patients who received HLA-mismatched transplants, T-cell depletion, or with ongoing abnormal T-cell responses against Epstein–Barr virus, including augmented immunosuppression for the treatment of GVHD.[47] Although the detection of Epstein–Barr virus in whole blood is sensitive and has been shown to increase before PTLD disease onset, it is not specific for Epstein–Barr virus–associated PTLD; thus, diagnosis requires histopathologic evidence of Epstein–Barr virus–associated PTLD. A reduction in immunosuppression is the mainstay of therapy, although this measure may not always be possible. Antiviral agents do not demonstrate efficacy for the treatment of proven Epstein–Barr virus PTLD. Anti-CD20 monoclonal antibodies such as rituximab are increasingly being used preemptively and also as treatment for PTLD.[48] Restoring the immune response using Epstein–Barr virus–specific T cells remains experimental at many centers.

Human herpes virus 6 (HHV 6), most frequently HHV 6B, may reactivate during this time, occurring in up to 70% of HCT recipients with increasing risk in allo-HCT recipients of mismatched/unrelated donors or UCB transplants. HHV 6 most frequently manifests as DNAemia, but has also been associated with encephalitis in HCT recipients.[49] Patients may present with altered mentation, including anterograde amnesia and subclinical seizures. Diagnosis requires exclusion of other causes of encephalitis and HHV 6 detection in the cerebrospinal fluid in the presence of cerebrospinal fluid pleocytosis and abnormal neuroimaging on MRI. HHV 6 has also been associated with pneumonitis, hepatitis, GVHD, and delayed engraftment or graft failure; however, causality remains less well-established.[50]

Fungal infections may occur during this phase, caused by yeasts and molds. *Pneumocystis jirovecii* pneumonia also remains a concern in HCT recipients, although it occurs less frequently in the era of prophylaxis. Primary prophylaxis with trimethoprim/sulfamethoxazole given 2 to 3 times weekly is the preferred regimen to start after neutrophil engraftment and continued for 6 months or while immunosuppressive therapy is given, whichever is longer.[4,51] For patients intolerant of trimethoprim/sulfamethoxazole, prophylaxis alternatives include pentamidine, atovaquone, or dapsone, keeping in mind the higher incidence of breakthrough *P jirovecii* pneumonia infections with non–trimethoprim/sulfamethoxazole prophylaxis regimens.

INFECTIONS OCCURRING LATE AFTER HEMATOPOIETIC CELL TRANSPLANTATION

Infections after day 100 are rare in HCT recipients with immune reconstitution. However, the risk for and severity of infections during this time period are directly related to GVHD in allo-HCT recipients. Immune defects associated with GVHD include those related to humoral, cellular immunity, and functional hyposplenism. Thus, patients are at greater risk for infections with viruses, fungi, and encapsulated bacteria. In addition, steroid-refractory GVHD is treated with multiple immunosuppressive agents with distinct immune targets, further altering the risk for and clinical manifestations of infections. Data from the Childhood Cancer Survivor Study demonstrated that long-term HCT survivors experience excess morbidity and mortality from infectious diseases[52,53] and may require additional infectious disease surveillance and prophylaxis strategies.[54]

Reactivation of VZV occurs late after HCT. In VZV R+ patients, antiviral prophylaxis has been shown to be effective in preventing infection and is recommended for the first year after HCT.[55] Continuation beyond 1 year after HCT should be considered in patients receiving ongoing immunosuppression.[56] Late-onset CMV infection may also occur, particularly in patients with GVHD, ongoing lymphopenia, and those who have received universal antiviral prophylaxis.

The high incidence of invasive pneumococcal disease (IPD) late after HCT is due to persistence of inadequate antibody production and functional hyposplenism. In a recent analysis of IPD from the US Pediatric Multicenter Pneumococcal Surveillance network, pediatric HCT recipients developed IPD at a median of 11 months after HCT and presented most frequently with bacteremia followed by pneumonia.[57] Vaccine serotypes caused 37% to 49% of IPD cases from 2000 to 2014 and 5% of HCT recipients had 2 or more episodes of microbiologically proven IPD.

In patients with ongoing GVHD or hypogammaglobulinemia, antibiotic prophylaxis against encapsulated bacteria is recommended for the duration of immunosuppression.[4,58] Penicillin VK is appropriate in institutions where the local epidemiology demonstrates low resistance to penicillin. Optimizing pneumococcal vaccination dosing and timing may allow for improved IPD prevention. It is recommended that pneumococcal vaccination begin 3 to 6 months after HCT.[4,7] Three doses of pneumococcal conjugate vaccine (PCV13) should be provided, followed by pneumococcal polysaccharide vaccine (PPSV23) in all HCT recipients 2 years of age or older who are 12 months past HCT, if they have no evidence of GVHD; if GVHD is present, a fourth dose of PCV13 should be considered.[7,59] Vaccination against influenza should be given to children 6 months of age or older. Inactivated influenza vaccine may be given as early as 3 to 4 months after HCT in the setting of a community influenza outbreak, with a second vaccine dose given 4 weeks afterward.[60] Vaccination with other inactivated vaccines may start 6 to 12 months after HCT.[4,7,61,62] Vaccination with injectable live virus vaccines (MMR, varicella) is considered safe beginning at 24 or more months after HCT, provided the recipient has not been receiving systemic immunosuppression for 1 year or longer, and 8 months have passed since last intravenous immunoglobulin supplementation. More detailed vaccine recommendations for specific populations are available elsewhere.[63,64]

FUTURE DIRECTIONS

Given the ongoing challenges in treating infections after HCT and limited prospects in the antimicrobial pipeline, research endeavors continue to evaluate novel diagnostic and treatment strategies. An improved understanding of the pathogenesis of distinct infections and host–pathogen interactions has resulted in the identification of potential novel host-directed therapies and targeted host microbiome interventions.[65] The discovery and validation of surrogate biomarkers of immune recovery may allow for their application in predicting outcomes after HCT, provide a more individualized approach to antimicrobial prophylaxis and vaccination strategies, and the discovery of novel transplant strategies and therapies.[66] Immunotherapy proof-of-principle studies have already demonstrated the efficacy of donor derived or matched third party virus-specific T cells in preventing and treating multiple viral infections and accelerating immune reconstitution after HCT.[67–70] These advances and ongoing research endeavors hold promise in enhancing the clinical management and improving outcomes in children with infections after HCT.

SUMMARY

HCT are increasingly being performed in children for the treatment of malignant and nonmalignant diseases. Transplant, host, and pathogen-specific factors impact the risk of developing infectious complications after HCT. The timing of infections caused by bacteria, viruses, and fungi may be more frequent during certain timepoints, but may occur at any time until there is successful immune reconstitution. Optimizing preventative strategies and further research into possible novel therapies and immune monitoring hold promise for the prevention and treatment of infections in children after HCT.

REFERENCES

1. Gooley TA, Chien JW, Pergam SA, et al. Reduced mortality after allogeneic hematopoietic-cell transplantation. N Engl J Med 2010;363(22):2091–101.

2. D'Souza A, PM, Zhu X. Current use and outcome of hematopoietic stem cell transplantation: CIBMTR summary slides, 2016. 2016. Available at: http://www.cibmtr.org. Accessed July 1, 2017

3. Bosch M, Khan FM, Storek J. Immune reconstitution after hematopoietic cell transplantation. Curr Opin Hematol 2012;19(4):324–35.

4. Tomblyn M, Chiller T, Einsele H, et al. Guidelines for preventing infectious complications among hematopoietic cell transplantation recipients: a global perspective. Biol Blood Marrow Transplant 2009;15(10):1143–238.

5. US Food and Drug Administration. Testing HCT/P donors: specific requirements. 2017. Available at: https://www.fda.gov/BiologicsBloodVaccines/SafetyAvailability/TissueSafety/ucm151757.htm. Accessed May 25, 2017.

6. Confer D, Gress R, Tomblyn M, et al. Hematopoietic cell graft safety. Bone Marrow Transplant 2009;44(8):463–5.

7. Rubin LG, Levin MJ, Ljungman P, et al. 2013 IDSA clinical practice guideline for vaccination of the immunocompromised host. Clin Infect Dis 2014;58(3):e44–100.

8. Yokoe D, Casper C, Dubberke E, et al. Safe living after hematopoietic cell transplantation. Bone Marrow Transplant 2009;44(8):509–19.

9. Pappas PG, Kauffman CA, Andes DR, et al. Clinical practice guideline for the management of candidiasis: 2016 update by the Infectious Diseases Society of America. Clin Infect Dis 2016;62(4):e1–50.

10. Patterson TF, Thompson GR 3rd, Denning DW, et al. Practice guidelines for the diagnosis and management of aspergillosis: 2016 update by the Infectious Diseases Society of America. Clin Infect Dis 2016;63(4):e1–60.

11. Martino R, Parody R, Fukuda T, et al. Impact of the intensity of the pretransplantation conditioning regimen in patients with prior invasive aspergillosis undergoing allogeneic hematopoietic stem cell transplantation: a retrospective survey of the Infectious Diseases Working Party of the European Group for Blood and Marrow Transplantation. Blood 2006;108(9):2928–36.

12. Cordonnier C, Rovira M, Maertens J, et al. Voriconazole for secondary prophylaxis of invasive fungal infections in allogeneic stem cell transplant recipients: results of the VOSIFI study. Haematologica 2010;95(10):1762–8.

13. Fries BC, Riddell SR, Kim HW, et al. Cytomegalovirus disease before hematopoietic cell transplantation as a risk for complications after transplantation. Biol Blood Marrow Transplant 2005;11(2):136–48.

14. Rowe RG, Guo D, Lee M, et al. Cytomegalovirus infection in pediatric hematopoietic stem cell transplantation: risk factors for primary infection and cases of recurrent and late infection at a single center. Biol Blood Marrow Transplant 2016;22(7):1275–83.

15. Hirsch HH, Martino R, Ward KN, et al. Fourth European Conference on Infections in Leukaemia (ECIL-4): guidelines for diagnosis and treatment of human respiratory syncytial virus, parainfluenza virus, metapneumovirus, rhinovirus, and coronavirus. Clin Infect Dis 2013;56(2):258–66.

16. Campbell AP, Guthrie KA, Englund JA, et al. Clinical outcomes associated with respiratory virus detection before allogeneic hematopoietic stem cell transplant. Clin Infect Dis 2015;61(2):192–202.

17. Peck AJ, Corey L, Boeckh M. Pretransplantation respiratory syncytial virus infection: impact of a strategy to delay transplantation. Clin Infect Dis 2004;39(5):673–80.

18. Dandoy CE, Ardura MI, Papanicolaou GA, et al. Bacterial bloodstream infections in the allogeneic hematopoietic cell transplant patient: new considerations for a persistent nemesis. Bone Marrow Transplant 2017;52(8):1091–106.

19. Srinivasan A, Wang C, Srivastava DK, et al. Timeline, epidemiology, and risk factors for bacterial, fungal, and viral infections in children and adolescents after allogeneic hematopoietic stem cell transplantation. Biol Blood Marrow Transplant 2013;19(1):94–101.

20. Poutsiaka DD, Price LL, Ucuzian A, et al. Blood stream infection after hematopoietic stem cell transplantation is associated with increased mortality. Bone Marrow Transplant 2007;40(1):63–70.

21. Dandoy CE, Haslam D, Lane A, et al. Healthcare burden, risk factors, and outcomes of mucosal barrier injury laboratory-confirmed bloodstream infections after stem cell transplantation. Biol Blood Marrow Transplant 2016;22(9):1671–7.

22. Raanani P, Gafter-Gvili A, Paul M, et al. Immunoglobulin prophylaxis in hematopoietic stem cell transplantation: systematic review and meta-analysis. J Clin Oncol 2009;27(5):770–81.

23. Bucaneve G, Micozzi A, Menichetti F, et al. Levofloxacin to prevent bacterial infection in patients with cancer and neutropenia. N Engl J Med 2005;353(10): 977–87.

24. Freifeld AG, Bow EJ, Sepkowitz KA, et al. Clinical practice guideline for the use of antimicrobial agents in neutropenic patients with cancer: 2010 update by the Infectious Diseases Society of America. Clin Infect Dis 2011;52(4):e56–93.

25. Avery RK, Marty FM, Strasfeld L, et al. Oral maribavir for treatment of refractory or resistant cytomegalovirus infections in transplant recipients. Transpl Infect Dis 2010;12(6):489–96.

26. Mikulska M, Del Bono V, Raiola AM, et al. Blood stream infections in allogeneic hematopoietic stem cell transplant recipients: reemergence of Gram-negative rods and increasing antibiotic resistance. Biol Blood Marrow Transplant 2009; 15(1):47–53.

27. Robenshtok E, Gafter-Gvili A, Goldberg E, et al. Antifungal prophylaxis in cancer patients after chemotherapy or hematopoietic stem-cell transplantation: systematic review and meta-analysis. J Clin Oncol 2007;25(34):5471–89.

28. Marr KA, Seidel K, Slavin MA, et al. Prolonged fluconazole prophylaxis is associated with persistent protection against candidiasis-related death in allogeneic marrow transplant recipients: long-term follow-up of a randomized, placebo-controlled trial. Blood 2000;96(6):2055–61.

29. Kontoyiannis DP, Marr KA, Park BJ, et al. Prospective surveillance for invasive fungal infections in hematopoietic stem cell transplant recipients, 2001-2006: overview of the Transplant-Associated Infection Surveillance Network (TRANS-NET) Database. Clin Infect Dis 2010;50(8):1091–100.

30. Ethier MC, Science M, Beyene J, et al. Mould-active compared with fluconazole prophylaxis to prevent invasive fungal diseases in cancer patients receiving chemotherapy or haematopoietic stem-cell transplantation: a systematic review and meta-analysis of randomised controlled trials. Br J Cancer 2012;106(10): 1626–37.

31. O'Donnell PH, Swanson K, Josephson MA, et al. BK virus infection is associated with hematuria and renal impairment in recipients of allogeneic hematopoietic stem cell transplants. Biol Blood Marrow Transplant 2009;15(9):1038–48.e1031.

32. Harkensee C, Vasdev N, Gennery AR, et al. Prevention and management of BK-virus associated haemorrhagic cystitis in children following haematopoietic stem cell transplantation–a systematic review and evidence-based guidance for clinical management. Br J Haematol 2008;142(5):717–31.

33. Satwani P, Freedman JL, Chaudhury S, et al. A multicenter study of bacterial blood stream infections in pediatric allogeneic hematopoietic cell transplantation

recipients: the role of acute gastrointestinal graft-versus-host disease. Biol Blood Marrow Transplant 2017;23(4):642–7.

34. Staffas A, Burgos da Silva M, van den Brink MR. The intestinal microbiota in allogeneic hematopoietic cell transplant and graft-versus-host disease. Blood 2017; 129(8):927–33.

35. Shono Y, Docampo MD, Peled JU, et al. Increased GVHD-related mortality with broad-spectrum antibiotic use after allogeneic hematopoietic stem cell transplantation in human patients and mice. Sci Transl Med 2016;8(339):339ra371.

36. Zaia J, Baden L, Boeckh MJ, et al. Viral disease prevention after hematopoietic cell transplantation. Bone Marrow Transplant 2009;44(8):471–82.

37. Teira P, Battiwalla M, Ramanathan M, et al. Early cytomegalovirus reactivation remains associated with increased transplant-related mortality in the current era: a CIBMTR analysis. Blood 2016;127(20):2427–38.

38. Boeckh M, Ljungman P. How we treat cytomegalovirus in hematopoietic cell transplant recipients. Blood 2009;113(23):5711–9.

39. Green ML, Leisenring W, Stachel D, et al. Efficacy of a viral load-based, risk-adapted, preemptive treatment strategy for prevention of cytomegalovirus disease after hematopoietic cell transplantation. Biol Blood Marrow Transplant 2012;18(11):1687–99.

40. Chemaly RF, Ullmann AJ, Stoelben S, et al. Letermovir for cytomegalovirus prophylaxis in hematopoietic-cell transplantation. N Engl J Med 2014;370(19): 1781–9.

41. Marty FM, Ljungman P, Papanicolaou GA, et al. Maribavir prophylaxis for prevention of cytomegalovirus disease in recipients of allogeneic stem-cell transplants: a phase 3, double-blind, placebo-controlled, randomised trial. Lancet Infect Dis 2011;11(4):284–92.

42. Lankester AC, Locatelli F, Bader P, et al. Will post-transplantation cell therapies for pediatric patients become standard of care? Biol Blood Marrow Transplant 2015;21(3):402–11.

43. Nesher L, Shah DP, Ariza-Heredia EJ, et al. Utility of the enzyme-linked immunospot interferon-gamma-release assay to predict the risk of cytomegalovirus infection in hematopoietic cell transplant recipients. J Infect Dis 2016;213(11):1701–7.

44. Admiraal R, de Koning CCH, Lindemans CA, et al. Viral reactivations and associated outcomes in the context of immune reconstitution after pediatric hematopoietic cell transplantation. J Allergy Clin Immunol 2017. [Epub ahead of print].

45. Lindemans CA, Leen AM, Boelens JJ. How I treat adenovirus in hematopoietic stem cell transplant recipients. Blood 2010;116(25):5476–85.

46. Grimley MS, Chemaly RF, Englund JA, et al. Brincidofovir for asymptomatic adenovirus viremia in pediatric and adult allogeneic hematopoietic cell transplant recipients: a randomized placebo-controlled phase II trial. Biol Blood Marrow Transplant 2017;23(3):512–21.

47. Heslop HE. How I treat EBV lymphoproliferation. Blood 2009;114(19):4002–8.

48. Garcia-Cadenas I, Castillo N, Martino R, et al. Impact of Epstein Barr virus-related complications after high-risk allo-SCT in the era of pre-emptive rituximab. Bone Marrow Transplant 2015;50(4):579–84.

49. Ogata M, Fukuda T, Teshima T. Human herpesvirus-6 encephalitis after allogeneic hematopoietic cell transplantation: what we do and do not know. Bone Marrow Transplant 2015;50(8):1030–6.

50. Zerr DM, Boeckh M, Delaney C, et al. HHV-6 reactivation and associated sequelae after hematopoietic cell transplantation. Biol Blood Marrow Transplant 2012;18(11):1700–8.

51. Maertens J, Cesaro S, Maschmeyer G, et al. ECIL guidelines for preventing Pneumocystis jirovecii pneumonia in patients with haematological malignancies and stem cell transplant recipients. J Antimicrob Chemother 2016;71(9):2397–404.
52. Kurt BA, Nolan VG, Ness KK, et al. Hospitalization rates among survivors of childhood cancer in the Childhood Cancer Survivor Study cohort. Pediatr Blood Cancer 2012;59(1):126–32.
53. Perkins JL, Chen Y, Harris A, et al. Infections among long-term survivors of childhood and adolescent cancer: a report from the Childhood Cancer Survivor Study. Cancer 2014;120(16):2514–21.
54. Majhail NS, Rizzo JD, Lee SJ, et al. Recommended screening and preventive practices for long-term survivors after hematopoietic cell transplantation. Hematol Oncol Stem Cell Ther 2012;5(1):1–30.
55. Boeckh M, Kim HW, Flowers ME, et al. Long-term acyclovir for prevention of varicella zoster virus disease after allogeneic hematopoietic cell transplantation–a randomized double-blind placebo-controlled study. Blood 2006;107(5):1800–5.
56. Erard V, Guthrie KA, Varley C, et al. One-year acyclovir prophylaxis for preventing varicella-zoster virus disease after hematopoietic cell transplantation: no evidence of rebound varicella-zoster virus disease after drug discontinuation. Blood 2007;110(8):3071–7.
57. Olarte L, Lin PL, Barson WJ, et al. Invasive pneumococcal infections in children following transplantation in the pneumococcal conjugate vaccine era. Transpl Infect Dis 2017;19(1):1–7.
58. Chow EJ, Anderson L, Baker KS, et al. Late effects surveillance recommendations among survivors of childhood hematopoietic cell transplantation: a Children's Oncology Group report. Biol Blood Marrow Transplant 2016;22(5):782–95.
59. Cordonnier C, Ljungman P, Juergens C, et al. Immunogenicity, safety, and tolerability of 13-valent pneumococcal conjugate vaccine followed by 23-valent pneumococcal polysaccharide vaccine in recipients of allogeneic hematopoietic stem cell transplant aged >/=2 years: an open-label study. Clin Infect Dis 2015;61(3): 313–23.
60. Ljungman P, Avetisyan G. Influenza vaccination in hematopoietic SCT recipients. Bone Marrow Transplant 2008;42(10):637–41.
61. Carpenter PA, Englund JA. How I vaccinate blood and marrow transplant recipients. Blood 2016;127(23):2824–32.
62. Ljungman P, Cordonnier C, Einsele H, et al. Vaccination of hematopoietic cell transplant recipients. Bone Marrow Transplant 2009;44(8):521–6.
63. Heimall J, Buckley RH, Puck J, et al. Recommendations for screening and management of late effects in patients with severe combined immunodeficiency after allogenic hematopoietic cell transplantation: a consensus statement from the Second Pediatric Blood and Marrow Transplant Consortium International Conference on late effects after pediatric HCT. Biol Blood Marrow Transplant 2017;23(8): 1229–40.
64. Dietz AC, Mehta PA, Vlachos A, et al. Current knowledge and priorities for future research in late effects after hematopoietic cell transplantation for inherited bone marrow failure syndromes: consensus statement from the Second Pediatric Blood and Marrow Transplant Consortium International Conference on late effects after pediatric hematopoietic cell transplantation. Biol Blood Marrow Transplant 2017; 23(5):726–35.
65. Zumla A, Rao M, Wallis RS, et al. Host-directed therapies for infectious diseases: current status, recent progress, and future prospects. Lancet Infect Dis 2016; 16(4):e47–63.

66. Forcina A, Noviello M, Carbone MR, et al. Predicting the clinical outcome of allogeneic hematopoietic stem cell transplantation: the long and winding road toward validated immune biomarkers. Front Immunol 2013;4:71.
67. Leen AM, Christin A, Myers GD, et al. Cytotoxic T lymphocyte therapy with donor T cells prevents and treats adenovirus and Epstein-Barr virus infections after haploidentical and matched unrelated stem cell transplantation. Blood 2009;114(19): 4283–92.
68. Papadopoulou A, Gerdemann U, Katari UL, et al. Activity of broad-spectrum T cells as treatment for AdV, EBV, CMV, BKV, and HHV6 infections after HSCT. Sci Transl Med 2014;6(242):242ra283.
69. Leen AM, Bollard CM, Mendizabal AM, et al. Multicenter study of banked third-party virus-specific T cells to treat severe viral infections after hematopoietic stem cell transplantation. Blood 2013;121(26):5113–23.
70. Gerdemann U, Katari UL, Papadopoulou A, et al. Safety and clinical efficacy of rapidly-generated trivirus-directed T cells as treatment for adenovirus, EBV, and CMV infections after allogeneic hematopoietic stem cell transplant. Mol Ther 2013;21(11):2113–21.

Moving?

Make sure your subscription moves with you!

To notify us of your new address, find your **Clinics Account Number** (located on your mailing label above your name), and contact customer service at:

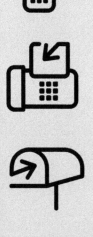

Email: journalscustomerservice-usa@elsevier.com

800-654-2452 (subscribers in the U.S. & Canada)
314-447-8871 (subscribers outside of the U.S. & Canada)

Fax number: 314-447-8029

Elsevier Health Sciences Division
Subscription Customer Service
3251 Riverport Lane
Maryland Heights, MO 63043

*To ensure uninterrupted delivery of your subscription, please notify us at least 4 weeks in advance of move.

Printed and bound by CPI Group (UK) Ltd, Croydon, CR0 4YY

08/05/2025

01864709-0001